# Designing Clinical Research

## An Epidemiologic Approach

Second Edition

# Designing
# Clinical Research
## An Epidemiologic Approach

Second Edition

**By**

**STEPHEN B. HULLEY, M.D., M.P.H.**
*Professor and Chair, Department of Epidemiology & Biostatistics*
*University of California, San Francisco*

**STEVEN R. CUMMINGS, M.D.**
*Professor of Medicine and of Epidemiology & Biostatistics*
*Assistant Dean for Clinical Research*
*University of California, San Francisco*

**WARREN S. BROWNER, M.D., M.P.H.**
*Professor of Medicine and of Epidemiology & Biostatistics*
*Chief, General Internal Medicine Section*
*San Francisco Veterans Affairs Medical Center*
*University of California, San Francisco*

**DEBORAH GRADY, M.D., M.P.H.**
*Professor of Epidemiology & Biostatistics and of Medicine*
*Staff Physician, Medical Service*
*San Francisco Veterans Affairs Medical Center*
*University of California, San Francisco*

**NORMAN HEARST, M.D., M.P.H.**
*Professor of Family & Community Medicine and of*
*Epidemiology & Biostatistics*
*Attending Physician, Department of Family &*
*Community Medicine*
*University of California, San Francisco*

**THOMAS B. NEWMAN, M.D., M.P.H.**
*Professor of Epidemiology & Biostatistics, of Pediatrics, and of*
*Laboratory Medicine*
*Attending Physician, Department of Pediatrics*
*University of California, San Francisco*

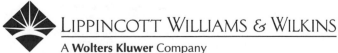

LIPPINCOTT WILLIAMS & WILKINS
A **Wolters Kluwer** Company
Philadelphia • Baltimore • New York • London
Buenos Aires • Hong Kong • Sydney • Tokyo

Acquisitions Editor: Timothy Y. Hiscock
Developmental Editor: Joyce A. Murphy
Production Editor: John C. Vassiliou
Manufacturing Manager: Benjamin Rivera
Cover Designer: Mark Lerner
Compositor: The PRD Group/Bi-Comp.
Printer: R. R. Donnelley

© 2001 by LIPPINCOTT WILLIAMS & WILKINS
530 Walnut Street
Philadelphia, PA 19106 USA
LWW.com

**Library of Congress Cataloging-in-Publication Data**

Designing clinical research : an epidemiologic approach / by Stephen B. Hulley
... [et al.].—2nd ed.
    p. ; cm.
   Includes bibliographical references and index.
   ISBN 0-7817-2218-7
   1. Clinical trials—Technique. 2. Medicine—Research—Methodology. 3.
Epidemiology—Research—Methodology. I. Hulley, Stephen B.
   [DNLM: 1. Epidemiologic Methods. 2. Research Design. WA 950 D457
2001]
   R853.C55 D47 2001
   610'.72—dc21                                                      00-042418

Care has been taken to confirm the accuracy of the information presented
and to describe generally accepted practices. However, the authors, editors, and
publisher are not responsible for errors or omissions or for any consequences
from application of the information in this book and make no warranty,
expressed or implied, with respect to the currency, completeness, or accuracy of
the contents of the publication. Application of this information in a particular
situation remains the professional responsibility of the practitioner.

The authors, editors, and publisher have exerted every effort to ensure that
drug selection and dosage set forth in this text are in accordance with current
recommendations and practice at the time of publication. However, in view of
ongoing research, changes in government regulations, and the constant flow of
information relating to drug therapy and drug reactions, the reader is urged to
check the package insert for each drug for any change in indications and dosage
and for added warnings and precautions. This is particularly important when the
recommended agent is a new or infrequently employed drug.

Some drugs and medical devices presented in this publication have Food and
Drug Administration (FDA) clearance for limited use in restricted research
settings. It is the responsibility of the health care provider to ascertain the FDA
status of each drug or device planned for use in their clinical practice.

10 9 8 7 6 5 4 3

To our families and our students.

# Contents

13  Research Using Existing Data: Secondary Data Analysis, Ancillary Studies, and Systematic Reviews . . . . . . . . . . 195

*Norman Hearst, Deborah Grady, Hal V. Barron, and Karla Kerlikowske*

## Section III: Implementation

14  Addressing Ethical Issues . . . . . . . . . . . . . . 215

*Bernard Lo*

15  Designing Questionnaires and Data Collection Instruments . . 231

*Steven R. Cummings, Anita L. Stewart, and Stephen B. Hulley*

16  Data Management . . . . . . . . . . . . . . . . 247

*Deborah Grady, Thomas B. Newman, and Eric Vittinghoff*

# Contributing Authors

**Hal V. Barron,** M.D., F.A.C.C.
*Assistant Clinical Professor of Medicine and of Epidemiology & Biostatistics*
*University of California, San Francisco*
*Director of Cardiovascular Clinical Research, Genentech Inc.*
*San Francisco, California*

**Elizabeth A. Holly,** Ph.D., M.P.H.
*Professor of Epidemiology & Biostatistics*
*University of California, San Francisco*

**Karla Kerlikowske,** M.D.
*Assistant Professor of Medicine and of Epidemiology & Biostatistics*
*Director, Women Veterans Comprehensive Health Center*
*San Francisco Veterans Affairs Medical Center*
*University of California, San Francisco*

**Bernard Lo,** M.D.
*Professor of Medicine*
*Director, The Program in Medical Ethics*
*Attending Physician, Department of Medicine, Moffit-Long Hospital*
*University of California, San Francisco*

**Jeffrey N. Martin,** M.D., M.P.H.
*Assistant Professor of Epidemiology & Biostatistics and of Medicine*
*Attending Physician, Department of Medicine*
*San Francisco General Hospital*
*University of California, San Francisco*

**Anita L. Stewart,** Ph.D.
*Professor in Residence*
*Institute for Health & Aging, School of Nursing*
*University of California, San Francisco*

**Eric Vittinghoff,** Ph.D., M.P.H.
*Assistant Adjunct Professor*
*Department of Epidemiology & Biostatistics*
*University of California, San Francisco*

# Introduction

This book is designed to help beginning investigators get started in the world of clinical research. This includes patient-oriented and translational research, epidemiologic and behavioral studies, and public health and health services research. There is a national mandate to enhance activities in this arena, in order to provide the knowledge base for evidence-based medicine and health policy (1–4).

The first edition was useful in this role, judging by comments we have received and steady sales. But a dozen years have passed since it was written, and although the fundamental approaches to designing clinical research have not changed, there have been important developments. Moreover, our thinking as authors has matured, in part from another decade of designing, funding, and implementing our own clinical research, and in part from the experience of teaching 100 physicians and health professionals in our Research Methods Workshop each summer. It was time for renewal.

Even so, the decision to write a second edition was not easy. Each of the authors is now a busy professor, still at UCSF but overcommitted in other areas. The logistics of reassembling our team to spend meaningful time together were daunting, and there was the unsettling possibility that messing with a book that worked could produce one that didn't. Our goal in writing a second edition was to preserve the virtues of the earlier version while correcting its deficiencies.

## ■ PRESERVING VIRTUES AND CORRECTING DEFICIENCIES

We have retained the virtue of keeping it simple. For example, the book provides thoughtful but reader-friendly tools for estimating sample size. Leaving out unnecessary complexities makes it short and easy to read, and allows the investigator to focus on the most important things: finding a good research question and planning the most appropriate design. The book remains a guide for helping an investigator to bring **common sense** to the many difficult choices involved in designing a successful study.

Correcting the book's deficiencies was more involved. We injected new ideas and fresh examples and references throughout, added exercises and whole new segments, and reordered the chapters into what had become the preferred sequence in the Research Methods Workshop.* There are now three parts:

- **Section I** begins with a chapter on how research works and then turns to the basic ingredients: research question, study subjects, measurements, hypotheses,

---

*The syllabus for the Research Methods Workshop may be useful to others interested in teaching clinical research. The current version, which shepherds chapter-by-chapter development of the pieces of a clinical research protocol, is on the UCSF Department of Epidemiology and Biostatistics Website. Incidentally, our Departmental Website also contains links to current sites that provide tools, such as sample size calculators, that are useful for designing clinical research.

and sample size. Of note are the simplified approaches to selecting and recruiting subjects (Chapter 3), the improved sections on Bayesian thinking about multiple and post hoc hypotheses (Chapter 5), and the approaches to estimating sample sizes for a broader set of design options (Chapter 6). Sample size also appears much earlier in the book so that students who are developing a protocol as they read will discover early on whether the study they plan has feasible sample size requirements.

- **Section II** presents the design options: cohort, cross-sectional, case-control and diagnostic test studies, clinical trials, a chapter on confounding, and another on the use of existing data. Of note is the greatly expanded treatment of clinical trials (Chapters 10 and 11). Chapter 12, on the growing domain of diagnostic test studies, is entirely rewritten. The expanded chapter on using existing data (Chapter 13), of particular interest to new investigators because of the low cost in time and money of this approach, includes two new topics: ancillary studies and systematic reviews (meta-analysis).

- **Section III** presents updated versions of additional skills needed for designing and implementing clinical research. Chapter 14, on ethics, is considerably expanded to incorporate society's growing ideas about the responsible conduct of research. The description of questionnaires (Chapter 15) takes note of the utility of e-mail and the Internet, and the chapter on data management (Chapter 16) is entirely rewritten to present the current state of computerized and Internet technologies. A new chapter on community and international studies (Chapter 18) reflects our experience with research in diverse communities and countries, and we have updated the final chapter on getting funded.

This is still not a book about statistics. Planning for statistical analyses is an important clinical research domain that investigators must find other ways to master. This is also not a book on presenting and publishing the findings of clinical research, for which we recommend a companion text (5).

# ■ BENEDICTION

New investigators often find the choice of a research question to be the most difficult step in designing a study (Chapter 2). Fortunately, most studies generate more questions than they answer, and many scientists find that their awareness of researchable questions grows as they gain experience.

There are other benefits that come with experience. Clinical research becomes easier and more rewarding as investigators gain familiarity with the particulars of recruitment, measurement, and design that pertain to their area of specialization. A higher percentage of their applications for funding are successful. They acquire a staff and junior colleagues and develop lasting friendships with scientists working on the same topic in distant places. And because most increments in knowledge are small and uncertain—major scientific breakthroughs are rare—they begin to see substantial advances in the state of medicine as an aggregate result of their efforts.

These are reassuring thoughts when we set out to design a research project. There is no need to solve the whole puzzle all at once. It will suffice to join the many first-rate scientists at work, adding small but true pieces of knowledge, one at a time.

## References

1. Report of NIH Director's Panel on Clinical Research, 1997.
2. Fletcher RH, Fletcher SW, Wagner EH. *Clinical epidemiology: the essentials*, 3rd ed. Baltimore: Williams & Wilkins, 1996.
3. Sackett DL, Haynes RB, Guyatt GH, Tugwell P. *Clinical epidemiology: a basic science for clinical medicine*, 2nd ed. Boston: Little, Brown and Company, 1991.
4. Friedland D. *Evidence-based medicine*. Stamford: Appleton & Lange, 1998.
5. Browner WS. *Publishing and presenting clinical research*. Baltimore: Lippincott Williams & Wilkins, 1999.

# Acknowledgments

We acknowledge the exceptional role played by Maya Dulay, who spent a year as project assistant in our department while awaiting medical school. Maya exercised extraordinary efficiency and accuracy with the innumerable details of multiple authors producing numerous drafts, and she evolved into our graphic designer and software expert. But most important was her enthusiasm for the many review sessions and retreats, and the contributions she made as scientific reviewer.

We are also grateful to the Andrew P. Mellon Foundation for bringing us together and stimulating the first edition, to our publisher for steadily inviting a second edition until resistance became futile, and to our students over the years, whose accomplishments have been fun to watch and who continue to sharpen our thinking.

# Section I
# Basic Ingredients

# Getting Started: The Anatomy and Physiology of Clinical Research

## Stephen B. Hulley, Thomas B. Newman, and Steven R. Cummings

This chapter introduces clinical research from two viewpoints, setting up themes that run together through the book. One theme is the anatomy of research—what it's made of. This includes the tangible elements of the study plan: the research question, design, subjects, measurements, sample size calculation, and so forth. An investigator's goal is to create these elements in a form that will make the project fast, inexpensive, and easy.

The other theme is the physiology of research—how it works. Studies are useful to the extent that they yield valid inferences, first about what happened in the study sample and then about generalizing these events to people outside the study. The goal is to minimize the errors, random and systematic, that threaten conclusions based on these inferences.

Separating these two themes is artificial in the same way that the anatomy of the human body does not make much sense without some understanding of its physiology. But the separation has the same advantage: It clarifies our thinking about a complex topic.

## ■ THE ANATOMY OF RESEARCH: WHAT IT'S MADE OF

The structure of a research project is set out in its protocol, the written plan of the study. Protocols are well known as devices for seeking grant funds, but they also have a vital scientific function: helping the investigator to organize her research in a logical, focused, and efficient way. Table 1.1 outlines the components of a protocol. We will introduce the whole set here, expand on each of them in the ensuing chapters of the book, and return to put the completed pieces together in Chapter 19.

### The Research Question

The research question is the objective of the study, the uncertainty that the investigator wants to resolve. Research questions often begin with a general concern that must be narrowed down to a concrete, researchable issue. For example,

| ■ TABLE 1.1 Outline of the Study Protocol | |
| --- | --- |
| **Element** | **Purpose** |
| Research questions | What questions will the study address? |
| Significance (background) | Why are these questions important? |
| Design<br>  Time frame<br>  Epidemiologic approach | How is the study structured? |
| Subjects<br>  Selection criteria<br>  Sampling design | Who are the subjects and how will they be selected? |
| Variables<br>  Predictor variables<br>  Confounding variables<br>  Outcome variables | What measurements will be made? |
| Statistical issues<br>  Hypotheses<br>  Sample size<br>  Analytic approach | How large is the study and how will it be analyzed? |

*Initial research question:* Should women take hormones after menopause?

This is a good place to start, very practical and important, but the question must be focused before planning efforts can begin. Often this involves breaking the whole question into its constituent parts and singling out one or two of these to build the protocol around.

*More specific research questions:*

How commonly women take estrogen after menopause?
Does taking estrogen after menopause lower the likelihood of developing coronary heart disease (CHD)?
Are there other benefits and harms of estrogen treatment?

A good research question should pass the "So what?" test. Getting the answer should contribute usefully to our state of knowledge. The acronym *FINER* denotes five essential characteristics of a good research question: that it be *feasible, interesting, novel, ethical,* and *relevant* (Chapter 2).

## Significance

The significance section of a protocol sets the proposed study in context and gives its rationale: What is known about the topic at hand? Why is the research question important? What kind of answers will the study provide? This section cites previous research that is relevant (including the investigator's own work) and indicates the problems with that research and what questions remain. It makes clear how the findings of the proposed study will help resolve these uncertainties, leading to new scientific understanding and influencing clinical and public health policy.

## The Design

The design of a study is a complex issue. A fundamental decision is whether to take a passive role in observing the events taking place in the study subjects in an **observational study** or to apply an intervention and examine its effects on these events in a **clinical trial** (Table 1.2). Among observational studies, two of the most common designs are **cohort** studies, in which a group of subjects is followed over time, and **cross-sectional** studies, in which the observations are made on a single occasion. A third common option is the **case-control** design, in which the investigator compares a group of subjects who have a disease or condition with another group of subjects who do not. Another design decision is whether to deal with past events in a retrospective study or to follow study subjects prospectively for events that have not yet occurred. Among clinical trial options, the **randomized blinded trial** is often the best design but unblinded or time-series designs may be more suitable for some research questions.

No one approach is always better than the others, and each research question requires a judgment about which design is the most efficient way to get a satisfactory answer. The randomized blinded trial is often held up as the gold standard for establishing causality and the effectiveness of interventions, but there are many situations for which an observational study is a better choice or the only feasible option. The relatively low cost of case-control studies and their suitability for uncommon outcomes makes them attractive for many questions. Special considerations apply to choosing designs for studying diagnostic tests. These issues are discussed in Chapters 7 through 12.

A typical sequence for studying a topic begins with observational studies of a type that is often called **descriptive**. These studies explore the lay of the land—for example, describing distributions of diseases and health-related characteristics in the population (*How common is estrogen treatment in women after menopause?*) or the sensitivity and specificity of a diagnostic test. Descriptive studies are usually

### ■ TABLE 1.2
Examples of Common Clinical Research Designs Used to Study Whether Hormone Therapy After Menopause Prevents Coronary Heart Disease

| Study Design | Key Feature | Example |
| --- | --- | --- |
| **Observational Designs** | | |
| Cohort study | A group followed over time | The investigator examines a cohort of women yearly for several years, observing the incidence of heart attacks in hormone users and nonusers. |
| Cross-sectional study | A group examined at one point in time | She examines the group of women once, observing the prevalence of a history of heart attacks in hormone users and nonusers. |
| Case-control study | Two groups, based on the outcome | She examines a group of women with heart attacks (the ''cases'') and compares them with a group of healthy women (the controls), asking about hormone use. |
| **Experimental Design** | | |
| Randomized blinded trial | Two groups created by a random process, and a blinded intervention | She randomly assigns women to receive hormone or identical placebo, then follows both treatment groups for several years to observe the incidence of heart attacks. |

followed or accompanied by **analytic** studies that evaluate associations to discover cause-and-effect relationships (*Is taking estrogen after menopause associated with lower risk of CHD?*). The final step is often a clinical trial to establish the effects of an intervention (*Does hormone treatment alter the incidence of CHD?*). Experiments usually occur later in the sequence of research studies, because they tend to be more difficult and expensive, and answer more narrowly focused questions that arise from the findings of observational studies.

It is useful to characterize the design in a single sentence that begins with its name. Some studies do not easily fit into these molds, however, and classifying them can be a surprisingly difficult exercise. It is worth the effort—a precise description of the type of study clarifies the investigator's thoughts and is useful for orienting colleagues and consultants. (This single sentence is the research analog to the opening sentence of a medical resident's report on a new hospital admission: "This 62-year-old white policewoman was well until 2 hours before admission, when she developed crushing chest pain radiating to the left shoulder.") If the study has two major phases, the design for each should be mentioned.

> *Research design:* This is a cross-sectional study of the prevalence of estrogen treatment among women aged 50 to 69 years, followed by a prospective cohort study of whether estrogen treatment is associated with low risk of subsequent heart attacks.

## The Study Subjects

Two major decisions must be made in choosing the study subjects (Chapter 3). The first is to specify selection criteria that define the target population: the *kinds* of patients best suited to the research question. The second decision concerns how best to recruit enough women from an accessible aspect of this population who will be the actual subjects of the study. For example, the study of hormones and CHD in women might select women aged 50 to 69 years attending primary care clinic at the investigator's hospital, and the investigator might decide to invite the next 1,000 such patients. These design choices represent trade-offs; studying a random sample of all U.S. women of that age would enhance generalizability but be formidably difficult and costly.

## The Variables

Another major set of decisions in designing any study concerns the choice of which variables (characteristics that vary from one study subject to another) to measure (Chapter 4). In a descriptive study the investigator looks at individual variables one at a time. A study of the prevalence of hormone treatment, for example, might record the presence or absence of the self-report of taking estrogen.

In an analytic study the investigator studies the associations among two or more variables in order to predict outcomes and to draw inferences about cause and effect. In considering the association between two variables, the one that precedes (or is presumed on biologic grounds to be antecedent) is called the **predictor variable;** the other is called the **outcome variable.*** Most observational

---

* Predictor variables are often termed independent and outcome variables are termed dependent, but we find this usage confusing, particularly since independent means something quite different in the context of multivariate analyses.

studies have many predictor variables (e.g., estrogen treatment, blood cholesterol, age, race), and several outcome variables (e.g., heart attacks, strokes).

Experiments study an **intervention** (a special kind of predictor variable that the investigator manipulates), such as treatment with estrogen or placebo. This design allows her to observe the effects on the outcome variable, often using randomization to control for the influence of confounding variables (other predictors such as age that could confuse the interpretation of the findings).

## Statistical Issues

The investigator must develop plans for managing and analyzing the study data. For experiments this always involves specifying a **hypothesis,** a version of the research question that provides the basis for testing the statistical significance of the findings (Chapter 5).

> *Hypothesis:* Women who receive estrogen treatment after menopause will have fewer heart attacks than those who do not.

The hypothesis also allows the investigator to estimate the **sample size,** the number of subjects needed to observe the expected difference in outcome between study groups with a reasonable degree of probability, or **power** (Chapter 6).

Most observational studies have an analytic component that also benefits from having a prior hypothesis. For purely descriptive studies (e.g., the prevalence of CHD in women 50 to 69 years of age), an analogous approach estimates the number of subjects needed to produce an acceptable level of precision when confidence intervals are calculated for the means, proportions, or other descriptive statistics.

## ■ THE PHYSIOLOGY OF RESEARCH: HOW IT WORKS

The goal of clinical research is to draw *inferences* from the study results about the nature of truth in the universe (Fig. 1.1). With this in mind, the process of doing research reverses this sequence. Beginning with a decision about what health problem the investigator wishes to address, the investigator undertakes a study that will answer this research question.

This undertaking involves two distinct steps (Fig. 1.2). The first is to *design* a study plan with subjects and measurements chosen to enhance the process of appropriately answering the research question and generalizing these conclusions to the people and phenomena addressed by the research question. The second step is to *carry out* the study in a fashion that enhances the likelihood of getting

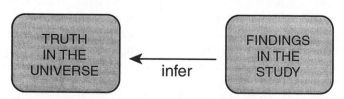

## ■ FIGURE 1.1

The findings of a study lead to inferences about the universe outside.

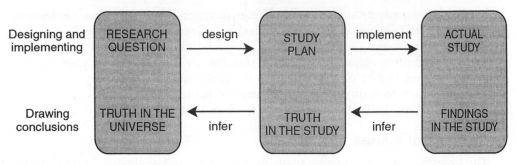

**■ FIGURE 1.2**

The process of designing and implementing a research project sets the stage for drawing conclusions from the findings.

the right answer; in other words, to draw the correct conclusions about what actually happened in the study.

In this section we will first address the design side of Fig. 1.2, then the implementation side. We will then turn to the errors that threaten the validity of clinical research inferences.

## Designing the Study

The research question, as noted earlier, is what the investigator really wants to answer. For the purpose of illustration, we will use a simple descriptive question: *How common is it for women to take estrogen after menopause?*

This question cannot be answered with perfect accuracy because it would be impossible to study all postmenopausal women and because our instruments for discovering whether a woman is taking estrogen are imperfect. So the investigator must settle for a related question that can be answered by the study, such as the following: *"Among postmenopausal women seen for the first time in her primary care clinic, what proportion report on a questionnaire that they are taking estrogen?"* The transformation from research question to study plan is illustrated in Fig. 1.3.

One major component of this transformation is the choice of a sample of subjects that will represent the population. The group of subjects specified in the protocol can only be a sample of the population of interest because there are practical barriers to studying the entire population. The decision to study patients entering the UCSF primary care clinics is a compromise. This is a sample that is feasible to study but one that may produce a different prevalence of estrogen treatment than that found in all women.

The other major component of the transformation is the choice of variables that will represent the phenomena of interest. The variables specified in the study plan are usually proxies for these phenomena. The decision to use a self-report questionnaire to assess estrogen treatment is a fast and inexpensive way to collect information, but it will not be perfectly accurate. Some women will not give the right answer because they know they're taking hormones but don't recognize the phrase *estrogen treatment* that appears in the questionnaire, or because they may have forgotten what they are taking.

In short, each of the differences in Fig. 1.3 between the research question and the study plan has the purpose of making the study more practical. The cost of this increase in practicality, however, is the risk that the study may produce a

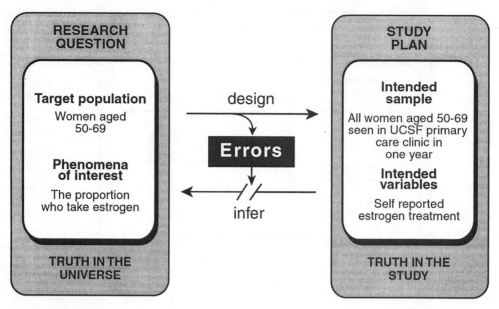

■ **FIGURE 1.3**

Design errors. If the intended sample and variables do not represent the target population and phenomena of interest, these errors may distort inferences about the answer to the research question.

wrong answer to the research question. Figure 1.3 illustrates the important fact that errors in designing the study are a common reason for getting the wrong answer to the research question.

## Implementing the Study

Returning to Fig. 1.2, the right-hand side is concerned with implementation, and the degree to which the actual study matches the study plan. At issue here is the problem of a wrong answer to the research question because the way the sample was actually drawn and the measurements made differed in important ways from the way they were designed (Fig. 1.4).

The actual sample of study subjects is almost always different from the intended sample. The plans to study all age-eligible women entering primary care clinics, for example, would probably be disrupted by incomplete attendance (say only 150 of the 278 patients who are scheduled for first visits ever show up during the year of the study) and by refusal to participate (say only 100 of these consent to be studied). The 100 patients who agree to be studied may have a different prevalence of estrogen treatment from those who do not show up or refuse. In addition to these problems with the subjects, the actual measurements can differ from the intended measurements. If the format of the questionnaire is unclear, the women may get confused and check the wrong box, for example, or they may simply omit the question by mistake.

These differences between the study plan and the actual study can alter the answer to the research question. Figure 1.4 illustrates the important fact that errors in implementing the study are the other common reasons (besides errors of design) for getting the wrong answer to the research question.

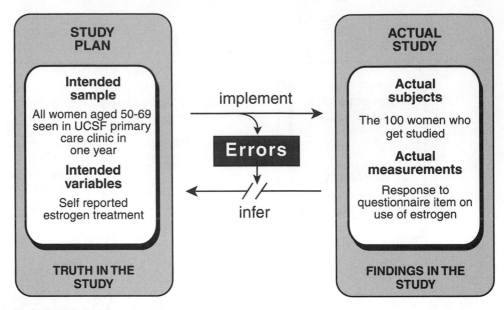

■ **FIGURE 1.4**

Implementation errors. If the actual subjects and measurements do not represent the intended sample and variables, these errors may distort inferences about what actually happened in the study.

## Drawing Causal Inference

A special kind of validity problem arises in studies that examine the **association** between a predictor and an outcome variable in order to draw causal inference. If the study finds an association between hormone therapy and heart attacks, does this represent cause and effect, or is there some other explanation? Reducing the likelihood of confounding and other rival explanations is one of the major challenges in designing an observational study (Chapter 9).

## The Errors of Research

No study is free of errors, and the inferences that have been described are never perfectly valid. The goal is simply to maximize the validity of drawing inferences from what happened in the study sample to reach conclusions about the nature of things in the population. Erroneous inferences can be addressed in the analysis phase of research, but the best strategies are focused on design and implementation (Fig. 1.5): Preventing errors from occurring in the first place, to the extent that it is practical and economic to do so.

The two main kinds of error that interfere with research inferences are random error and systematic error. The distinction is important because the strategies for minimizing them are quite different.

**Random error** is a wrong result due to **chance**—unknown sources of variation that are equally likely to distort the sample in either direction. If the true prevalence of estrogen treatment in 50- to 69-year-old women is 20%, a well-designed sample of 100 patients from that population might contain exactly 20 patients with this disease. More likely, however, the sample would contain a nearby number such as 18, 19, 21, or 22. Occasionally, chance would produce a substantially different number, such as 12 or 28. Among several techniques for reducing the influence

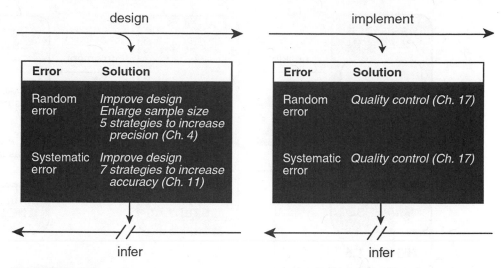

■ **FIGURE 1.5**

Research errors. These can have both random and systematic elements, as indicated in this blown-up version of the error boxes in Figs. 1.3 and 1.4. The boxes summarize the design and implementation strategies for minimizing the effects of these errors.

of random error, the simplest and best known is to increase the sample size. The use of a larger sample diminishes the likelihood of a wrong result by increasing the **precision** of the estimate—the degree to which the observed prevalence approximates 20% each time a sample is drawn.

**Systematic error** is a wrong result due to **bias** (sources of variation that distort the study findings in one direction). An illustration is the decision in Fig. 1.3 to use patients who come to the primary care clinic, who might be more likely than average to adopt medical treatments. Increasing the sample size has no effect on systematic error. The only way to improve the **accuracy** of the estimate (the degree to which it approximates the true value) is to design the study in a way that either reduces the size of the various biases or gives some information about them. An example would be to draw a second sample of women from a setting that may be less likely to bias the proportion of women treated with estrogen (e.g., employees in a corporation), and to compare the observed prevalence in the two samples.

The examples of random and systematic error in the preceding two paragraphs are components of sampling error, which threatens inferences from the study subjects to the population. Both random and systematic errors can also contribute to measurement error, threatening the inferences from the study measurements to the phenomena of interest. An illustration of random measurement error is the variation in the response when a questionnaire is administered on several occasions. An example of systematic measurement error is the underestimation of the prevalence of estrogen treatment due to lack of clarity in how the question is phrased. Additional strategies for controlling all these sources of error are presented in Chapters 3 and 4.

The concepts presented in the last several pages are summarized in Fig. 1.6. Here is an important bottom line: Getting the right answer to the research question is a matter of designing and implementing the study in a fashion that keeps the extent of inferential errors at an acceptable level.

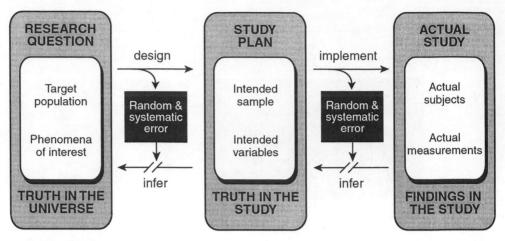

■ **FIGURE 1.6**

Summary of how research works.

## ■ DESIGNING THE STUDY

### Developing the Study Protocol

The first step in designing a study is to establish the research question. This task is discussed at length in Chapter 2. Once the research question is in hand, the process of developing the study plan can begin. There are three versions of the study plan that are produced in sequence, each larger and more detailed than the preceding one.

- A **one- to two-page outline** of the elements of the study. We recommend the sequence in Table 1.1. It serves as a standardized checklist to remind the investigator to include all the components. Just as important, the sequence has an orderly logic that helps clarify the investigator's thinking on the topic.
- The **study protocol,** an expansion on the one- to two-page outline that can range from five to 25 or more pages. The full protocol is the main document used to plan the study and to apply for grant support; we discuss parts of it throughout this book and put them all together in Chapter 19.
- The **operations manual,** a collection of specific procedural instructions, questionnaires, and other materials designed to ensure a uniform and standardized approach to carrying out the study with good quality control (Chapters 4 and 17).

The study question and one- to two-page outline should be written out at an early stage. Putting thoughts down on paper leads the way from vague ideas to specific plans and provides a concrete basis for getting advice from colleagues and consultants. It is a challenge to do it (ideas are easier to talk about than to write down), but the rewards are a faster start and a better project.

Appendix 1.1 provides an example of a one-page study plan. As usual, this plan deals more with the anatomy of research (Table 1.1) than with its physiology (Fig. 1.6), so the investigator must remind herself to worry about the errors that may result when it comes time to draw inferences about what happened in the study sample and formulate conclusions for the population. A study's virtues and problems can be revealed by explicitly considering how the question the study is likely to answer differs from the research question, given the plans for acquiring subjects and making measurements, and given the likely problems of implementation.

With the one- to two-page outline in hand and the intended inferences in mind, the investigator can proceed with the details of her protocol. This includes getting advice from colleagues, drafting specific recruitment and measurement methods, considering scientific and ethical appropriateness, changing the study question and outline, pretesting specific recruitment and measurement methods, making more changes, getting more advice, and so forth. This iterative process is the nature of research design and the topic of the rest of this book.

## Trade-offs

Errors are an inherent part of all studies. The main issue is whether the errors will be large enough to change the conclusions in important ways. When designing a study, the investigator is in much the same position as a labor union official bargaining for a new contract. The union official begins with a wish list—shorter hours, more pay, parking spaces, and so forth. She must then make concessions, holding on to the things that are most important and relinquishing those that are not essential. At the end of the negotiations is a vital step: She must look at the best contract she could negotiate and decide if it has become so bad that it is no longer worth having.

The same sort of concessions must be made by an investigator when she transforms the research question to the study plan and considers the potential problems in implementation. On one side is the issue of scientific validity; on the other, feasibility. The vital last step of the union negotiator is all too often omitted. Once the study plan has been formulated, the investigator must decide whether it adequately addresses the research question and whether it can be implemented with acceptable levels of error. Often the answer is no, and the investigator must begin the process anew. But take heart! Good scientists distinguish themselves not so much by their uniformly good research ideas as by their tenacity in turning over those that won't work at an early stage and trying again.

## ■ SUMMARY

1. The **anatomy of research** is the set of tangible elements that make up the study plan: the **research question, design, study subjects,** and **measurement approaches**. The challenge is to design a study plan with elements that are fast, inexpensive, and easy to implement.

2. The **physiology of research** is how the study works. The study findings are used to draw **inferences** about what actually happened in the study sample and about events in the universe outside. The challenge here is to design and implement a study plan with adequate control over two major threats to these inferences: **random error** (chance) and **systematic error** (bias).

3. A good way to develop the **study plan** is to write a one-sentence summary and to expand this into a **one- to two-page outline** that sets out the study elements in a standardized sequence. Later on the study plan will be expanded into the **protocol** and the **operations manual**.

4. The next step is to consider the main **inferences** that will be drawn from the study subjects to the population and from the study measurements to the

phenomena of interest. At issue here are the relationships between the **research question** (what the investigator really wants to answer in the universe), the **study plan** (what the study is designed to answer), and the **actual study** (what the study will actually answer, given the errors of implementation that can be anticipated).

5. Good judgment by the investigator and advice from colleagues are needed for the many **trade-offs** involved and for determining the overall viability of the project.

# EXERCISES

**1.** For each of the following abstracts, state the research question in a single sentence that specifies the predictor and outcome variables, and population sampled. What is the study design? Think about the main inference that can be drawn from the study, to whom can it be generalized, and what are the potential errors in drawing and applying these inferences?

**a.** Giving vitamin D to patients with vitamin D deficiency can improve strength. To find out whether the ordinary weakness of aging could be treated with vitamin D, we selected 38 men and women 70 years of age and greater from a hypertension treatment clinic and randomly assigned them to receive either vitamin $D_3$ or identical placebo. Muscle strength of the quadriceps, measured with an isokinetic dynamometer after 6 months of treatment, was similar in the two groups.

**b.** We examined the use of estrogen replacement therapy in relation to breast cancer in postmenopausal women. During 367,187 person-years of follow-up, there were 722 new cases of breast cancer. The risk of breast cancer was significantly elevated among current estrogen users (relative risk, 1.36; 95% confidence interval (CI) 1.11 to 1.67), but not among former users.

**c.** To assess whether the sedative effects of psychotropic drugs might cause hip fractures, we studied 1,021 men and women with hip fractures and 5,606 without hip fracture among elderly Medicaid enrollees. Persons treated with short-acting tranquilizers had no increased risk of hip fracture. By contrast, there was an increased risk associated with current use of tranquilizers having half-lives of more than 24 hours (odds ratio, 1.8; 95% CI 1.3 to 2.4).

**d.** Knowledge about acquired immmunodeficiency syndrome (AIDS) was studied among 893 teen-aged boys and 633 girls drawn from 12 secondary schools in Zimbabwe. Ninety-three percent of the children thought that it was an infection caused by having sexual relations, and 10% believed that it could be contracted from toilet seats.

# ■ APPENDIX 1.1

## Outline of a Study*

| Element | Example |
|---|---|
| **Title** | Effects of Hormone Treatment after Menopause on Lipoprotein (a) (Lp(a)) |
| **Research question** | What are the effects of treatment with estrogen plus progestin (compared with placebo) on Lp(a) levels in postmenopausal women? |
| **Significance** | 1. Epidemiologic studies suggest that hormone treatment after menopause may help prevent coronary heart disease, the largest cause of death in women. |
| | 2. Lp(a) is an understudied lipoprotein that has been found to be an independent risk factor for coronary disease in several studies. |
| | 3. Among conventional lipid-lowering drugs, only nicotinic acid in high doses lowers Lp(a) levels; however, previous studies have suggested that hormone treatment may have this effect. |
| | 4. There is a need to confirm this finding for the estrogen plus progestin treatment that is now commonly used after menopause, and to extend it to women with existing coronary disease. |
| **Design** | Randomized blinded trial with one year of follow-up. |
| **Subjects** | |
| Entry criteria | Postmenopausal women with documented coronary disease (evidence for prior myocardial infarction or coronary artery surgery, or 50% obstruction on angiography). |
| Recruitment | Consecutive sample of all women who qualify in 20 clinical centers, recruited in cardiology clinics and by mailings and advertisements. |
| **Variables** | |
| Predictor | Randomization to a daily tablet containing conjugated equine estrogen (0.65 mg) and medroxy-progesterone acetate (2.5 mg), or to a placebo identical in appearance. |
| Outcome | Change in serum level of Lp(a) between baseline and 1 year after randomization, measured immunochemically with a sandwich ELISA assay that uses a monoclonal antibody to apo(a) as the capture antibody (Strategic Diagnostics, Newark, DE). |
| **Statistical issues** | |
| Hypothesis | There will be a greater decrease in Lp(a) levels in the hormone-treated group than in the placebo group. |
| Sample size and power | The number of women in the existing HERS trial available for this ancillary study was 2,763. This allows detection of a reduction in Lp(a) of 2 mg/dL with a power of 90%, using a t-test and two-tailed alpha of 0.05. |

*This is part of an actual ancillary study (see Chapter 16) to the Heart and Estrogen/Progestin Replacement Study (HERS), an existing secondary prevention trial. The ancillary study was conceived, designed, and implemented by a UCSF fellow. Reprinted with permission from Shlipak MG, Simon JA, Vittinghoff E, et al. Estrogen and progestin, lipoprotein (a), and the risk of recurrent coronary heart disease events after menopause. *JAMA* 2000;283:1845.

# 2 Conceiving the Research Question

## Steven R. Cummings, Warren S. Browner, and Stephen B. Hulley

**T**he research question is the uncertainty about something in the population that the investigator wants to resolve by making measurements on her study subjects. There is no shortage of questions. Even as we succeed in producing good answers to some questions, we remain surrounded by others. Recent clinical trials, for example, have established that the estrogen-like drug tamoxifen reduces the risk of breast cancer during 4 years of use by women at high risk of breast cancer (1). But now there are new questions: Does tamoxifen reduce the risk of death due to breast cancer? How long should treatment be continued? Might other estrogen-like drugs have the same beneficial effects without tamoxifen's propensity for thromboembolism?

The challenge in searching for a research question is not a shortage of uncertainties; it is the difficulty of finding an important one that can be transformed into a feasible and valid study plan.

## ■ ORIGINS OF A RESEARCH QUESTION

For an established investigator the best research questions usually emerge from the findings and problems she has observed in her own prior studies and in those of other workers in the field. A new investigator has not yet developed this base of experience. Although a fresh perspective can sometimes be useful by allowing a creative person to conceive new approaches to old problems, lack of experience is largely an impediment.

### Mastering the Literature

It is important to master the published literature in an area of study; **scholarship** is a necessary ingredient to good research. A new investigator should conduct a thorough search of published literature in the area of study. Carrying out a systematic review such as a meta-analysis of a question is a great first step in developing and establishing expertise, and the literature review can serve as a source of background for grant proposals and research reports. Recent advances may be presented at research meetings or just be known to active investigators in a particular field long before they are published. Thus mastery of a subject entails participating in meetings and building relationships with experts in the field.

No amount of reading can substitute for firsthand experience in guiding the many judgments of clinical research. Therefore an essential strategy for a young investigator is to apprentice herself to an experienced **mentor** who has the time and interest to work with her regularly. A good relationship of this sort also provides the tangible resources a young investigator needs—office space, computer facilities, support for supplies and laboratory tests, and so on. The choice of one or two senior scientists who will be her mentor is the single most important decision a new investigator makes.

## Being Alert to New Ideas and Techniques

In addition to the medical literature as a source of ideas for research questions, all investigators find it very helpful to **attend conferences** in which recent work is presented. The discussion of the work in the meeting can be supplemented by informal conversations with other scientists during the breaks. A new investigator who overcomes her shyness and engages a speaker at the coffee break will often find the experience richly rewarding.

A **skeptical attitude** about prevailing beliefs can stimulate good research questions. For example, in the past, surgery was recommended for patients with asymptomatic gallstones because studies indicated that up to 50% of such patients eventually developed symptoms or complications. However, one research group critically reviewed these studies and observed that some had included patients with symptomatic gallstones and others had counted symptoms that were probably not due to gallstones. Using better criteria for gallstone-related symptoms in a well-defined cohort of patients with asymptomatic gallstones, the investigators found that only 15% of the patients suffered any biliary pain during 15 years of follow-up (2).

The application of **new technologies** often generates new insights and questions about familiar clinical problems (3). Recent advances in imaging and in techniques for molecular and genetic analyses, for example, have spawned many new clinical research studies. Similarly, taking a new concept or finding from one field and applying it to a problem in a different field can lead to good research questions. Higher levels of bone density, for example, have come to be seen as a marker that reflects a woman's lifelong exposure to estrogen. Investigators applied this technology to problems besides bone disease to demonstrate that women with low bone density have a lower risk of breast cancer (4) and higher rates of cognitive decline (5), perhaps due to low levels of estrogen over a lifetime.

## Keeping the Imagination Roaming

Careful **observation** of patients has led to many descriptive studies and is a fruitful source of research questions. **Teaching** is also an excellent source of inspiration; ideas for studies often occur while preparing presentations or during discussions with inquisitive students. Because there is usually not enough time to develop these ideas on the spot, it is useful to keep them in a computer file or a notebook for future reference.

There is a major role for **creativity** in the process of conceiving research questions, imagining new answers to old questions, and having fun with ideas. There is also a need for **tenacity,** for returning to a troublesome problem repeatedly until a resolution is reached that feels comfortable. Some creative ideas come to mind during informal conversations with colleagues over lunch; others occur in brainstorming sessions. Many inspirations are solo affairs that strike while preparing a lecture, showering, perusing the Internet, or just sitting and thinking. The trick is to put an unresolved problem clearly in view and turn on the mental switch that lets the mind run freely toward it.

# ■ CHARACTERISTICS OF A GOOD RESEARCH QUESTION

The characteristics of a good research question are that it be feasible, interesting, novel, ethical, and relevant (which forms the mnemonic *FINER*; Table 2.1).

## Feasible

It is best to know the practical limits and problems of studying a question early on, before wasting much time and effort along unworkable lines.

***Number of Subjects.***   Many studies do not achieve their intended purposes because they cannot enroll enough subjects. The first step is to make a preliminary estimate of the sample size requirements of the study (Chapter 6). The next step is to estimate the number of subjects likely to be available for the study, the number who would be excluded or refuse to participate, and the number who would be lost to follow-up. Even careful planning often produces estimates that are overly optimistic, and the investigator should be very certain that there are enough willing subjects. It is sometimes necessary to carry out a pilot survey to be sure. If the number of subjects appears insufficient, the investigator can consider a number of strategies. These include expanding the inclusion criteria, eliminating unnecessary exclusion criteria, lengthening the time frame for enrolling subjects, acquiring additional sources of subjects, developing more precise measurement approaches (Chapter 4), and using a different study design.

***Technical Expertise.***   The investigators must have the skills, equipment, and experience needed for recruiting the subjects, measuring the variables, and managing and analyzing the data. The easiest strategy is to use familiar and established approaches, because the process of developing new methods and skills is time-consuming and uncertain. When it is necessary to develop an approach such as a new questionnaire for the study, expertise in how to accomplish the innovation

---

**■ TABLE 2.1**
FINER Criteria for a Good Research Question

**Feasible**
   Adequate number of subjects
   Adequate technical expertise
   Affordable in time and money
   Manageable in scope

**Interesting**
   To the investigator

**Novel**
   Confirms or refutes previous findings
   Extends previous findings
   Provides new findings

**Ethical**

**Relevant**
   To scientific knowledge
   To clinical and health policy
   To future research directions

should be available. Consultants can help to shore up technical aspects that are unfamiliar to the investigators, but for major areas of the study it is better to have an experienced colleague as a coinvestigator. For example, it is often wise to include a statistician as a member of the research team from the beginning of the planning process.

**Cost in Time and Money.**   It is important to estimate the costs of each component of the project, bearing in mind that the time and money needed will generally exceed the amounts projected at the outset. If the costs are prohibitive, the only options are to consider a less expensive design or to develop additional sources of funding. If the study will be too expensive or time-consuming, it is best to know this early, when the question can be modified or abandoned before expending a great deal of effort.

**Scope.**   Problems often arise when an investigator attempts to accomplish too much, making many measurements at repeated contacts with a large group of subjects in an effort to answer too many research questions. The solution is to narrow the scope of the study and focus only on the most important goals. Many scientists find it difficult to give up the opportunity to answer interesting side questions, but the reward will be a better answer to the main question at hand.

## Interesting

An investigator may have many motivations for pursuing a particular research question: because it will provide financial support, because it is a logical or important next step in building a career, or because getting at the truth of the matter seems interesting. We like this last reason; it is one that grows as it is exercised and that provides the intensity of effort needed for overcoming the many hurdles and frustrations of the research process. However, it is wise to confirm the interest of a question with mentors and outside experts before devoting substantial energy to developing a research plan or grant proposal that peers and funding agencies may find dull.

## Novel

Good clinical research contributes new information. A study that merely reiterates what is already established is not worth the effort and cost. The novelty of a proposed study can be determined by thoroughly reviewing the literature, consulting with experts who are familiar with ongoing research, and searching lists of projects that have been funded by agencies. (See, for example, the NIH Computer Retrieval of Information on Scientific Projects [CRISP] website.) A question need not be totally original. It may ask whether a previous observation can be replicated, whether the findings in one population also apply to others, or whether improved measurement techniques can clarify the relationship between known risk factors and a disease. A confirmatory study is particularly useful if it avoids the weaknesses of previous studies.

## Ethical

A good research question must be ethical. If the study poses unacceptable physical risks or invasion of privacy (Chapter 14), the investigator must seek other ways to answer the question. If there is uncertainty about whether the study is ethical, it is important to discuss it at an early stage with the institutional review board.

## Relevant

Among the characteristics of a good research question, none is more important than its relevance. A good way to decide about relevance is to imagine the various outcomes that are likely to occur and consider how each possibility might advance scientific knowledge, influence clinical management and health policy, or guide further research.

# ■ DEVELOPING THE RESEARCH QUESTION AND STUDY PLAN

It helps a great deal to write down the research question and a brief (one- or two-page) outline of the study plan at an early stage. This requires some self-discipline, but it forces the investigator to clarify her own ideas about the plan and to discover specific problems that need attention. The outline also provides a basis for colleagues to react to with specific suggestions.

## Problems and Solutions

The potential problems in choosing the research question and developing the study plan are recapped, with solutions, in Table 2.2. Two general kinds of solutions deserve special emphasis. The first is the importance of getting good advice.

### ■ TABLE 2.2
The Research Question and Study Plan: Problems and Solutions

| Potential Problem | Solutions |
|---|---|
| A. The research question is not FINER | |
|   1. Not feasible | |
|     Too broad | Specify a smaller set of variables<br>Narrow the question |
|     Not enough subjects available | Expand the inclusion criteria<br>Eliminate or modify exclusion criteria<br>Add other sources of subjects<br>Lengthen the time frame for entry into study<br>Use strategies to decrease sample size (Chapter 6) |
|     Methods beyond the skills of the investigator | Collaborate with colleagues who have the skills<br>Consult experts and review the literature for alternative methods<br>Learn the skills |
|     Too expensive | Consider less costly study designs<br>  Fewer subjects and measurements<br>  Less extensive measurements<br>  Fewer follow-up visits |
|   2. Not interesting, novel, or relevant | Consult with mentor<br>Modify the research question |
|   3. Uncertain ethical suitability | Consult with institutional review board<br>Modify the research question |
| B. The study plan is vague | Write the research question at an early stage<br>Get specific in the one- to two-page study plan<br>  How the subjects will be sampled<br>  How the variables will be measured |

We recommend a research team that includes representatives of each of the major aspects of the study and that includes at least one senior scientist. In addition, it is a good idea to consult with specialists who can guide the discovery of previous research on the topic and the choice and design of measurement techniques. Sometimes a local expert will do, but it is often useful to contact individuals in other institutions who have published pertinent work on the subject. A new investigator may be intimidated by the prospect of writing or calling someone she knows only as an author in the *Journal of the American Medical Association*, but most scientists respond favorably to such requests for advice.

The second thing to emphasize is the way the study plan should gradually emerge from an iterative process of designing, reviewing, pretesting, and revising (Chapter 17). Once the one- to two-page study plan is written, advice from colleagues will usually result in important changes. As the protocol gradually takes shape, a small pretest of the number and willingness of the potential subjects may lead to changes in the recruitment plan. The preferred imaging test may turn out to be prohibitively costly and a less expensive alternative may be sought. And so on.

## Primary and Secondary Questions

Many studies have more than one research question. Experiments often address the effect of the intervention on several outcomes; for example, the Women's Health Initiative was designed to determine whether reducing dietary fat intake would reduce the risks of coronary heart disease, of breast cancer, and of fractures (6). The advantage of designing a study with several research questions is the efficiency that can result, with several answers emerging from a single study. The disadvantages are the increased complexity of designing and implementing the study and of drawing statistical inferences from a study with multiple hypotheses (Chapter 5). A sensible strategy is to establish a single primary research question around which to focus the development of the study plan and sample size estimate. This can be supplemented with secondary research questions that may also produce valuable conclusions.

## ■ SUMMARY

1. All studies should start with a **research question** that addresses what the investigator would like to know. The goal is to find an important one that can be developed into a feasible and valid study plan.
2. One key ingredient for developing a research question is **scholarship** that is acquired by a thorough and continuing review of the work of others, both published and unpublished. Another key ingredient is **experience,** and the single most important decision a new investigator makes is her choice of one or two senior scientists who will be her **mentor.**
3. Good research questions arise from medical articles and conferences, from critical thinking about clinical practices and problems, from applying new concepts or methods to old issues, and from ideas that emerge from teaching.
4. Before committing much time and effort to writing a proposal or carrying out a study, the investigator should consider whether the research question and study plan are "FINER": **feasible, interesting, novel, ethical,** and **relevant.**
5. Early on, the research question should be developed into a brief **written study plan** that specifically describes how many subjects will be needed, and how the subjects will be selected and the measurements made.

6. Developing the research question and study plan is an **iterative process** that includes consultations with advisors and friends, a growing familiarity with the literature, and pilot studies of the recruitment and measurement approaches. The qualities needed in the investigator are **judgment, tenacity, and creativity.**

7. Most studies have more than one question, but it is useful to focus on a **single primary question** in designing and implementing the study

## EXERCISES

1. Consider the following research questions. First, write each question in a single sentence that specifies a predictor, outcome, and population. Then discuss whether it meets the FINER criteria (feasible, interesting, novel, ethical, relevant). Rewrite the question in a form that overcomes any problems in meeting their criteria.
   a. What is the relationship between depression and health?
   b. Does eating red meat cause cancer?
   c. Does lowering serum cholesterol prevent heart disease?
   d. Can a relaxation exercise decrease the anxiety associated with the mammography?
   e. Do contraceptive vaginal sponges prevent HIV infection?

## References

1. Fisher B, Costantino JP, Wickerham DL, et al. Tamoxifen for prevention of breast cancer: report of the National Surgical Adjuvant Breast and Bowel Project P-1 Study. *J Natl Cancer Inst* 1998;90:1371–88.
2. Gracie WA, Ransohoff DF. The natural history of silent gallstones: the innocent gallstone is not a myth. *N Engl J Med* 1982;307:798–800.
3. Kuhn TS. *The structure of scientific revolutions.* Chicago: University of Chicago Press, 1962.
4. Cauley JA, Lucas FL, Kuller LH, et al. Bone mineral density and risk of breast cancer in older women: the study of osteoporotic fractures. Study of Osteoporotic Fractures Research Group. *JAMA* 1996;276:1404–8.
5. Yaffe K, Browner W, Cauley J, Launer L, Harris T. Association between bone mineral density and cognitive decline in older women. *J Am Geriatr Soc* 1999;47:1176–82.
6. Design of the Women's Health Initiative clinical trial and observational study. The Women's Health Initiative Study Group. *Control Clin Trials* 1998;19:61–109.

#  Choosing the Study Subjects: Specification, Sampling, and Recruitment

### Stephen B. Hulley, Thomas B. Newman, and Steven R. Cummings

**A** good choice of study subjects serves the vital purpose of ensuring that the findings in the study accurately represent what is going on in the **population** of interest. The protocol must specify a **sample** of subjects that can be studied at an acceptable cost in time and money, yet one that is large enough to control random error in generalizing the study findings to the population and representative enough to control systematic error in these inferences.

These are conflicting goals that challenge the judgment of the investigator. We will come to the issue of choosing the appropriate *number* of study subjects in Chapter 6. In this chapter we address the process of specifying and sampling the *kinds* of subjects who will be representative and feasible. We also discuss strategies for recruiting these subjects to participate in the study.

## ■ BASIC TERMS AND CONCEPTS

### Target Population and Sample

A population is a complete set of people with a specified set of characteristics, and a sample is a subset of the population. In the lay usage, the characteristics that define a population are geographic; we speak, for example, of the "population of Canada." In research the defining characteristics are also clinical, demographic, and temporal:

- Clinical and demographic characteristics define the **target population,** the large set of people throughout the world to which the results will be generalized (e.g., all teenagers with asthma).
- The **study sample** is the subset of the target population available for study (e.g., teenagers with asthma living in the investigator's town in 2002).

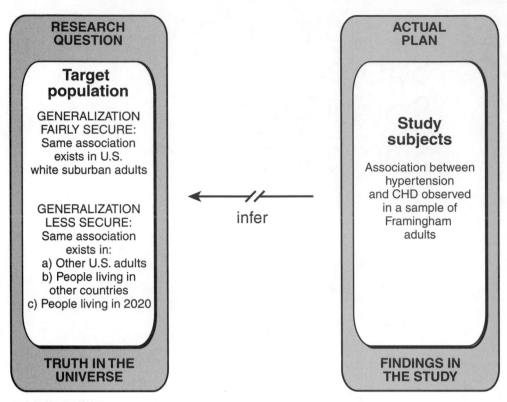

RESEARCH QUESTION — ACTUAL PLAN

**Target population**

GENERALIZATION FAIRLY SECURE: Same association exists in U.S. white suburban adults

GENERALIZATION LESS SECURE: Same association exists in:
a) Other U.S. adults
b) People living in other countries
c) People living in 2020

infer

**Study subjects**

Association between hypertension and CHD observed in a sample of Framingham adults

TRUTH IN THE UNIVERSE — FINDINGS IN THE STUDY

■ **FIGURE 3.1**
Inferences in generalizing from the study subjects to the target populations.

## Generalizing the Study Findings

The target population and study sample are illustrated in Fig. 3.1 with a finding in the Framingham Study—the association between hypertension and coronary heart disease (CHD).

In deciding whether this finding represents an association in the general population, the investigator must first consider whether the sample of study subjects differs from the population of Framingham, Massachusetts. The sampling design called for listing all the adult residents of this town and then asking every second person to participate. Unfortunately, one-third of the Framingham residents selected for the study refused to participate, and in their place the investigators accepted other residents who had heard about the study and volunteered (1). Because respondents are often more healthy than nonrespondents, especially if they are volunteers, the characteristics of the actual sample probably differ from those of the intended sample. Every sample has some errors, however, and the issue is whether they are large enough to cause a wrong answer to the research question. The Framingham Study sampling errors do not seem large enough to invalidate the conclusion that hypertension is a risk factor for CHD, and other studies that do not have the same errors support this conclusion.

The investigator must next consider the validity of generalizing from Framingham adults to the target population. This inference is more subjective. The town of Framingham was selected from the universe of towns in the world, not with a scientific sampling design, but because it seemed a fairly typical middle-class

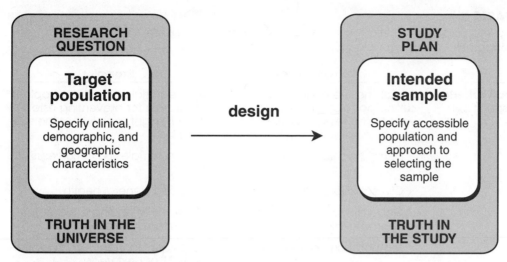

**■ FIGURE 3.2**
Steps in designing the protocol for choosing the study subjects.

residential community and it was convenient to the investigators. The validity of generalizing the results to other populations is based on the general knowledge that relationships tend to be similar in demographically similar populations; and on the findings of other studies.

In general, analytic studies and clinical trials that address biologic relationships produce more widely generalizable results than descriptive studies that address distributions of characteristics. For example, the strength of hypertension as a risk factor for CHD tends to be more consistent among diverse populations than the prevalence of hypertension. The uncertainty of drawing inferences to other populations illustrates the fact that in clinical research, generalizability is not a simple yes-or-no matter; it is a complex and largely qualitative judgment.

### Steps in Designing the Protocol for Acquiring Study Subjects

The inferences in Fig. 3.1 are presented from right to left, the sequence used for interpreting the findings of a completed study. An investigator who is planning a study reverses this sequence (Fig. 3.2). She begins by specifying the clinical and demographic characteristics of the target population that will serve the research question well. She then uses geographic and temporal criteria to specify the choice of a study sample that is representative and practical.

## ■ SELECTION CRITERIA

Suppose an investigator wants to study the efficacy of calcium supplements for preventing osteoporosis. She begins by creating selection criteria that define the population to be studied.

### Establishing Inclusion Criteria

The inclusion criteria define the main characteristics of the target population (Table 3.1). The task of specifying the clinical characteristics often involves difficult judgments about what factors are important to the research question and how to

| | Considerations | Examples |
|---|---|---|
| **Inclusion criteria** (be specific) | Specifying the characteristics that define populations that are relevant to the research question and efficient for study: | A 5-year trial of calcium supplementation for preventing osteoporosis might specify that the subjects be: |
| | Demographic characteristics | • White females 50 to 60 years old |
| | Clinical characteristics | • In good general health |
| | Geographic (administrative) characteristics | • Patients attending clinic at the investigator's hospital |
| | Temporal characteristics | • Between January 1 and December 31 of next year |
| **Exclusion criteria** (be parsimonious) | Specifying subsets of the population that will *not* be studied because of: | The calcium supplementation trial might exclude subjects who are: |
| | • A high likelihood of being lost to follow-up | • Alcoholic or plan to move out of state |
| | • An inability to provide good data | • Disoriented or have a language barrier* |
| | • Being at high risk of side effects | • Sarcoidosis due to propensity for hypercalcemia |
| | • Characteristics that make it unethical to withhold the study treatment | • Taking corticosteroids |

**■ TABLE 3.1**
Designing Selection Criteria for a Clinical Trial of Calcium Supplements to Prevent Osteoporosis

*Alternatives to exclusion (when these subgroups are important to the research question) would be collecting nonverbal data or using bilingual staff and questionnaires.

define them. How, for example, would an investigator put into practice the criterion that the subjects be in "good general health"? She might decide to include patients with diseases that are not strongly related to osteoporosis or immediately life-threatening (e.g., hypertension) but not to include patients with diseases that might cause osteoporosis (e.g., paraplegia) or interfere with follow-up (e.g., metastatic lung cancer). The task of specifying the demographic characteristics (age, sex, and race) is even tougher, often involving trade-offs that balance generalizability against efficiency. Including men and black women in the study of osteoporosis, for example, would expand generalizability at the cost of an increase in the size or duration of the study (because osteoporosis develops more slowly in these populations).

On these issues there is no single course of action that is clearly right or wrong; the important thing is to make decisions that are sensible, that can be used consistently throughout the study, and that will provide a basis for applying the published conclusions to other populations. This is accomplished by thinking about these issues during the design process and resolving them with explicit criteria in the protocol.

The selection criteria that address the geographic and temporal characteristics of the accessible population also involve trade-offs between scientific and practical goals. The investigator may find that patients at her own hospital are the most available and inexpensive source of subjects. The decision about whether peculiarities of the local population or environment might interfere with generalizing the results to all patients with the disease depends on the nature of the research question.

## Establishing Exclusion Criteria

Exclusion criteria indicate subsets of individuals who would be suitable for the research question were it not for characteristics that might interfere with the quality of the data or with the acceptability of randomization interpretation of the findings (Table 3.1). Exclusion criteria may improve the feasibility of a study at the cost of generalizability, so the investigator should use them sparingly. Including alcoholics in the osteoporosis study would expand generalizability, for example, and allow the investigator to study excess alcohol consumption as a cause of demineralization. However, these advantages could come at the cost of greater problems with follow-up, and the investigator may decide to exclude alcoholics if she believes that preventing loss to follow-up is the more important consideration. (She will then face the problem of developing specific criteria for classifying whether or not an individual is alcoholic.) Clinical trials differ somewhat from observational studies in the nature of their exclusion criteria—for example, being more likely to have exclusions mandated by ethical considerations (Chapter 10).

The investigator must consider whether subjects excluded for these reasons will threaten the validity of generalizing the findings to the population. If the number or kind of such exclusions becomes excessive (and what is excessive depends a good deal on the research question), the generalizability of the study may be compromised.

## Clinical versus Community Populations

If the research question involves patients with a disease, hospitalized or clinic-based patients are inexpensive and easy to recruit, but selection factors that determine who comes to the hospital or clinic may have an important effect. For example, a specialty clinic at a tertiary care medical center tends to accumulate patients with serious forms of the disease who give a distorted impression of the commonplace features and prognosis. For research questions that pertain to diagnosis, treatment, and prognosis of patients in medical settings, however, clinic-based samples can be an excellent choice.

Another common option in choosing the sample is to select subjects in the community who will represent a nonclinical population. Such "population-based" samples can be difficult and expensive to recruit, but they are particularly useful for guiding public health and clinical practice in the community. One of the largest and best examples is the National Health and Nutrition Examination Survey (NHANES), which used a probability sample of all U.S. residents (search for NHANES on the web).

The size and diversity of a sample can be increased by collecting data by mail or telephone, by collaborating with colleagues in other cities, or by using preexisting data sets such as the NHANES and Medicare. Electronically accessible populations have come into widespread use in clinical research and are often more representative and less time-consuming than other possibilities (Chapter 13).

# ■ SAMPLING

Often, the population of people who meet the selection criteria is too large, and there is a need to select a **sample** (a subset of the population) for study.

## Convenience Samples

In clinical research the study sample is usually made up of people who meet the entry criteria and are easily accessible to the investigator. This is termed a **convenience sample**. It has obvious advantages in cost and logistics, and is a good choice for many research questions.

A convenience sample can minimize volunteerism and other selection biases by consecutively selecting every accessible person who meets the entry criteria. A **consecutive sample** is especially desirable when it amounts to taking the entire accessible population over a long enough period to include seasonal variations or other changes over time considered important to the research question. The validity of a sample as a basis for study is the implicit assumption that, for the purpose of answering the research question at hand, it sufficiently represents the target population. With convenience samples this is a matter of judgment.

## Probability Samples

Sometimes, particularly with descriptive research questions, there is a need for a scientific basis for generalizing the findings in the study sample to the population. Probability sampling, the gold standard for ensuring generalizability, uses a random process to guarantee that each unit of the population has a specified chance of selection. It is a scientific approach and provides a rigorous basis for estimating the fidelity with which phenomena observed in the sample represent those in the population, and for computing statistical significance and confidence intervals. There are several versions of this approach.

A **simple random sample** is drawn by enumerating the units of the population and selecting a subset at random. The most common use of this approach in clinical research is when the investigator wishes to select a representative subset from a population that is larger than she needs. To take a random sample of the gallbladder surgery patients at her hospital, for example, the investigator could list all such patients on the operating room schedules for the period of study, then use a table of random numbers to select individuals for study (Appendix 3.1).

A **stratified random sample** involves dividing the population into subgroups according to characteristics such as sex or race and taking a random sample from each of these "strata." The subsamples in a stratified sample can be weighted to draw disproportionately from subgroups that are less common in the population but of special interest to the investigator. In studying the incidence of toxemia in pregnancy, for example, it would be possible to stratify the population according to race and then to sample equal numbers from each one. This would yield incidence estimates for blacks and whites that have comparable precision.

A **cluster sample** is a random sample of natural groupings (*clusters*) of individuals in the population. Cluster sampling is very useful when the population is widely dispersed and it is impractical to list and sample from all its elements. Consider, for example, the problem of reviewing the hospital records of patients with lung cancer selected randomly from a statewide list of discharge diagnoses; patients could be studied at lower cost by choosing a random sample of the hospitals and taking the cases from these. Community surveys often use a two-stage cluster sample: A random sample is drawn from city blocks enumerated on a map and a field team visits the blocks in the sample, lists all the addresses in each, and selects a subsample for study by a second random process.

The advantages of cluster sampling are illustrated by the national NHANES noted earlier, but they come at the cost of adding to the complexity of data analysis. Another disadvantage is the fact that naturally occurring groups are often homogeneous (relative to the population) for the variables of interest; each city block, for example, tends to have people of uniform socioeconomic status.

A **systematic sample** resembles a simple random sample in first enumerating the population but differs in that the sample is selected by a preordained periodic process (e.g., the Framingham approach of taking every second person from a list of town residents). Systematic sampling is susceptible to errors caused by natural periodicities in the population, and it allows the investigator to predict and perhaps manipulate those who will be in the sample. It offers no logistic advantages over simple random sampling, and in clinical research it is rarely a better choice.

## Summarizing the Sampling Design Options

The use of descriptive statistics and tests of statistical significance to draw inferences about the population from observations in the study sample is based on the assumption that a probability sample has been used. But in clinical research a random sample of the target population is rarely possible. Convenience sampling, preferably with a consecutive design, is a practical approach that can be suitable for most clinical research projects. The decision about whether the proposed sampling design is satisfactory requires that the investigator make a judgment: For the research question at hand, will the conclusions of the study be similar to those that would result from studying a true probability sample of the target population?

## ■ RECRUITMENT

### The Goals of Recruitment

An important factor to consider in choosing the accessible population and sampling approach is the feasibility of recruiting the subjects into the study. There are two main goals: (a) to recruit a sample that adequately represents the target population; and (b) to recruit enough subjects to meet the sample size requirements of the study.

### Achieving a Representative Sample

The goal of recruiting a representative sample begins in the design phase with choosing populations and sampling methods wisely, as discussed earlier in this chapter. It ends with implementation, guarding against errors in applying the entry criteria to prospective study participants, and monitoring adherence to these criteria as the study progresses.

A particular concern, especially in observational studies, is the problem of **nonresponse**. The proportion of eligible subjects who agree to enter the study (the **response rate**) influences the validity of inferring that the sample represents the population. People who are difficult to reach and those who refuse to participate once they are contacted tend to be different from people who do enroll. The level of nonresponse that will compromise the generalizability of the study depends on the research question and on the reasons for not responding. A nonresponse rate of 25%, although a good achievement in many settings, can seriously distort the observed prevalence of a disease when the disease itself is a cause of nonresponse. The degree to which this bias may influence the conclusions of a study can sometimes be estimated during the study with an intensive effort to acquire additional information on a sample of nonrespondents. The best way to deal with nonresponse bias, however, is to minimize it at the outset.

The problem of failure to make contact with individuals who have been chosen for the sample can be reduced by designing a systematic series of repeated contact attempts and by using alternative methods (mail, telephone, home visit). Among those who are contacted, refusal to participate can be minimized by improving the efficiency and attractiveness of the study (especially the initial encounter), by choosing a design that avoids invasive and uncomfortable tests, by using brochures and individual discussion to allay anxiety and discomfort, and by providing incentives such as reimbursing the costs of transportation and providing the results of tests. If language barriers are prevalent, they can be circumvented by using bilingual staff and translated questionnaires.

## Recruiting Sufficient Numbers of Subjects

Falling short in the rate of recruitment is one of the commonest problems in clinical research (2). In planning a study it is safe to assume that the number of subjects who meet the entry criteria and agree to enter the study will be fewer, often by several fold, than the number projected at the outset. The solutions to this problem are to estimate the magnitude of the recruitment problem empirically with a pretest, to plan the study with an accessible population that is larger than believed necessary, and to make contingency plans should the need arise for additional subjects. While the study is in progress it is important to closely monitor progress in meeting the recruitment goals and tabulate reasons for falling short of the goals; understanding the proportions of potential subjects lost to the study at various stages can lead to strategies for enhancing recruitment by reducing some of these losses.

Sometimes recruitment involves selecting patients who are already known to the members of the research team (e.g., in a study of a new treatment in patients who are attending the investigator's clinic). Here the chief concern is to present the opportunity for participation in the study fairly, making clear the advantages and disadvantages. (In discussing the desirability of participation, the investigator must recognize the special ethical dilemmas that arise when her advice as the patient's physician might conflict with her preferences as an investigator [Chapter 14].)

Often recruitment involves contacting populations that are not known to the members of the research team. Especially in this endeavor, it is helpful if at least one member of the research team has previous experience with the approaches for contacting the prospective subjects. These include screening in work settings or public places such as shopping malls; sending out large numbers of mailings to listings such as driver's license holders; advertising on the Internet; inviting referrals from clinicians; carrying out retrospective record reviews; and examining lists of patients seen in clinic and hospital settings. Some of these approaches, particularly the latter two, involve concerns with privacy invasion that must be reviewed by the institutional review board.

It may be helpful to prepare for recruitment by getting the support of important organizations. For example, the investigator can meet with hospital administrators to discuss a clinic-based sample, and with the leadership of the medical society and county health department to plan a community screening operation or mailing to physicians. Written endorsements can be included as an appendix in applications for funding. For large studies it may be useful to create a favorable climate in the community by giving public lectures or by advertising through radio, TV, newspaper, fliers, websites, or mass mailings.

# ■ SUMMARY

1. All clinical research is based, philosophically and practically, on the use of a **sample** to represent a **population**.
2. The advantage of sampling is efficiency; it allows the investigator to draw inferences about a large population by examining a **sample** at relatively small cost in time and effort. The disadvantage is the source of error it introduces. If the sample is not sufficiently representative for the research question at hand, the findings may not **generalize** well to the population.
3. In designing a study the first step is to conceptualize the **target population,** formulating a specific set of **inclusion criteria** that establish the demographic and clinical characteristics of subjects well suited to the research question, and a parsimonious set of **exclusion criteria** that eliminate subjects who are unethical or inappropriate to study.
4. The next step is to design an approach to **sampling** the population. A **convenience** sample is often a good choice in clinical research, especially if it is drawn **consecutively. Simple random sampling** can be used to reduce the size of a convenience sample if necessary, and **other probability samples** (stratified and cluster) are useful in certain situations.
5. Finally, the investigator must design and implement strategies for **recruiting** a sample of subjects that is large enough to meet the study needs.

# EXERCISES

1. The research question is to determine factors that cause people to start smoking. The investigator decides to invite all eleventh graders in her suburban high school and to study those who volunteer. Discuss the suitability of this sample for the target population of interest.
2. Suppose that the investigator decided to avoid the bias associated with choosing volunteers by designing a 25% random sample of the entire eleventh grade, and that the actual sample turns out to be 70% female. If it is known that roughly equal numbers of boys and girls are enrolled in the school, then the disproportion in the sex distribution represents an error in drawing the sample. Could this have occurred through random error, systematic error, or both?
3. The research question is, ''What is the prevalence of alcohol and drug use among persons who attend rock concerts?'' You plan a cross-sectional study. Classify the following sampling schemes, commenting on feasibility and whether the results will be generalizable to all people who attend rock concerts.
    a. As each patron entered the theater, you asked him or her to throw a die. All patrons who threw a 6 were asked to fill out a brief questionnaire.

**b.** As each patron entered the theater, you asked him or her to throw a die. Men who threw a 1 and women who threw an even number were asked to fill out a brief questionnaire.

**c.** Tickets to the concert were numbered serially. You asked any patron whose ticket number ended in 1 to fill out a brief questionnaire.

**d.** After all the patrons were seated, you picked five rows at random by drawing from a set of cards, with each card corresponding to one of the rows. You asked all patrons in those five rows to fill out a brief questionnaire.

**e.** You interviewed the first 27 patrons who entered the theater.

**f.** Some tickets were sold by mail and some were sold at the box office just before the performance. Whenever there were three or more people waiting in line to buy tickets at the box office, you asked the last person in line (who had the most time available) to fill out a brief questionnaire while waiting.

**g.** When patrons began to leave after the performance, you interviewed those who were willing and able to answer questions.

## References

1. Dawber TR. *The Framingham Study*. Cambridge, MA: Harvard University Press, 1980:14–29.
2. Friedman LM, Furberg CD, DeMets DL. *Fundamentals of clinical trials*, 3rd ed. St. Louis: Mosby, 1996:30–40.

# ■ APPENDIX 3.1

## Selecting a Random Sample from a Table of Random Numbers

| | | | | | |
|---|---|---|---|---|---|
| 10480 | 15011 | 01536 | 81647 | 91646 | 02011 |
| 22368 | 46573 | 25595 | 85393 | 30995 | 89198 |
| 24130 | 48390 | 22527 | 97265 | 78393 | 64809 |
| 42167 | 93093 | 06243 | 61680 | 07856 | 16376 |
| 37570 | 33997 | 81837 | 16656 | 06121 | 91782 |
| 77921 | 06907 | 11008 | 42751 | 27756 | 53498 |
| 99562 | 72905 | 56420 | 69994 | 98872 | 31016 |
| 96301 | 91977 | 05463 | 07972 | 18876 | 20922 |
| 89572 | 14342 | 63661 | 10281 | 17453 | 18103 |
| 85475 | 36857 | 53342 | 53998 | 53060 | 59533 |
| 28918 | 79578 | 88231 | 33276 | 70997 | 79936 |
| 63553 | 40961 | 48235 | 03427 | 49626 | 69445 |
| 09429 | 93969 | 52636 | 92737 | 88974 | 33488 |
| 10365 | 61129 | 87529 | 85689 | 48237 | 52267 |
| 07119 | 97336 | 71048 | 08178 | 77233 | 13916 |
| 51085 | 12765 | 51821 | 51259 | 77452 | 16308 |
| 02368 | 21382 | 52404 | 60268 | 89368 | 19885 |
| 01011 | 54092 | 33362 | 94904 | 31273 | 04146 |
| 52162 | 53916 | 46369 | 58569 | 23216 | 14513 |
| 07056 | 97628 | 33787 | 09998 | 42698 | 06691 |
| 48663 | 91245 | 85828 | 14346 | 09172 | 30163 |
| 54164 | 58492 | 22421 | 74103 | 47070 | 25306 |
| 32639 | 32363 | 05597 | 24200 | 38005 | 13363 |
| 29334 | 27001 | 87637 | 87308 | 58731 | 00256 |
| 02488 | 33062 | 28834 | 07351 | 19731 | 92420 |
| 81525 | 72295 | 04839 | 96423 | 24878 | 82651 |
| 29676 | 20591 | 68086 | 26432 | 46901 | 20949 |
| 00742 | 57392 | 39064 | 66432 | 84673 | 40027 |
| 05366 | 04213 | 25669 | 26422 | 44407 | 44048 |
| 91921 | 26418 | 64117 | 94305 | 26766 | 25940 |

To select a 10% random sample, begin by enumerating (listing and numbering) every element of the population to be sampled. Then decide on a rule for obtaining an appropriate series of numbers; for example, if your list has 741 elements, your rule might be to go vertically down each column using the first three digits of each number (beginning at the upper left, the numbers are 104, 223, etc.) and to select the first 74 different numbers that fall in the range of 1 to 741. Finally, pick a starting point by an arbitrary process. (Closing your eyes and putting your pencil on some number in the table is one way to do it.)

# Planning the Measurements: Precision and Accuracy

## Stephen B. Hulley, Jeffrey N. Martin, and Steven R. Cummings

**M**easurements describe phenomena in terms that can be analyzed statistically. The validity of a study depends on how well the variables designed for the study represent the phenomena of interest. How well does a fasting blood sugar level represent control of diabetes, for example, or a question about insomnia represent actual sleeping habits?

This chapter begins by considering how the choice of measurement **scale** influences the information content of the measurement. We then turn to the central goal of minimizing measurement error: how to design measurements that are relatively **precise** (free of random error) and **accurate** (free of systematic error), thereby enhancing the validity of drawing inferences from the study to the universe. We conclude with some considerations for measurements in clinical research, noting especially the advantages of storing specimens for later measurement.

## ■ MEASUREMENT SCALES

Table 4.1 presents a simplified classification of measurement scales and the information that results. The classification is important because some types of variables yield more informative statistics than others, adding power to the study and reducing sample size requirements.

### Continuous Variables

Continuous variables have quantified intervals on an infinite scale of values. The number of possible values of body weight, for example, is limited only by the sensitivity of the machine that is used to measure it. Continuous variables are rich in information.

A scale that has a finite number of intervals (such as the number of cigarettes smoked per day) is termed **discrete.** Discrete variables that have a considerable number of possible values resemble continuous variables in statistical analyses and are equivalent for the purpose of designing measurements.

■ **TABLE 4.1**
Measurement Scales

| Type of Measurement | Characteristics of Variable | Example | Descriptive Statistics | Information Content |
|---|---|---|---|---|
| Categorical* Nominal | Unordered categories | Sex; blood type; vital status | Counts, proportions | Lower |
| Ordinal | Ordered categories with intervals that are not quantifiable | Degree of pain | In addition to the above: medians | Intermediate |
| Continuous or Ordered discrete† | Ranked spectrum with quantifiable intervals | Weight; number of cigarettes/day | In addition to the above: means, standard deviations | Higher |

*Categorical measurements that contain only two classes (e.g., sex) are termed **dichotomous.**

†Continuous variables have an infinite number of values (e.g., weight), whereas discrete variables have a finite scale (e.g., number of cigarettes/day). Discrete variables that are ordered (i.e., arranged in sequence from few to many) and that have a large number of possible values resemble continuous variables for practical purposes of measurement and analysis.

## Categorical Variables

Phenomena that are not suitable for quantification can often be measured by classifying them in categories. Categorical variables with two possible values (e.g., dead or alive) are termed **dichotomous.** Categorical variables with more than two categories (polychotomous) can be further characterized according to the type of information they contain. Nominal variables have categories that are not ordered; type O blood, for example, is neither more nor less than type B. **Nominal** variables tend to have a qualitative and absolute character that makes them straightforward to measure. **Ordinal** variables have categories that do have an order, such as severe, moderate, and mild pain. This is an advantage over nominal variables, but because ordinal variables do not specify a numerical or uniform difference between one category and the next, the information content is less than that of discrete variables.

## Choosing a Measurement Scale

A good general rule is to prefer continuous variables, because the additional information they contain improves efficiency. In a study comparing the antihypertensive effects of several treatments, for example, measuring blood pressure in millimeters of mercury allows the investigator to observe the magnitude of the change in every subject, whereas measuring it as a dichotomous variable (hypertensive vs. normotensive) would limit the assessment. The continuous variable contains much more information, and the result is a study with more power and/or a smaller sample size (Chapter 6).

The rule has some exceptions. If the research question involves the determinants of low birth weight, for example, the investigator would be more concerned with babies whose weight is so low that their health is compromised than with differences observed over the full spectrum of birth weights. In this case she is better off with a large enough sample to be able to analyze the results with a dichotomous outcome like the proportion of babies whose weight is below 2,500 g. Even when the categorical data are more meaningful, however, it is still best to collect the data as a continuous variable. This leaves the analytic options open: to change the cutoff point that defines low birth weight (she may later decide that 2,350 g is a better value for identifying babies at increased risk of developmental abnormalities), or to fall back on the more powerful analysis of the predictors of the full spectrum of weight.

Similarly, when there is the option of designing the number of response categories in an ordinal scale, as in a question about food preferences, it is often useful to provide a half-dozen categories that range from "strongly dislike" to "extremely fond of." The results can later be collapsed into a dichotomy (dislike and like), but not vice versa.

Many characteristics, particularly symptoms (e.g., pain) or aspects of lifestyle (e.g., quality of life), are difficult to describe with categories or numbers. But these phenomena often have important roles in diagnostic and treatment decisions, and the attempt to measure them is an essential part of the scientific approach to description and analysis. This is illustrated by the SF-36, a standardized questionnaire for assessing quality of life (1). The processes of classification and measurement, if done well, can increase the objectivity of our knowledge, reduce bias, and provide a means of communication.

## ■ PRECISION

A very precise measurement is one that is **reproducible**; it has nearly the same value each time it is measured. A beam scale can measure body weight with great precision, whereas an interview to measure quality of life is more likely to produce values that vary from one observer to the next. Precision has a very important influence on the power of a study. The more precise a measurement, the greater the statistical power at a given sample size to estimate mean values and to test hypotheses (Chapter 6).

Precision (also called reproducibility, reliability, and consistency) is affected by *random* error (chance); the greater the error, the less precise the measurement. There are three main sources of error in making measurements: observer variability, subject variability, and instrument variability. **Observer variability** refers to variability in measurement that is due to the observer, and includes such things as choice of words in an interview and skill in using a mechanical instrument. **Instrument variability** refers to variability in the measurement due to changing environmental factors such as temperature, or to aging mechanical components, etc. **Subject variability** refers to intrinsic biologic variability in the study subjects due to such things as fluctuations in mood, and time since last medication.

### Assessing Precision

Precision is assessed as the consistency of repeated measurements.

- **Within-observer reproducibility**: a single observer performs repeated measurements on a set of subjects or specimens
- **Between-observer reproducibility**: different observers perform measurements on a set of subjects or specimens

- **Within-instrument reproducibility**: a single instrument is used for repeated measurements on a set of subjects or specimens
- **Between-instrument reproducibility**: different instruments are used for measurements on a set of subjects or specimens

The reproducibility of continuous variables is often expressed as the **within-subject standard deviation**. However, if a "Bland-Altman" plot (2) of the within-subject standard deviation versus that subject's mean demonstrates a linear association, then the preferred approach is the **coefficient of variation** (within-subject standard deviation divided by the mean). Correlation coefficients should be avoided (2). For categorical variables, **percent agreement** and the **kappa** statistic (3) are often used (Chapter 12).

## Strategies for Enhancing Precision

There are five approaches to minimizing random variation and increasing the precision of measurements (Table 4.2):

1. **Standardizing the measurement methods.** All study protocols should include operational definitions (i.e., specific instructions for making the measurements). This includes written directions for how to prepare the environment and the subject, how to carry out and record the interview, how to calibrate the instrument, and so forth (Appendix 4.1). This set of materials, part of the **operations manual,** is essential for large and complex studies and highly recommended for smaller ones. Even when there is only a single observer, specific written guidelines for making each measurement will help her performance to be uniform over the duration of the study and serve as the basis for describing the methods when the results are reported.
2. **Training and certifying the observers.** Training will improve the consistency of measurement techniques, especially when several observers are involved. It is often important to test the mastery of the techniques specified in the operations manual and to certify that observers have achieved the prescribed level of performance (Chapter 17).
3. **Refining the instruments.** Mechanical and electronic instruments can be engineered to reduce variability. Similarly, questionnaires and interviews can be written to increase clarity and avoid potential ambiguities (Chapter 15).
4. **Automating the instruments.** Variations in the way human observers make measurements can be eliminated with automatic mechanical devices and self-response questionnaires. Of course, this strategy will improve precision only if the automatic device produces more precise measurements than human observers do.
5. **Repetition.** The effect of random error from any source is reduced by repeating the measurement and using the mean of the two or more readings. Precision can be substantially increased by this strategy, the primary limitation being the added cost and practical difficulties of repeating the measurements.

For each measurement in the study, the investigator must decide how vigorously to pursue each of these strategies. This decision can be based on the importance of the variable, the magnitude of the potential problem with precision, and the feasibility and cost of the strategy. In general, the first two strategies

■ **TABLE 4.2**

Strategies for Reducing Random Error in Order to Increase Precision, with Illustrations from a Study of Antihypertensive Treatment

| Strategy to Reduce Random Error | Source of Random Error | Example of Random Error | Example of Strategy to Prevent the Error |
|---|---|---|---|
| 1. Standardizing the measurement methods in an operations manual | Observer | Variation in blood pressure (BP) measurement due to variable rate of cuff deflation (sometimes faster than 2 mm Hg/sec and sometimes slower) | Specify that the cuff be deflated at 2 mm Hg/sec |
| | Subject | Variation in BP due to variable length of quiet sitting | Specify that subject sit in a quiet room for 5 minutes before BP measurement |
| 2. Training and certifying the observer | Observer | Variation in BP due to variable observer technique | Train observer in standard techniques |
| 3. Refining the instrument | Instrument or observer | Variation in BP due to digit preference (e.g., the tendency to round numbers to a multiple of 5) | Use random zero sphygmomanometry to conceal BP reading until after it has been recorded |
| 4. Automating the instrument | Observer | Variation in BP due to variable observer technique | Use automatic BP measuring device |
| | Subject | Variation in BP due to variable reaction to observer by subject | Use automatic BP measuring device |
| 5. Repeating the measurement | Observer, subject, and instrument | All measurements and all sources of variation | Use mean of two or more BP measurements |

(standardizing and training) should always be used, and the fifth (repetition) is an option that is guaranteed to improve precision when it is feasible and affordable.

## ■ ACCURACY

The accuracy of a variable is the degree to which it actually represents what it is intended to represent. This has a very important influence on the internal and external validity of the study—the degree to which the observed findings lead to the correct inferences about phenomena taking place in the study sample and in the universe.

Accuracy is different from precision in the ways shown in Table 4.3, and the two are not necessarily linked. If serum cholesterol were measured repeatedly using standards that had inadvertently been diluted twofold, for example, the result would be inaccurate but it could still be precise (i.e., consistently off by a factor of 2). This concept is further illustrated in Fig. 4.1. Accuracy and precision

**■ TABLE 4.3**
The Precision and Accuracy of Measurement

|  | **Precision** | **Accuracy** |
| --- | --- | --- |
| Definition | The degree to which a variable has nearly the same value when measured several times | The degree to which a variable actually represents what it is supposed to represent |
| Best way to assess | Comparison among repeated measures | Comparison with a reference standard |
| Value to study | Increase power to detect effects | Increase validity of conclusions |
| Threatened by | Random error (chance) contributed by<br>　The observer<br>　The subject<br>　The instrument | Systematic error (bias) contributed by<br>　The observer<br>　The subject<br>　The instrument |

usually go hand in hand, however, and many of the strategies for increasing precision will also improve accuracy.

Accuracy is a function of *systematic* error; the greater the error, the less accurate the variable. The three main classes of measurement error noted in the earlier section on precision each have counterparts here.

- **Observer bias** is a distortion, conscious or unconscious, in the perception or reporting of the measurement by the observer. It may represent systematic errors in the way an instrument is operated, such as a tendency to round down blood pressure measurements, or in the way an interview is carried out, as in the use of leading questions.

- **Subject bias** is a distortion of the measurement by the study subject. This may represent systematic bias in reporting an event (respondent bias). Breast cancer patients who believe that dietary fat is a cause of cancer, for example, may recall exaggerated amounts of fat eaten when younger.

- **Instrument bias** can result from faulty function of a mechanical instrument. A scale that has not been calibrated recently may drift downward, for example, and begin to produce consistently lower body weight readings.

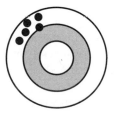
Good precision
Poor accuracy

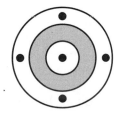
Poor precision
Good accuracy

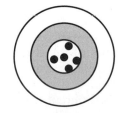
Good precision
Good accuracy

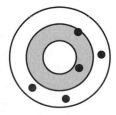
Poor precision
Poor accuracy

**■ FIGURE 4.1**
The difference between precision and accuracy.

## Assessing Accuracy

The accuracy of a measurement is best assessed by comparing it to a "**gold standard**", a reference technique that is considered accurate. For measurements on a continuous scale, the mean difference between the measurement under investigation and the gold standard across study subjects can be determined. For measurements on a categorical scale, accuracy in comparison to a gold standard can be described in terms of sensitivity and specificity (see Chapter 12). When a gold standard is not available, the researcher must rely upon other approaches to assess accuracy (see discussion on validity below).

## Strategies for Enhancing Accuracy

The major approaches to increasing accuracy include the first four of the strategies listed earlier for precision, and three additional ones (Table 4.4):

1. **Standardizing the measurement methods**
2. **Training and certifying the observers**
3. **Refining the instruments**
4. **Automating the instruments**
5. **Making unobtrusive measures.** It is sometimes possible to design measurements that the subjects are not aware of, thereby eliminating the possibility that they will consciously bias the variable. A study of advice on healthy eating patterns for schoolchildren, for example, could measure the number of candy bar wrappers in the trash.
6. **Blinding.** This classic strategy does not ensure the overall accuracy of the measurements, but it can eliminate **differential bias** that affects one study group more than another. In a double-blind experiment, neither the observer nor the subject knows whether active medicine or placebo has been assigned, ensuring that outcome measurements will not have different degrees of accuracy in the two groups. Observational studies also use blinding to conceal values of predictor variables from those who will be measuring outcomes.
7. **Calibrating the instrument.** The accuracy of many instruments, especially those that are mechanical or electrical, can be increased by periodic calibration using a gold standard.

The decision on how vigorously to pursue each of these seven strategies for each measurement rests, as noted earlier for precision, on the judgment of the investigator. The considerations are the *importance of the variable*, the *magnitude of the potential impact* that the anticipated degree of inaccuracy will have on the conclusions of the study, and the *feasibility and cost* of the strategy. The first two strategies (standardizing and training) should always be used, blinding is essential when feasible, and calibration is needed for any instrument that has the potential to change over time.

## Validity

Whether a variable represents what is intended is difficult to assess when measuring subjective and abstract phenomena, such as pain or quality of life, for which there is no concrete gold standard. At issue here is a particular type of accuracy that is usually termed **validity**—how well the measurement represents the phenomenon of interest. The assessment of validity has three main aspects:

■ **TABLE 4.4**

Strategies for Reducing Systematic Error in Order to Increase Accuracy, with
Illustrations from a Study of Antihypertensive Treatment

| Strategy to Reduce Systematic Error | Source of Systematic Error | Example of Systematic Error | Example of Strategy to Prevent the Error |
|---|---|---|---|
| 1. Standardizing the measurement methods in an operations manual | Observer | Consistently high diastolic blood pressure (BP) readings due to using the point at which sounds become muffled | Specify the operational definition of diastolic BP as the point at which sounds cease to be heard |
| | Subject | Consistently high readings due to measuring BP right after walking upstairs to clinic | Specify that subject sit in quiet room for 5 minutes before measurement |
| 2. Training and certifying the observer | Observer | Consistently high BP readings due to failure to follow procedures specified in operations manual | Trainer checks accuracy of observer's reading with a double-headed stethoscope |
| 3. Refining the instrument | Instrument | Consistently high BP readings with standard cuff in subjects with very large arms | Use extra-wide BP cuff in obese patients |
| 4. Automating the instrument | Observer | Conscious or unconscious tendency for observer to read BP lower in treatment group | Use automatic BP measuring device |
| | Subject | BP increase due to proximity of attractive technician | Use automatic BP measuring device |
| 5. Making unobtrusive measurements | Subject | Tendency of subject to overestimate compliance with study drug | Measure study drug level in urine |
| 6. Blinding | Observer | Conscious or unconscious tendency for observer to read BP lower in active treatment group | Use double-blind placebo to conceal study group assignment |
| | Subject | Tendency of subject to over-report side effects if he knew he was on active drug | Use double-blind placebo to conceal study group assignment |
| 7. Calibrating the instrument | Instrument | Consistently high BP readings due to anaeroid manometer being out of adjustment | Calibrate against mercury manometer each month |

■ **Content validity** has two components. **Face validity** is a subjective judgment
about whether a measurement makes sense intuitively, whether it is reasonable.
**Sampling validity** refers to whether the measurement incorporates all or most
of the aspects of the phenomenon under study; for example, a valid measure
of quality of life should include questions on social, physical, emotional, and
intellectual functioning.

■ **Construct validity** refers to how well a measurement conforms to theoretical concepts (constructs) concerning the entity under study. For example, if a particular trait is theoretically believed to differ between two groups of individuals a measurement with construct validity would show this difference.

■ **Criterion-related validity** is the degree to which the measurement correlates with an external criterion of the phenomenon under investigation. A variation is **predictive validity**, the ability of the measurement to predict the future occurrence of that criterion; for example, an investigator could validate a measure of depression by examining its ability to predict suicide.

The general approach to validating an abstract measure is to begin by searching the literature and consulting with experts in an effort to find a suitable instrument that has already been validated. If one can be found, its use may bypass the need to study the validity of the measurement approach. This strategy also has the advantage of making the results of the new study comparable with earlier work in the area and may simplify and strengthen the process of applying for grants and publishing the results. Its disadvantage, however, is that an instrument taken off the shelf may be outmoded or not appropriate for the research question.

If existing instruments are not suitable for the needs of the study, then the investigator will need to develop a new measurement approach and validate it herself. This can be an interesting, creative challenge (Chapter 15) and a worthwhile contribution in itself, but it is fair to say that the process is often less scientific and conclusive than the word *validation* connotes. Criterion-related validity, the most substantive and convincing strategy, is often not feasible. In this situation, the investigator may have to fall back on construct or face validity.

# ■ OTHER FEATURES OF MEASUREMENT APPROACHES

Measurements should be **sensitive** enough to detect differences in a characteristic that are important to the investigator. Just how much sensitivity is needed depends on the research question. For example, a study of whether a new medication helps people to quit smoking can use an outcome measure that is relatively insensitive to the precise number of cigarettes smoked each day. On the other hand, if the question is the effect of reducing the nicotine content of cigarettes on the number of cigarettes smoked, the method would need to be sensitive to differences in daily habits of just a few cigarettes.

An ideal measurement is **specific,** representing only the characteristic of interest. The carbon monoxide level in expired air is a measure of smoking habits that is fairly specific but that can also be affected by exposure to automobile exhaust. The overall specificity of assessing smoking habits can be increased by supplementing the carbon monoxide data with other measurements (such as self-report and serum cotinine level) that are not affected by air pollution.

Measurements should be **appropriate** to the objectives of the study. A study of stress as an antecedent to myocardial infarction, for example, would need to consider which kind of stress (psychologic or physical, acute or chronic) was of interest before setting out the operational definitions for measuring it.

Measurements should provide an adequate **distribution of responses** in the study population. A measure of functional status is most useful if it produces values that range from high in some subjects to low in others. One of the main functions of pretesting is to ensure that the actual responses do not all cluster around one end of the possible range of response (Chapter 17).

Finally, there is the issue of **objectivity.** This is achieved by reducing the involvement of the observer and by increasing the structure of the instrument and the degree to which it addresses specific detail. The danger in these strategies, however, is the consequent tunnel vision that limits the scope of the observations and the ability to discover unanticipated phenomena. The best design is often a compromise, including an opportunity for acquiring subjective and qualitative data with the main set of objective and quantitative measurements.

# ■ MEASUREMENTS ON STORED MATERIALS

Clinical research involves measurements on people that range across a broad array of domains (Table 4.5). Some of these measurements can only be made during a contact with the study subject, but many can be carried out later on **banks of specimens** stored for chemical or genetic analysis, or of images such as radiographic procedures filed electronically.

One advantage of such storage is the opportunity to reduce the cost of the study by making measurements on individuals who turn out during follow-up to develop the condition of interest. A terrific approach to doing this is the nested case-control design (Chapter 7), which can also increase power by allowing paired blinded measurements to be made in the same analytic batch (thus eliminating the batch-to-batch component of random error). A major advantage is that scientific advances may lead to new ideas and measurement techniques that can be employed years after the study is completed.

Measurements have become available that have greatly expanded clinical research in the areas of **genetic and molecular epidemiology** (4,5). Measurements on specimens that contain DNA (e.g., cells from saliva or a drop of blood on filter paper, or the buffy coat of a tube of anticoagulated blood) can contribute information on genotypes that modify a patient's response to treatment. Advances in imaging technology have improved our ability to detect candidates for preven-

---

**■ TABLE 4.5**
Common Types of Measurements that Can Be Made on Stored Materials

| Type of Measurement | Examples | Bank for Later Measurement |
|---|---|---|
| Medical history | Medications, operations, symptoms | Clinical charts |
| Psychosocial factors | Depression, family history | Voice recordings |
| Anthropometric | Height, weight, body composition | Photographs |
| Clinical signs | Skin turgor, heart sounds, weakness | Clinical charts |
| Biochemical measures | Serum cholesterol, plasma fibrinogen | Serum, plasma, urine, pathology specimens |
| Genetic/molecular tests | HLA type | Blood on filter paper, DNA, immortal cell line |
| Imaging | Bone density, coronary calcium | X-rays, digital images |
| Electromechanical | Arrhythmia, congenital heart disease | ECG, echocardiogram |

tive medicine interventions because, for example, they have low bone mineral content of the femoral neck (6) or calcium in the walls of the coronary arteries (7).

# ■ IN CLOSING

Table 4.5 reviews the many kinds of measurements that can be included in a study. Some of these are the topic of later chapters in this book. In Chapter 9 we will address the issue of how to choose the particular set of measurements that will facilitate inferences about confounding and causality. And in Chapter 15 we will address the topic of questionnaires and other instruments for measuring information supplied verbally by the study subject.

An important consideration, however, is the issue of **efficiency.** The full set of measurements should collect useful data at an affordable cost in time and money. Efficiency can be improved by increasing the quality of each item and by reducing the number of items measured. Collecting more data than are needed is a common error that can tire the subjects, overwhelm the research team, and clutter data management and analysis. The result may be a more expensive study that paradoxically is less successful in answering the main research questions.

# ■ SUMMARY

1. Variables are either **continuous** (quantified on an infinite scale), **discrete** (quantified on a finite scale), or **categorical** (classified in categories). Categorical variables are further classified as **nominal** (unordered) or **ordinal** (ordered); those that have only two categories are termed **dichotomous**.
2. Clinical investigators prefer variables that contain more information and thereby permit smaller sample sizes: continuous variables > discrete variables > ordered categorical variables > nominal and dichotomous variables.
3. The **precision** of a measurement (i.e., the reproducibility of replicate measures) is another major determinant of power and sample size. Precision is reduced by **random error** (i.e., chance) from three sources of variability: the observer, the instrument, and the subject.
4. Two **strategies for increasing precision** that should be part of every study are to operationally define and standardize methods in an operations manual, and to train and certify observers. Other strategies that are often useful are refining the instruments, automating the instruments, and using the mean of repeated measurements.
5. The **accuracy** of a measurement (i.e., the degree to which it actually measures the characteristic it is supposed to measure) is a major determinant of inferring correct conclusions. **Validity** is a form of accuracy commonly used for abstract variables. Accuracy is reduced by **systematic error** (i.e., bias) from the same three sources: the observer, the subject, and the instrument.
6. The **strategies for increasing accuracy** include all those listed for precision with the exception of repetition. In addition, accuracy is enhanced by calibration, by unobtrusive measures, and (in comparisons between groups) by blinding.
7. Individual measurements should be **sensitive, specific, appropriate,** and **objective,** and they should produce a **range of values.** In the aggregate, they should be broad but parsimonious, serving the research question at moderate cost in time and money.

8. Investigators should consider **storing banks of materials** for later measurements using nested case-control designs.

# EXERCISES

1. Classify the following variables as dichotomous, nominal, ordinal, continuous, or ordered discrete. Could any of them be modified to increase power, and how?
   a. Sex
   b. Age
   c. Education (high school degree/no degree)
   d. Education (highest year of schooling)
   e. History of heart attack present/absent
   f. Number of drinks containing alcohol per day
   g. Depression (none, mild, moderate, severe)
   h. Percent occlusion of coronary arteries
   i. Hypercholesterolemia (>250, <250)
2. The research question is, "Does body weight at age 1 year predict the number of drop-in clinic visits during the following year?" You plan a prospective cohort study, measuring body weight using an infant scale. You note the following problems while pretesting your measurements. Are these problems due to lack of accuracy, lack of precision, or both? Is the problem mainly due to observer, subject, or instrument variability, and what could be done about it?
   a. When babies are scared, they try to climb off of the scale and the observer must hold them on the scale to complete the measurement.
   b. If the baby is "squirmy," the pointer on the scale swings up and down wildly.
   c. When you weigh a 10-pound reference weight on the infant scale 20 times, the mean weight is 10.01 ± 1.00 pounds (mean ± SD).
   d. When you weigh a 10-pound reference weight on the infant scale 20 times, the mean weight is 10.60 ± 0.01 pounds (mean ± SD).
   e. Some of the babies arrive for the examination immediately after being fed, whereas others are hungry; some of the babies had wet diapers.

## References

1. Ware JE, Jr, Gandek B. Overview of the SF-36 Health Survey and the International Quality of Life Assessment (IQOLA) Project. *J Clin Epidemiol* 1998;51:903–12.
2. Bland JM, Altman DG. Measurement error and correlation coefficients. *BMJ* 1996;313:41–2; also, Measurement error proportional to the mean. *BMJ* 1996;313:106.
3. Cohen J. A coefficient of agreement for nominal scales. *Educ Psychol Meas* 1960;20:37–46.
4. Ellsworth DL, Manolio TA. The emerging importance of genetics in epidemiologic research II. Issues in study design and gene mapping. *Ann Epidemiol* 1999;9:75–90.
5. Ellsworth DL, Manolio TA. The emerging importance of genetics in epidemiologic research III: bioinformatics and statistical genetic methods. *Ann Epidemiol* 1999;9:207–24.
6. Cummings SR, Marcus R, Palermo L, Ensrud KE, Genant HK. Does estimating volumetric bone density of the femoral neck improve the prediction of hip fracture? A prospective study. Study of Osteoporotic Fractures Research Group. *J Bone Miner Res* 1994;9:1429–32.

7. Arad Y, Spadaro LA, Goodman K, et al. Predictive value of electron beam computed tomography of the coronary arteries. 19-Month follow-up of 1173 asymptomatic subjects. *Circulation* 1996;93:1951–3.

# ■ APPENDIX 4.1

## Operations Manual: Operational Definition of a Measurement of Grip Strength

The operations manual describes the method for conducting and recording the results of all the measurements made in the study. This example is taken from the operations manual of our Study of Osteoporotic Fractures. It describes the use of a dynamometer to measure grip strength. To standardize the instructions from examiner to examiner and from subject to subject, the protocol includes a script of instructions to be read to the participant verbatim.

## Protocol for Measuring Grip Strength with the Dynamometer

Grip strength will be measured in both hands. The handle should be adjusted so that the participant holds the dynamometer comfortably. Place the dynamometer in the right hand with the dial facing the palm. The participant's arm should be flexed 90° at the elbow with the forearm parallel to the floor.

1. Demonstrate the test to the subject: As you demonstrate, instruct the individual to squeeze the hand as hard as she can while simultaneously lowering the arm on a 3-second count. Her grip should be released when her arm is completely extended, hanging straight at her side. While demonstrating, use the following description: "This device measures your arm and upper body strength. We will measure your grip strength in both arms. I will demonstrate how it is done. Bend your elbow at a 90° angle, with your forearm parallel to the floor. Don't let your arm touch the side of your body. Lower the device slowly as you squeeze as hard as you can. Once your arm is fully extended, you can loosen your grip."
2. Allow one practice trial for each arm. On the second trial, record the kilograms of force from the dial to the nearest 0.5 kg.
3. Reset the dial. Repeat the procedure for the left arm.

## Precautions

The arm should not contact the body. The gripping action should be a slow, sustained squeeze rather than an explosive jerk.

# 5 Getting Ready to Estimate Sample Size: Hypotheses and Underlying Principles

Warren S. Browner,
Thomas B. Newman,
Norman Hearst, and
Stephen B. Hulley

**A**fter an investigator has decided who and what she is going to study and the design to be used, she must decide how many subjects to sample. Even the most rigorously executed study may fail to answer its research question if the sample size is too small. On the other hand, a study with too large a sample will be more difficult and costly than necessary. The goal of sample size planning is to estimate an *appropriate* number of subjects for a given study design.

Although a useful guide, sample size calculations give a deceptive impression of statistical objectivity. They are only as accurate as the data and estimates on which they are based, which are often just informed guesses. Sample size planning is a mathematical way of making a ballpark estimate. It often reveals that the research design is not feasible or that different predictor or outcome variables are needed. Thus sample size should be estimated early in the design phase of a study, when major changes are still possible.

Before setting out the specific cookbook approaches to calculating sample size for several common research designs in Chapter 6, we will spend some time considering the underlying principles. Readers who find some of these principles confusing will enjoy discovering that sample size planning does not require their total mastery. However, just as a recipe makes more sense if the cook is somewhat familiar with the ingredients, sample size calculations are easier if the investigator is acquainted with the basic concepts.

## ■ HYPOTHESES

In Chapter 1 we introduced the research question and discussed its transformation into an operational analog, the study question. Many study questions undergo a further transformation into a final and most specific version, termed the **research hypothesis,** that summarizes the elements of the study: the sample, the design, and the predictor and outcome variables. The primary purpose of the hypothesis is to establish the basis for tests of statistical significance.

Hypotheses are not needed in descriptive studies, which describe how characteristics are distributed in a population, such as a study of the prevalence of a particular genotype among patients with hip fractures. Hypotheses are needed for studies that will use tests of statistical significance to compare findings among groups, such as a study of whether that particular genotype is more common among patients with hip fractures than among controls. Because most observational studies and all experiments address research questions that involve making comparisons, most studies need to specify at least one hypothesis. If any of the following terms appear in the research question, then the study is not simply descriptive, and a hypothesis should be formulated: *greater than, less than, causes, leads to, compared with, more likely than, associated with, related to, similar to,* or *correlated with.*

## Characteristics of a Good Hypothesis

A good hypothesis must be based on a good research question. It should also be simple, specific, and stated in advance.

***Simple versus Complex.***    A simple hypothesis contains one predictor and one outcome variable (*a sedentary lifestyle is associated with an increased risk of proteinuria in patients with diabetes*). A complex hypothesis contains more than one predictor variable (*a sedentary lifestyle and alcohol consumption are associated with an increased risk of proteinuria in patients with diabetes*) or more than one outcome variable (*alcohol consumption is associated with an increased risk of proteinuria and neuropathy in patients with diabetes*). Complex hypotheses like these are not readily tested with a single statistical test and are more easily approached as two or more simple hypotheses.

Sometimes, however, a combined predictor or outcome variable can be used (*smoking cigarettes, cigars, or a pipe is associated with an increased risk of proteinuria in patients with diabetes*). In this example the investigator has decided that what matters is whether a participant smokes tobacco, not what type she smokes.

***Specific versus Vague.***    A specific hypothesis leaves no ambiguity about the subjects and variables or about how the test of statistical significance will be applied. It uses concise operational definitions that summarize the nature and source of the subjects and how variables will be measured (*a history of using tricyclic antidepressant medications, as measured by review of pharmacy records, is more common in patients hospitalized with an admission diagnosis of myocardial infarction at Longview Hospital in the past year than in controls hospitalized for pneumonia*). This is a long sentence, but it communicates the nature of the study in a clear way that minimizes any opportunity for testing something a little different once the study findings have been examined. It would be incorrect to substitute a different measurement of the predictor, such as the self-report of pills for depression, without considering the issue of multiple hypothesis testing (a topic we discuss at the end of the chapter). Sometimes these details are explicit in the study plan and need not be stated in the research hypothesis. But they should always be clear in the investigator's conception of the study.

It is often obvious from the research hypothesis whether the predictor variable and the outcome variable are dichotomous, continuous, or categorical. If it is not clear, then the type of variables may need to be specified (*alcohol consumption [in mg/day] is associated with an increased risk of proteinuria [>30 mg/dL] in patients with diabetes*). If the research hypothesis begins to get too cumbersome, the definitions can be left out, as long as they are clarified elsewhere in the protocol.

***In Advance versus After-the-Fact.***    The hypothesis should be stated in writing at the outset of the study. Most important, this will keep the research effort focused on the primary objective. A single prestated hypothesis also creates a stronger basis for interpreting the study results than several hypotheses that emerge as a result of inspecting the data. Hypotheses that are formulated after examination of the data are a form of multiple hypothesis testing that often leads to over-interpreting the importance of the findings.

## Types of Hypotheses

For the purpose of testing statistical significance, the research hypothesis must be restated in forms that categorize the expected difference between the study groups.

***Null and Alternative Hypotheses.***    The **null hypothesis** states that there is no association between the predictor and outcome variables in the population (*there is no difference in the frequency of drinking well water between subjects who develop peptic ulcer disease and those who do not*). The null hypothesis is the formal basis for testing statistical significance. Assuming that there really is no association in the population, statistical tests help to estimate the probability that an association observed in a study is due to chance.

The proposition that there is an association (*the frequency of drinking well water is different in subjects who develop peptic ulcer disease than in those who do not*) is called the **alternative hypothesis**. The alternative hypothesis cannot be tested directly; it is accepted by default if the test of statistical significance rejects the null hypothesis (see later).

***One- and Two-Sided Alternative Hypotheses.***    A one-sided hypothesis specifies the direction of the association between the predictor and outcome variables. The prediction that drinking well water is more common among subjects who develop peptic ulcers is a one-sided hypothesis. A two-sided hypothesis states only that an association exists; it does not specify the direction. The prediction that subjects who develop peptic ulcer disease have a different frequency of drinking well water than those who do not is a two-sided hypothesis.

One-sided hypotheses are clearly appropriate in selected circumstances, such as when only one direction for an association is important or biologically meaningful. An example is the one-sided hypothesis that a new drug for hypertension is more likely to cause rashes than a placebo; the possibility that the drug causes fewer rashes than the placebo is not usually worth testing. A one-sided hypothesis may also be appropriate when there is good evidence from prior studies that an association is unlikely to occur in one of the two directions, such as a hypothesis that tested whether cigarette smoking affects the risk of brain cancer. Prior evidence that smoking is unlikely to decrease the incidence of brain cancer, because smoking has been associated with an increased risk of many different types of cancers, might justify the use of a one-sided hypothesis. However, investigators should be aware that many well-supported hypotheses (e.g., that beta-carotene therapy will reduce the risk of lung cancer or that treatment with drugs that reduce the number of ventricular ectopic beats will reduce sudden death among patients with ventricular arrhythmias) turn out to be very wrong when tested in randomized trials. Indeed, in these two examples, the results of well-done trials revealed a statistically significant effect that was opposite in direction from the one supported by previous data (1–3).

It is important, however, to keep in mind the difference between a **research hypothesis,** which is often one-sided, and the alternative hypothesis used when planning sample size, which is usually two-sided. For example, suppose the research hypothesis is that recurrent use of antibiotics during childhood is associated with an increased risk of inflammatory bowel disease. That hypothesis specifies the direction of the anticipated effect, so it is one-sided. Why use a two-sided alternative hypothesis when planning the sample size? The answer is that many grant and manuscript reviewers expect two-sided hypotheses, and are critical if they are one-sided. More importantly, statistical rigor requires the investigator to make the choice between one- and two-sided hypotheses before analyzing the data; switching to a one-sided alternative hypothesis to reduce the $P$ value (see below) is not correct.

## ■ UNDERLYING STATISTICAL PRINCIPLES

A hypothesis, such as that 5 minutes or more of exercise per day is associated with a lower mean fasting glucose level in middle-aged women with diabetes, is either true or false in the real world. Because an investigator cannot study all middle-aged women with diabetes, she must test the hypothesis in a sample of that target population. As noted in Figure 1.6, there will always be a need to draw inferences about phenomena in the population from events observed in the sample.

In some ways, the investigator's problem is similar to that faced by a jury judging a defendant (Table 5.1). The absolute truth about whether the defendant committed the crime cannot usually be determined. Instead, the jury begins by presuming innocence: The defendant did not commit the crime. The jury must decide whether there is sufficient evidence to reject the presumed innocence of the defendant; the standard is known as "beyond a reasonable doubt." A jury can err, however, by convicting an innocent defendant or by failing to convict a guilty one.

In similar fashion, the investigator starts by presuming the null hypothesis of no association between the predictor and outcome variables in the population. Based on the data collected in her sample, the investigator uses statistical tests to determine whether there is sufficient evidence to reject the null hypothesis in favor of the alternative hypothesis that there is an association in the population. The standard for these tests is known as the **level of statistical significance.**

### Type I and Type II Errors

Like a jury, an investigator may reach a wrong conclusion. Sometimes by chance alone a sample is not representative of the population. Thus the results in the sample do not reflect reality in the population and lead to an erroneous inference. A **Type I error** (false-positive) occurs if an investigator rejects a null hypothesis that is actually true in the population; a **Type II error** (false-negative) occurs if the investigator fails to reject a null hypothesis that is actually not true in the population. Although Type I and II errors can never be avoided entirely, the investigator can reduce their likelihood by increasing the sample size (the larger the sample, the less likely that it will differ substantially from the population) or by manipulating the design or the measurements in other ways that we will discuss.

■ **TABLE 5.1**

The Analogy Between Jury Decisions and Statistical Tests

| Jury Decision | Statistical Test |
|---|---|
| *Innocence:* The defendant did not counterfeit money. | *Null hypothesis:* There is no association between dietary carotene and the incidence of colon cancer in the population. |
| *Guilt:* The defendant did counterfeit money. | *Alternative hypothesis:* There is an association between dietary carotene and the incidence of colon cancer. |
| *Standard for rejecting innocence:* Beyond a reasonable doubt. | *Standard for rejecting null hypothesis:* Level of statistical significance ($\alpha$). |
| *Correct judgment:* Convict a counterfeiter. | *Correct inference:* Conclude that there is an association between dietary carotene and colon cancer when one does exist in the population. |
| *Correct judgment:* Acquit an innocent person. | *Correct inference:* Conclude that there is no association between carotene and colon cancer when one does not exist. |
| *Incorrect judgment:* Convict an innocent person. | *Incorrect inference (Type I error):* Conclude that there is an association between dietary carotene and colon cancer when there actually is none. |
| *Incorrect judgment:* Acquit a counterfeiter. | *Incorrect inference (Type II error):* Conclude that there is not an association between dietary carotene and colon cancer when there actually is one. |

False-positive and false-negative results can also occur because of bias. (Errors due to bias are not usually referred to as Type I and II errors.) Such errors are especially troublesome, because they may be difficult to detect and cannot usually be quantified using statistical methods or avoided by increasing the sample size. In this chapter and the next, we will deal only with ways to reduce error due to chance, also known as random error. (See Chapters 1, 3, 4, and 7 through 12 for ways to reduce errors due to bias.)

## Effect Size

The likelihood that a study will be able to detect an association between a predictor and an outcome variable depends on the actual magnitude of that association in the target population. If it is large (e.g., if mean fasting blood glucose levels are 20 mg/dL lower in diabetic women who exercise than in those who do not), it will be easy to detect in the sample. Conversely, if the size of the association is small (e.g., a difference of 2 mg/dL), it will be difficult to detect in the sample.

Unfortunately, the investigator does not usually know exactly how large (or small) the association is; one of the purposes of the study is to estimate it. Instead, the investigator must choose the size of the association that she would like to be able to detect in the sample or that would be clinically important. That quantity is known as the **effect size**. Selecting an appropriate effect size is the most difficult aspect of sample size planning (4). The investigator should first try to find data from prior studies in related areas to make an informed guess about a reasonable effect size. Alternatively, she can choose the smallest effect size that in her opinion would be clinically meaningful (e.g., a 10 mg/dL reduction in the fasting glucose level). When data are not available, it may be necessary to do a small pilot study.

Of course, from the public health point of view, even a reduction of 2 or 3 mg/dL in fasting glucose levels might be important, especially if it was easy to achieve. Thus the choice of the effect size is always arbitrary, and considerations of feasibility are often paramount. Indeed, when the number of available or affordable subjects is limited, the investigator may have to work backward (Chapter 6) to determine the effect size that her study will be able to detect.

There are many different ways to measure the size of an association, especially when the outcome variable is dichotomous. For example, consider a study of whether middle-aged men are more likely to have impaired hearing than middle-aged women. Suppose an investigator finds that 20% of women and 30% of men 50 to 65 years of age are hard of hearing. These results could be interpreted as showing that men are 10% more likely to have impaired hearing than women (30% − 20%, the absolute difference), or 50% more likely ([30% − 20%] ÷ 20%, the relative difference). For sample size planning, both of the proportions matter; the sample size tables in this book use the smaller proportion (in this case, 20%) and the absolute difference (10%) between the groups being compared.

Many studies measure several effect sizes, because they measure several different predictor and outcome variables. For sample size planning, the sample size using the desired effect size for the most important hypothesis should be determined; the effect sizes for the other hypotheses can then be estimated. If there are several hypotheses of similar importance, then the sample size for the study should be based on whichever hypothesis needs the largest sample.

## $\alpha, \beta$, and Power

After a study is completed, the investigator uses statistical tests to try to reject the null hypothesis in favor of its alternative, much in the same way that a prosecuting attorney tries to convince a jury to reject innocence in favor of guilt. Depending on whether the null hypothesis is true or false in the target population, and assuming that the study is free of bias, four situations are possible (Table 5.2). In two of these, the findings in the sample and reality in the population are concordant, and the investigator's inference will be correct. In the other two situations, either a Type I or Type II error has been made, and the inference will be incorrect.

The investigator establishes the maximum chance of making Type I and II errors in advance of the study. The probability of committing a Type I error

■ **TABLE 5.2**
Truth in the Population versus the Results in the Study Sample: The Four Possibilities

|  | Truth in the Population | |
| --- | --- | --- |
| **Results in the Study Sample** | **Association Between Predictor and Outcome** | **No Association Between Predictor and Outcome** |
| Reject null hypothesis | Correct | Type I error |
| Fail to reject null hypothesis | Type II error | Correct |

(rejecting the null hypothesis when it is actually true) is called $\alpha$ (**alpha**). Another name for $\alpha$ is the **level of statistical significance.**

If, for example, a study of the effects of exercise on fasting blood glucose levels is designed with an $\alpha$ of 0.05, then the investigator has set 5% as the maximum chance of incorrectly rejecting the null hypothesis (and inferring that exercise and fasting blood glucose levels are associated in the population when, in fact, they are not). This is the level of reasonable doubt that the investigator will be willing to accept when she uses statistical tests to analyze the data after the study is completed.

The probability of making a Type II error (failing to reject the null hypothesis when it is actually false) is called $\beta$ (**beta**). The quantity $[1 - \beta]$ is called **power,** the probability of rejecting the null hypothesis in the sample if the actual effect in the population equals the effect size.

If $\beta$ is set at 0.10, then the investigator has decided that she is willing to accept a 10% chance of missing an association of a given effect size. This represents a power of 0.90; that is, a 90% chance of finding an association of that size. For example, suppose that exercise really would lead to an average reduction of 20 mg/dL in fasting glucose levels among diabetic women in the entire population. Suppose that the investigator drew a sample of women from the population on numerous occasions, each time carrying out the same study (with the same measurements and the same sample size each time). Then in nine of 10 studies the investigator would be able to reject the null hypothesis that exercise has no effect on mean fasting glucose level. This does not mean, however, that the investigator will be unable to detect a smaller effect, say, a 10 mg/dL reduction; it means simply that she will have less than a 90% likelihood of doing so.

Ideally, $\alpha$ and $\beta$ would be set at zero, eliminating the possibility of false-positive and false-negative results. In practice they are made as small as possible. Reducing them, however, usually requires increasing the sample size; other strategies are discussed in Chapter 6. Sample size planning aims at choosing a sufficient number of subjects to keep $\alpha$ and $\beta$ at an acceptably low level without making the study unnecessarily expensive or difficult.

Many studies set $\alpha$ at 0.05 and $\beta$ at 0.20 (a power of 0.80). These are arbitrary values, and others are sometimes used: the conventional range for $\alpha$ is between 0.01 and 0.10, and that for $\beta$ is between 0.05 and 0.20. In general, the investigator should use a low $\alpha$ when the research question makes it particularly important to avoid a Type I (false-positive) error, such as if she is testing the efficacy of a potentially dangerous medication. She should use a low $\beta$ (and a small effect size) when it is especially important to avoid a Type II (false-negative) error, such as if she wants to provide evidence to reassure the public that living near a toxic waste dump is safe.

## P Value

The null hypothesis acts like a straw man: It is assumed to be true so that it can be knocked down as false with a statistical test. When the data are analyzed, such tests determine the **P value,** the probability of seeing an effect as big or bigger than that in the study by chance if the null hypothesis actually were true. The null hypothesis is rejected in favor of its alternative if the $P$ value is less than $\alpha$, the predetermined level of statistical significance.

A "nonsignificant" result (i.e., one with a $P$ value greater than $\alpha$) does not mean that there is no association in the population; it only means that the result observed in the sample is small compared with what could have occurred by chance alone. For example, an investigator might find that men with hypertension were twice as likely to develop prostate cancer as those with normal blood pressure, but because the number of cancers in the study was modest this large apparent effect had a $P$ value of only 0.08. This means that even if hypertension and prostatic carcinoma were not associated in the population, there would be an 8% chance of finding such an association due to random error in the sample. If the investigator had set the significance level as a two-sided $\alpha$ of 0.05, she would have to conclude that the association in the sample was "not statistically significant." It might be tempting for the investigator to change her mind about the level of statistical significance, reset the two-sided $\alpha$ to 0.10, and report, "The results showed a statistically significant association ($P < 0.10$)," or, even worse, switch to a one-sided $P$ value and report it as "$P = 0.04$." A better choice would be to report that,"The results, although suggestive of an association, did not achieve statistical significance ($P = 0.08$)." This solution acknowledges that statistical significance is not an all-or-none situation. In part because of this problem, many statisticians and epidemiologists are moving away from hypothesis testing, with its emphasis on $P$ values, to using confidence intervals to report the precision of the study results (5–7). However, for the purposes of sample size planning for analytic studies, hypothesis testing is still the standard.

## Sides of the Alternative Hypothesis

Recall that an alternative hypothesis actually has two sides, either or both of which can be tested in the sample by using **one- or two-sided statistical tests.** When a two-sided statistical test is used, the $P$ value includes the probabilities of committing a Type I error in each of two directions, which is about twice as great as the probability in either direction alone. Thus it is easy to convert from a one-sided $P$ value to a two-sided $P$ value, and vice versa. A one-sided $P$ value of 0.05, for example, is usually the same as a two-sided $P$ value of 0.10. (Some statistical tests are asymmetric, which is why we said "usually.")

In the situation in which an investigator is only interested in one of the sides and has so formulated the alternative hypothesis, sample size should be calculated accordingly. The investigator planning a sample size to test a one-sided hypothesis should be aware, however, that she will have less power to test a two-sided hypothesis should that eventually be required; she must therefore have a strong justification for her choice. A one-sided hypothesis should never be used just to reduce the sample size.

## Type of Statistical Test

The formulas used to calculate sample size are based on mathematical assumptions, which differ for each statistical test. Thus before the sample size can be calculated, the investigator must decide on the statistical approach to analyzing the data. That choice depends mainly on the type of predictor and outcome variables in the study. Table 6.1 lists some common statistics used in data analysis, and Chapter 6 provides simplified approaches to estimating sample size for studies that use these statistics.

## ■ ADDITIONAL POINTS

### Variability

It is not simply the size of an effect that is important; its variability also matters. Statistical tests depend on being able to show a difference between the groups being compared. The greater the variability (or spread) in the outcome variable among the subjects, the more likely it is that the values in the groups will overlap, and the more difficult it will be to demonstrate an overall difference between them. Because measurement error contributes to the overall variability, less precise measurements require larger sample sizes (8).

Consider a study of the effects of two isocaloric diets (low-fat and low-carbohydrate) in achieving weight loss in 20 obese patients. If all those on the low-fat diet lost about 5 kg and all those on the low-carbohydrate diet failed to lose any weight (an effect size of 5 kg), it is likely that the low-fat diet really is better (Fig. 5.1A). On the other hand, suppose that although the average weight loss is 5 kg in the low-fat group and 0 kg in the low-carbohydrate group, there is a great deal of overlap between the two groups. (The changes in weight vary from a loss of 8 kg to a gain of 8 kg.) In this situation (Fig. 5.1B), even though the effect size is still 5 kg, the greater variability will make it more difficult to detect a difference between the diets, and a larger sample size will be needed.

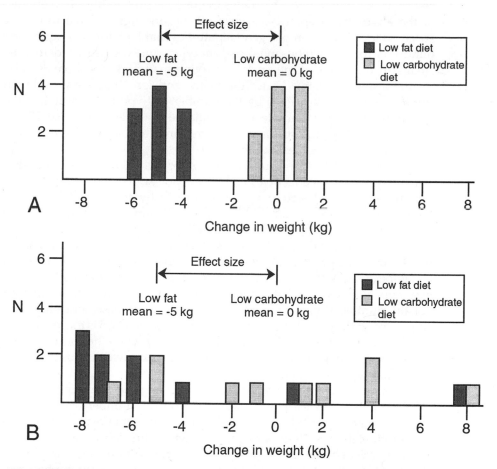

### ■ FIGURE 5.1

**A:** Weight loss achieved by two diets. Subjects on the low-fat diet all lost 4 to 6 kg, whereas the weight change of those on the low-carbohydrate diet ranged from −1 to +1 kg; the effect size is 5 kg. Because there is no overlap between the two groups, it is reasonable to infer that the low-fat diet really is better at achieving weight loss than the low-carbohydrate diet. **B:** Weight loss achieved by two diets. There is a great deal of overlap between the two groups, and some subjects in each group actually gained weight. Thus, even though the effect size is still 5 kg in favor of the low-fat diet, the study does not provide good evidence that the low-fat diet is really better than the low-carbohydrate diet at achieving weight loss.

When one of the variables used in the sample size estimate is continuous, the investigator will need to estimate its variability. (See the section on the *t* test in Chapter 6 for details.) In the other situations, variability is already included in the other parameters entered into the sample size formulas and tables, and need not be specified.

## Multiple and Post Hoc Hypotheses

When more than one hypothesis is tested in a study, especially if some of those hypotheses were formulated after the data were analyzed (post hoc hypotheses), the likelihood that at least one will achieve statistical significance on the basis of chance alone increases. For example, if 20 independent hypotheses are tested at an $\alpha$ of 0.05, the likelihood is substantial (64%; [$1 - 0.95^{20}$]) that at least one hypothesis will be statistically significant by chance alone. Some statisticians advocate adjusting the level of statistical significance when more than one hypothesis is tested in a study. This keeps the overall probability of accepting any one of the alternative hypotheses, when all the findings are due to chance, at the specified level. For example, genomic studies that look for an association between hundreds (or even thousands) of genotypes and disease need to use a much smaller $\alpha$ than 0.05, or they risk identifying many false-positive associations.

One approach, named after the mathematician **Bonferroni,** is to divide the significance level (say, 0.05) by the number of hypotheses tested. If there were four hypotheses, for example, each would be tested at an $\alpha$ of 0.0125 (i.e., 0.05 ÷ 4). This would require substantially increasing the sample size over that needed for testing each hypothesis at an $\alpha$ of 0.05.

We believe that a Bonferroni-type of approach to multiple hypothesis testing is usually too stringent. Investigators do not adjust the significance levels for hypotheses that are tested in separate studies. Why do so when several hypotheses are tested in the same study? In our view, adjusting $\alpha$ for multiple hypotheses is chiefly useful when the likelihood of making false-positive errors is high, because the number of tested hypotheses is substantial (say, more than 10) and the prior probability for each hypothesis is low (e.g., in screening a large number of genes for association with a phenotype). The first criterion is actually stricter than it may appear, because what matters is the number of hypotheses that are tested, not the number that are reported. Testing 50 hypotheses but only reporting or emphasizing the one or two *P* values that are less than 0.05 is misleading. Adjusting $\alpha$ for multiple hypotheses is especially important when the consequences of making a false-positive error are large, such as mistakenly concluding that an ineffective treatment is beneficial.

In general, the issue of what significance level to use depends more on the prior probability of each hypothesis than on the number of hypotheses tested. There is an analogy with the use of diagnostic tests that may be helpful (9). When interpreting the results of a diagnostic test, a clinician considers the likelihood that the patient being tested has the disease in question. For example, a modestly abnormal test result in a healthy person (e.g., a serum alkaline phosphatase level that is 15% greater than the upper limit of normal) is probably a false-positive test that is unlikely to have much clinical importance. Similarly, a *P* value of 0.05 for an unlikely hypothesis is probably also a false-positive result.

However, an alkaline phosphatase level that is 10 or 20 times greater than the upper limit of normal is unlikely to have occurred by chance (though it might be a laboratory error). So too a very small *P* value (say, < 0.001) is unlikely to have occurred by chance (though it could be due to bias). It is hard to dismiss very abnormal test results as being false-positives or to dismiss very low *P* values as being due to chance, even if the prior probability of the disease or the hypothesis was low.

Moreover, the number of tests that were ordered, or hypotheses that were tested, is not always relevant. The interpretation of an elevated serum uric acid level in a patient with a painful and swollen joint should not depend on whether the physician ordered just a single test (the uric acid level) or obtained the result as part of a panel of 20 tests. Similarly, when interpreting the $P$ value for testing a research hypothesis that makes good sense, it should not matter that the investigator also tested several unlikely hypotheses. What matters most is the reasonableness of the research hypothesis being tested: that it has a substantial prior probability of being correct. (Prior probability, in this "**Bayesian**" approach, is usually a subjective judgment based on evidence from other sources.) Most hypotheses that are formulated during the design of a study usually meet this requirement; after all, why else would the investigator put the time and effort into planning and doing the study?

What about unanticipated associations that appear during the collection and analysis of a study's results? This process is sometimes called **hypothesis generation** or, less favorably, "data-mining" or a "fishing expedition." The many informal comparisons that are made during data analysis are a form of multiple hypothesis testing. A similar problem arises when variables are redefined during data analysis, or when results are presented for a few subgroups of the sample. Significant $P$ values for data-generated hypotheses that were not considered during the design of the study are often due to chance. They should be viewed with skepticism and considered a fertile source of potential research questions.

Sometimes, however, an investigator fails to specify a particular hypothesis in advance, although that hypothesis seems reasonable when the data are being analyzed. This might happen, for example, if others discover a new risk factor while the study is going on, or if the investigator was initially unaware that a particular hypothesis made sense. The important issue is not whether the hypothesis was formulated before the study began, but whether there is a reasonable prior probability based on evidence from other sources that the hypothesis is true (9).

There are some definite advantages to formulating more than one hypothesis when planning a study. The use of multiple unrelated hypotheses increases the efficiency of the study, making it possible to answer more questions with a single research effort and to discover more of the true associations that exist in the population. It may also be a good idea to formulate several *related* hypotheses; if the findings are consistent, the study conclusions are made stronger. Several studies in patients with heart failure, for example, found that the use of angiotensin converting enzyme inhibitors is beneficial in reducing cardiac admissions, cardiovascular mortality, and total mortality. Had only one of these hypotheses been tested, the inferences from these studies would have been less definitive. Lunch may not be free, however, when multiple hypotheses are tested. Suppose that several prestated hypotheses are tested, only one or two of which turn out to be statistically significant. Then the investigator must decide (and try to convince reviewers, editors, and readers) whether the significant results, the nonsignificant results, or both sets of results are true.

A good rule is to establish in advance as many hypotheses as make sense, but specify just one as the primary hypothesis, which can be tested statistically without argument about whether to adjust for multiple hypothesis testing. More important, having a primary hypothesis helps to focus the study on its main objective and provides a clear basis for the main sample size calculation.

# ■ SUMMARY

1. **Sample size planning** is an important part of the design of both analytic and descriptive studies. The sample size should be estimated early in the process of developing the research design, so that appropriate modifications can be made.

2. Analytic studies and experiments need a **hypothesis** that specifies, for the purpose of subsequent **tests of significance,** the anticipated association between the main predictor and outcome variables. Purely descriptive studies, lacking the strategy of comparison, do not require a hypothesis.

3. Good hypotheses are **specific** about how the population will be sampled and the variables measured, **simple** (there is only one predictor and one outcome variable), and **formulated in advance**.

4. The **null hypothesis,** which proposes that the predictor and outcome variables are not associated, is the basis for tests of statistical significance. The **alternative hypothesis** proposes that they are associated. Statistical tests attempt to reject the null hypothesis of no association in favor of the alternative hypothesis that there is an association.

5. An alternative hypothesis is either **one-sided** (only one direction of association will be tested) or **two-sided** (both directions will be tested). One-sided hypotheses should only be used in the unusual circumstance that only one direction of the association is likely or biologically meaningful.

6. For analytic studies and experiments, the sample size is an estimate of the number of subjects required to detect an association of a given **effect size** and **variability** at a specified likelihood of making **Type I** (false-positive) and **Type II** (false-negative) **errors.** The maximum likelihood of making a Type I error is called $\alpha$; that of making a Type II error, $\beta$. The quantity $(1 - \beta)$ is **power,** the chance of observing an association of a given size or greater in a sample if one is actually present in the population.

7. It is often desirable to establish more than one hypothesis in advance, but the investigator should specify a single **primary hypothesis** as a focus and for sample size estimation. Interpretation of findings from testing **multiple hypotheses** in the sample, including unanticipated findings that emerge from the data, is based on a judgment about the **prior probability** that they represent a real event in the population.

# EXERCISES

**1.** Define the concepts in **boldface.**

An investigator is interested in designing a study with sufficient **sample size** to determine whether height is associated with stomach cancer among Japanese men. She is planning a case-control study with equal numbers of cases and controls. The **null hypothesis** is that there is no difference in mean height between cases of stomach cancer and controls; she has chosen an **alternative hypothesis** with two sides. She would like to have a **power** of 0.80, at a **level of statistical significance** ($\alpha$) of 0.05, to be able to detect an **effect size** of a difference in height of 5 cm between cases and controls. Review of the literature indicates that the **variability** of height among Japanese men is a standard deviation of 10 cm.

# References

1. The effect of vitamin E and beta carotene on the incidence of lung cancer and other cancers in male smokers. The Alpha-Tocopherol, Beta Carotene Cancer Prevention Study Group. *N Engl J Med* 1994;330:1029–35.
2. Echt DS, Liebson PR, Mitchell LB, et al. Mortality and morbidity in patients receiving encainide, flecainide, or placebo. The Cardiac Arrhythmia Suppression Trial. *N Engl J Med* 1991;324:781–8.
3. Effect of the antiarrhythmic agent moricizine on survival after myocardial infarction. The Cardiac Arrhythmia Suppression Trial II Investigators. *N Engl J Med* 1992;327:227–33.
4. Van Walraven C, Mahon JL, Moher D, Bohm C, Laupacis A. Surveying physicians to determine the minimal important difference: implications for sample-size calculation. *J Clin Epidemiol* 1999;52:717–23.
5. Daly LE. Confidence limits made easy: interval estimation using a substitution method. *Am J Epidemiol* 1998;147:783–90.
6. Goodman SN. Toward evidence-based medical statistics. 1: The *P* value fallacy. *Ann Intern Med* 1999;130:995–1004.
7. Goodman SN. Toward evidence-based medical statistics. 2: The Bayes factor. *Ann Intern Med* 1999;130:1005–13.
8. McKeown-Eyssen GE, Tibshirani R. Implications of measurement error in exposure for the sample sizes of case-control studies. *Am J Epidemiol* 1994;139:415–21.
9. Browner WS, Newman TB. Are all significant *P* values created equal? The analogy between diagnostic tests and clinical research. *JAMA* 1987;257:2459–63.

# 6 Estimating Sample Size and Power: The Nitty-gritty

Warren S. Browner,
Thomas B. Newman,
Steven R. Cummings, and
Stephen B. Hulley

**C**hapter 5 introduced the basic principles underlying sample size calculations. This chapter presents several cookbook techniques for using those principles to estimate the sample size needed for a research project. The first section deals with sample size estimates for an analytic study or experiment, including some special issues that apply to these studies, such as multivariate analysis. The second section considers studies that are primarily descriptive. Subsequent sections deal with studies that have a fixed sample size, strategies for maximizing the power of a study, and how to estimate the sample size when there appears to be insufficient information from which to work. The chapter concludes with common errors to avoid. There are tables and formulas in the appendixes for several basic methods of estimating sample size. In addition, there are many sites on the Web that can be helpful; search for "sample size" *and* "power."

## ■ SAMPLE SIZE TECHNIQUES FOR ANALYTIC STUDIES AND EXPERIMENTS

There are several variations on the recipe for estimating sample size in an analytic study or experiment, but they all have certain steps in common:

1. State the **null hypothesis** and either a **one-** or **two-sided alternative hypothesis.**
2. Select the appropriate **statistical test** from Table 6.1 based on the type of predictor variable and outcome variable in those hypotheses.
3. Choose a reasonable **effect size** (and **variability,** if necessary).
4. Set **α** and **β**. (Specify a two-sided α unless the alternative hypothesis is clearly one-sided.)
5. Use the appropriate table or formula in the appendix to estimate the sample size.

Even if the exact value for one or more of the ingredients is uncertain, it is important to estimate the sample size early in the design phase. Waiting until the last minute to prepare the sample size can be disastrous. It is often necessary to start over with new ingredients, which may mean redesigning the entire study. This is why this subject is covered so early in this book.

■ **TABLE 6.1**
Simple Statistical Tests for Use in Estimating Sample Size*

|                        | Outcome Variable       |                          |
| ---------------------- | ---------------------- | ------------------------ |
| **Predictor Variable** | **Dichotomous**        | **Continuous**           |
| Dichotomous            | Chi-squared test[†]    | *t* test                 |
| Continuous             | *t* test               | Correlation coefficient  |

*See text for what to do about categorical variables, dose-response studies, or if planning to analyze the data with another type of statistical test.
[†]The chi-squared test is always two-sided; a one-sided equivalent is the z statistic.

Not all analytic studies fit neatly into one of the three main categories that follow; a few of the more common exceptions are discussed in the section called "Other Considerations and Special Issues."

## The *t* Test

The *t* test (sometimes called Student's *t* test, after the pseudonym of its developer) is commonly used to determine whether the mean value of a continuous outcome variable in one group differs significantly from that in another group. For example, the *t* test would be appropriate to use when comparing the mean depression scores in patients treated with two different antidepressants, or the mean change in weight among two groups of participants in a placebo-controlled trial of a new drug for weight loss. The *t* test assumes that the distribution (spread) of the variable in each of the two groups approximates a normal (bell-shaped) curve. However, the *t* test is remarkably robust, so it can be used for almost any distribution unless the number of subjects is small (fewer than 30 to 40) or there are extreme outliers.

To estimate the sample size for a study that will be analyzed with a *t* test, the investigator must

1. State the null hypothesis and decide whether the alternative hypothesis is one- or two-sided.
2. Estimate the effect size ($E$) as the difference in the mean value of the outcome variable between the study groups.
3. Estimate the variability of the outcome variable as its standard deviation ($S$).
4. Calculate the standardized effect size ($E/S$), defined as the effect size divided by the standard deviation of the outcome variable.
5. Set $\alpha$ and $\beta$.

The effect size and variability can often be estimated from previous studies in the literature and consultation with experts. Occasionally, a small pilot study will be necessary to estimate the standard deviation of the outcome variable. When the outcome variable is the change in a continuous measurement (e.g., change in weight during a study), the investigator should use the standard deviation of the change in that variable (not the standard deviation of the variable itself) in the sample size estimates. The standard deviation of the change in a variable is usually smaller than the standard deviation of the variable; thus the sample size will also be smaller.

**Standardization** (i.e., dividing the effect size by the standard deviation of the outcome variable) simplifies comparisons between the effect sizes of different variables. The larger the standardized effect size, the smaller the required sample size. The standardized effect size for most studies is between 0.1 and 0.5; smaller effect sizes are difficult to detect, and larger ones are often obvious.

Appendix 6.A gives the sample size requirements for various combinations of $\alpha$ and $\beta$ for several standardized effect sizes. To use Table 6.A, look down its left-most column for the standardized effect size. Next, read across the table to the chosen values for $\alpha$ and $\beta$ for the sample size required per group. (The numbers in Table 6.A assume that the two groups being compared are of the same size; see the text below the table if that assumption is not true.)

---

**Example 6.1. Calculating Sample Size When Using the $t$ Test**

*Problem:* The research question is whether there is a difference in the efficacy of salbutamol and ipratropium bromide for the treatment of asthma. The investigator plans a randomized trial of the effect of these drugs on $FEV_1$ (forced expiratory volume in 1 second) after 1 week of treatment. A previous study has reported that the mean $FEV_1$ in persons with treated asthma was 2.0 liters, with a standard deviation of 1.0 liter. The investigator would like to be able to detect a difference of 10% or more in mean $FEV_1$ between the two treatment groups. How many patients are required in each group (salbutamol and ipratropium) at $\alpha$ (two-sided) = 0.05 and power = 0.80?

*Solution:* The ingredients for the sample size calculation are as follows:

1. *Null hypothesis:* Mean $FEV_1$ after 1 week of treatment is the same in asthmatic patients treated with salbutamol as in those treated with ipratropium.
   *Alternative hypothesis* (two-sided): Mean $FEV_1$ after 1 week of treatment is different in asthmatic patients treated with salbutamol from what it is in those treated with ipratropium.
2. Effect size = 0.2 liters (10% × 2.0 liters).
3. Standard deviation of $FEV_1$ = 1.0 liter.
4. Standardized effect size = effect size ÷ standard deviation = 0.2 liters ÷ 1.0 liter = 0.2.
5. $\alpha$ (two-sided) = 0.05; $\beta$ = 1 − 0.80 = 0.20. (Recall that $\beta$ = 1 − power.)

Looking across from a standardized effect size of 0.20 in the leftmost column of Table 6.A and down from $\alpha$ (two-sided) = 0.05 and $\beta$ = 0.20, 393 patients are required per group. This is the number of patients who need to complete the study; even more will need to be enrolled to account for dropouts. This sample size may not be feasible, and the investigator may need to reconsider the study design, or perhaps settle for only being able to detect a larger effect size. See the section on the $t$ test for paired samples (Example 6.8) for suggestions.

---

The $t$ test can also be used to estimate the sample size for a case-control study if the study has a continuous predictor variable. In this situation, the $t$ test compares the mean value of the predictor variable in the cases with that in the controls.

There is a convenient shortcut for approximating sample size using the $t$ test, when more than 30 subjects will be studied and the power is set at 0.80 ($\beta = 0.2$) and $\alpha$ (two-sided) is set at 0.05 (1). The formula is

$$\text{Sample size (per equal-sized group)} = 16 \div (E/S)^2$$

where $E/S$ is the standardized effect size. (For Example 6.1 the shortcut estimate of the sample size would be $16 \div 0.2^2 = 400$ per group.)

## The Chi-Squared Test

The chi-squared ($\chi^2$) test can be used to compare the proportion of subjects in each of two groups who have a dichotomous outcome. For example, the proportion of men who develop coronary heart disease (CHD) while treated with aspirin can be compared with the proportion who develop CHD while taking a placebo. The chi-squared test is always two-sided; an equivalent test for one-sided hypotheses is the one-sided Z test.

In an experiment or cohort study, effect size is specified by the difference between $P_1$, the proportion of subjects expected to have the outcome in one group, and $P_2$, the proportion expected in the other group. In a case-control study, $P_1$ represents the proportion of cases expected to have a particular risk factor, and $P_2$ represents the proportion of controls expected to have the risk factor. Variability is a function of $P_1$ and $P_2$, so it need not be specified.

To estimate the sample size for a study that will be analyzed with the chi-squared test, the investigator must

1. State the null hypothesis and decide whether the alternative hypothesis should be one- or two-sided.
2. Estimate the effect size and variability in terms of $P_1$, the proportion with the outcome in one group, and $P_2$, the proportion with the outcome in the other group.
3. Set $\alpha$ and $\beta$.

Appendix 6.B gives the sample size requirements for several combinations of $\alpha$ and $\beta$, and a range of values of $P_1$ and $P_2$. To estimate the sample size, look down the leftmost column of Tables 6.B.1 or 6.B.2 for the smaller of $P_1$ and $P_2$ (if necessary rounded to the nearest 0.05). Next, read across for the difference between $P_1$ and $P_2$. Based on the chosen values for $\alpha$ and $\beta$, the table gives the sample size required per group.

---

**Example 6.2. Calculating Sample Size When Using the Chi-Squared Test**

*Problem:* The research question is whether elderly smokers have a greater incidence of skin cancer than nonsmokers. A review of previous literature suggests that the 5-year incidence of skin cancer is about 0.20 in elderly nonsmokers. At $\alpha$ (two-sided) = 0.05 and power = 0.80, how many smokers and nonsmokers will need to be studied to determine whether the 5-year skin cancer incidence is at least 0.30 in smokers?

*Solution:* The ingredients for the sample size calculation are as follows:

1. *Null hypothesis:* The incidence of skin cancer is the same in elderly smokers and nonsmokers.
   *Alternative hypothesis* (two-sided): The incidence of skin cancer is different in elderly smokers and nonsmokers.
2. $P_2$ (incidence in nonsmokers) = 0.20; $P_1$ (incidence in smokers) = 0.30. The smaller of these values is 0.20, and the difference between them ($P_1 - P_2$) is 0.10.
3. $\alpha$ (two-sided) = 0.05; $\beta$ = 1 − 0.80 = 0.20.

Looking across from 0.20 in the leftmost column in Table 6.B.1 and down from an expected difference of 0.10, the middle number for $\alpha$ (two-sided) = 0.05 and $\beta$ = 0.20 is the required sample size of 293 smokers and 293 nonsmokers. If the investigator had chosen to use a one-sided alternative hypothesis, given that there is a great deal of evidence suggesting that smoking is a carcinogen and none suggesting that it prevents cancer, the sample size would be 231 smokers and 231 nonsmokers.

Often the investigator specifies the effect size in terms of the relative risk (risk ratio) of the outcome in two groups of subjects. For example, an investigator might study whether women who use oral contraceptives are at least twice as likely as nonusers to have a myocardial infarction. In a cohort study (or experiment), it is straightforward to convert back and forth between relative risk and the two proportions ($P_1$ and $P_2$), since the relative risk is just $P_1$ divided by $P_2$ (or vice versa).

For a case-control study, however, the situation is a little more complex because the relative risk must be approximated by the odds ratio, which equals $[P_1 \times (1 - P_2)] \div [P_2 \times (1 - P_1)]$. The investigator must specify the odds ratio (OR) and $P_2$ (the proportion of controls exposed to the predictor variable). Then $P_1$ (the proportion of cases exposed to the predictor variable) is

$$P_1 = \frac{OR \times P_2}{(1 - P_2) + (OR \times P_2)}$$

For example, if the investigator expects that 10% of controls will be exposed to the oral contraceptives ($P_2 = 0.1$) and wishes to detect an odds ratio of 3 associated with the exposure, then

$$P_1 = \frac{(3 \times 0.1)}{(1 - 0.1) + (3 \times 0.1)} = \frac{0.3}{1.2} = 0.25$$

## The Correlation Coefficient

Although the correlation coefficient ($r$) is not commonly used in sample size calculations, it can be useful when the predictor and outcome variables are both continuous. The correlation coefficient is a measure of the strength of the linear association between the two variables. It varies between $-1$ and $+1$. Negative values indicate that as one variable increases, the other decreases (like serum lead level and IQ in children). The closer the absolute value of $r$ is to 1, the stronger the association; the closer to 0, the weaker the association. Height and weight in adults, for example, are highly correlated in some populations, with $r \approx 0.9$. Such high values, however, are uncommon; many biologic associations have much smaller correlation coefficients.

Although the correlation coefficient is often used in some fields of clinical research, such as behavioral medicine and psychology, using it to estimate the sample size has a disadvantage: correlation coefficients have little intuitive meaning. When squared ($r^2$), a correlation coefficient represents the proportion of the variability in an outcome variable that can be explained by its linear association with a predictor variable (and vice versa). Thus $r = 0.4$ means that one of the variables "explains" 0.16 (or 16%) of the variance in the other. An alternative way to estimate the sample size for a study in which the predictor and outcome variables are both continuous is to dichotomize one of the two variables (say, at its median) and use the $t$ test calculations instead.

To estimate sample size for a study that will be analyzed with a correlation coefficient, the investigator must

1. State the null hypothesis, and decide whether the alternative hypothesis is one- or two-sided.
2. Estimate the effect size as the absolute value of the smallest correlation coefficient ($r$) that the investigator would like to be able to detect. (Variability is a function of $r$ and is already included in the table and formula.)
3. Set $\alpha$ and $\beta$.

In Appendix 6.C, look down the leftmost column of Table 6.C for the effect size ($r$). Next, read across the table to the chosen values for $\alpha$ and $\beta$, yielding the total sample size required. Table 6.C yields the appropriate sample size when the investigator wishes to reject the null hypothesis that there is no association between the predictor and outcome variables (e.g., $r = 0$). If the investigator wishes to determine whether the correlation coefficient in the study differs from a value other than zero (e.g., $r = 0.2$), she should see the text below Table 6.C for the appropriate methodology.

---

**Example 6.3. Calculating Sample Size When Using the Correlation Coefficient in a Cross-Sectional Study**

*Problem:* The research question is whether urinary cotinine levels (a measure of the intensity of current cigarette smoking) are correlated with bone density in smokers. A previous study found a modest correlation ($r = -0.3$) between reported smoking (in cigarettes per day) and bone density; the investigator anticipates that urinary cotinine levels will be at least as well correlated. How many smokers will need to be enrolled, at $\alpha$ (two-sided) $= 0.05$ and $\beta = 0.10$?
*Solution:* The ingredients for the sample size calculation are as follows:

1. *Null hypothesis:* There is no correlation between urinary cotinine level and bone density in smokers.
   *Alternative hypothesis:* There is a correlation between urinary cotinine level and bone density in smokers.
2. Effect size ($r$) $= |-0.3| = 0.3$.
3. $\alpha$ (two-sided) $= 0.05$; $\beta = 0.10$.

Using Table 6.C, reading across from $r = 0.30$ in the leftmost column and down from $\alpha$ (two-sided) $= 0.05$ and $\beta = 0.10$, 113 smokers will be required.

---

# ■ OTHER CONSIDERATIONS AND SPECIAL ISSUES

## Dropouts

Each sampling unit must be available for analysis; thus subjects who are enrolled in a study but in whom outcome status cannot be ascertained (such as dropouts) do not count in the sample size. If the investigator anticipates that any of her subjects will not be available for follow-up, she should increase the size of the enrolled sample accordingly. If, for example, the investigator estimates that 20% of her sample will be lost to follow-up, then the sample size should be increased by a factor of ($1 \div [1 - 0.20]$), or 1.25.

## Categorical Variables

Ordinal variables can often be treated as continuous variables, especially if the number of categories is relatively large (six or more) and if averaging the values of the variable makes sense. In other situations, the best strategy is to change the research hypothesis slightly by dichotomizing the categorical variable. As an example, suppose a researcher is studying whether gender is associated with the number of times that a diabetic patient visits a podiatrist in a year. The number of visits is unevenly distributed: many people will have no visits, some will make one visit, and only a few will make two or more visits. In this situation, the investigator could estimate the sample size as if the outcome were dichotomous (no visits versus one or more visits).

## Survival Analysis

When an investigator wishes to compare which of two treatments is more effective in prolonging life or in reducing the symptomatic phase of a disease, survival analysis will be the appropriate technique for analyzing the data (2,3). Although the outcome variable, say weeks of survival, appears to be continuous, the *t* test is not appropriate because what is actually being assessed is not time itself but the proportion of subjects who are still alive at each point in time. A reasonable approximation can be made by dichotomizing the outcome variable at the end of the anticipated follow-up period (e.g., the proportion surviving for 6 months or more), and estimating the sample size with the chi-squared test.

## Clustered Samples

Some research designs involve the use of clustered samples, in which subjects are sampled by groups (Chapter 11). Consider, for example, a study of whether an educational intervention directed at clinicians improves the use of pneumococcal vaccination. Suppose that 20 physician practices are randomly assigned to the group that receives the intervention and 20 practices are assigned to a control group and that the investigators plan to review the charts of a random sample of 50 patients in each practice. Does the sample size equal 20 (the number of practices per group) or 1000 (the number of patients)? The answer, which lies somewhere in between those two extremes, depends upon how similar the patients within a practice are (in terms of their vaccination status) compared with the similarity among all the patients. Estimating this quantity often requires obtaining pilot data, unless another investigator has previously done a similar study. There are several techniques for estimating the required sample size for a study using clustered samples (4–7), but they are challenging and usually require the assistance of a statistician.

A ballpark estimate can sometimes be made, assuming similar numbers of subjects in each cluster, by aggregating the outcomes within a cluster. For example, in the study of pneumococcal vaccination, each practice might be given a score representing the percentage of patients in that practice who were vaccinated. Then the *t* test will yield a (somewhat high) estimate of the number of practices needed.

## Matching

For a variety of reasons (Chapter 9), an investigator may choose to use a matched design. The techniques in this chapter, which ignore any matching, provide reasonable, although slightly high, estimates of the required sample size. More precise estimates can be made using approaches described by Schlesselman (8).

## Multivariate Adjustment and Other Special Statistical Analyses

When designing an observational study, an investigator may decide that one or more variables will confound the association between the predictor and outcome (Chapter 9), and plan to use statistical techniques to adjust for these confounders when she analyzes her results. When this adjustment will be included in testing the primary hypothesis, the estimated sample size needs to take this into account.

Analytic approaches that adjust for confounding variables often increase the required sample size (9,10). The magnitude of that increase depends on three factors: the prevalence of the confounder, the strength of the association between the predictor and the confounder, and the strength of the association between the confounder and the outcome. These effects are complex and no general rule covers all situations.

Statisticians have developed multivariate methods such as linear regression and logistic regression that allow the investigator to adjust for confounding variables. A particularly widely used statistical technique is **Cox proportional hazards** analysis, which can adjust both for confounders and for differences in length of follow-up. If one of these techniques is going to be used to analyze the data, there are corresponding approaches for estimating the required sample size (3,11–13). Sample size techniques are also available for other designs, such as studies of potential genetic risk factors or candidate genes (14–16), economic studies (17–19), dose-response studies (20), or studies that involve more than two groups (21).

But it is usually easier, at least for novice investigators, to estimate the sample size assuming a simpler method of analysis, such as the chi-squared test or the *t* test. Suppose, for example, an investigator is planning a case-control study of whether serum cholesterol level (a continuous variable) is associated with the occurrence of brain tumors (a dichotomous variable). Even if the eventual plan is to analyze the data with the logistic regression technique, a ballpark sample size can be estimated with the *t* test. It turns out that the simplified approaches usually produce sample size estimates that are similar to those generated by more sophisticated techniques. An experienced statistician may need to be consulted, however, if a grant proposal that involves substantial costs is being submitted for funding.

## Equivalence Studies

Sometimes the goal of a study is to show that the null hypothesis is correct and that there really is no association between the predictor and outcome variables (22–25). A common example is a clinical trial to test whether a new drug is as effective as an established drug. This situation poses a challenge when planning sample size, because the desired effect size is zero (i.e., the investigator would like to show that the two drugs are equally effective).

One acceptable method is to design the study to have substantial power (say, 0.90 or 0.95) to reject the null hypothesis when the effect size is small enough that it would not be clinically important (e.g., a difference of 5 mg/dL in the mean fasting glucose levels). If the new drug has practical advantages, such as being less expensive or safer, then a larger effect size may be acceptable. If the results of such a well-powered study are "negative" (i.e., no statistically significant difference is detected between the groups being compared), then the investigator can be reasonably confident that the two drugs are equivalent. One problem with equivalence studies, however, is that the additional power and the small effect size often require a large sample size.

Another problem involves the loss of the usual safeguards that are inherent in the paradigm of the null hypothesis, which protects a conventional study, such as one that compares an active drug with a placebo, against Type I errors (falsely rejecting the null hypothesis). The paradigm ensures that problems in the design or execution of a study, such as using inadequate measurements or losing subjects to follow-up, make it harder to reject the null hypothesis. That is because these defects usually blur the difference between the groups being compared. (It is harder to see clearly through a smudged window.) Thus investigators in a conventional study, who are trying to reject a null hypothesis, have a strong incentive to do the best possible study.

The same is not true for an equivalence study, in which the goal is not to find a difference, and the safeguards do not apply. Because a poorly done study with too small a sample size may miss a real difference, the investigators may have difficulty convincing others that "no difference" between two drugs in a study means that they will be "equivalent" in the real world.

# ■ SAMPLE SIZE TECHNIQUES FOR DESCRIPTIVE STUDIES

Estimating the sample size for descriptive studies, including studies of diagnostic tests, is based on somewhat different principles. Such studies do not have predictor and outcome variables, nor do they compare different groups. Thus the concepts of power and the null and alternative hypotheses do not apply. Instead, the investigator calculates descriptive statistics, such as means and proportions. Often, however, descriptive studies (*What is the prevalence of depression among elderly patients in a medical clinic?*) eventually ask analytic questions (*What are the predictors of depression among these patients?*). In this situation, sample size should be estimated for the analytic study as well, to avoid the common problem of having inadequate power for what turns out to be the question of greater interest.

Descriptive studies commonly report **confidence intervals,** a range of values about the sample mean or proportion. A confidence interval is a measure of the precision of a sample estimate. The investigator sets the confidence level, such as 95% or 99%. An interval with a greater confidence level (say 99%) is wider, and therefore more likely to include the true population value, than an interval with a lower confidence level (90%).

The width of a confidence interval depends on the sample size. For example, an investigator might wish to estimate the mean score on the U.S. Medical Licensing Examination in a group of medical students. From a sample of 200 students, she might estimate that the mean score in the population of all students is 215, with a 95% confidence interval from 190 to 240. A smaller study, say with 50 students, might have about the same mean score but would almost certainly have a wider 95% confidence interval.

When estimating sample size for descriptive studies, the investigator specifies the desired level and width of the confidence interval. The sample size can then be determined from the tables or formulas in the appendix.

## Continuous Variables

When the variable of interest is continuous, a confidence interval around the mean value of that variable is often reported. To estimate the sample size for that confidence interval, the investigator must

1. Estimate the standard deviation of the variable of interest.
2. Specify the desired precision (total width) of the confidence interval.
3. Select the confidence level for the interval (e.g., 95%, 99%).

To use Appendix 6.D, standardize the total width of the interval (divide it by the standard deviation of the variable), then look down the leftmost column of Table 6.D for the expected standardized width. Next, read across the table to the chosen confidence level for the required sample size.

---

**Example 6.4. Calculating Sample Size for a Descriptive Study of a Continuous Variable**

*Problem:* The investigator seeks to determine the mean IQ among third graders in an urban area with a 99% confidence interval of ±3 points. A previous study found that the standard deviation of IQ in a similar city was 15 points.
*Solution:* The ingredients for the sample size calculation are as follows:

1. Standard deviation of variable (SD) = 10 points.
2. Total width of interval = 6 points (3 points above and 3 points below). Thus the standardized width of interval = total width ÷ SD = 6 ÷ 15 = 0.4.
3. Confidence level = 99%.

Reading across from a standardized width of 0.4 in the leftmost column of Table 6.D and down from the 99% confidence level, the required sample size is 166 third graders.

---

## Dichotomous Variables

In a descriptive study of a dichotomous variable, results can be expressed as a confidence interval around the estimated proportion of subjects with one of the values. This includes, for example, studies of the sensitivity or specificity of a diagnostic test (Chapter 12). To estimate the sample size for that confidence interval, the investigator must

1. Estimate the expected proportion with the variable of interest in the population. (If more than half of the population is expected to have the characteristic, then plan sample size based on the proportion expected not to have the characteristic.)
2. Specify the desired precision (total width) of the confidence interval.
3. Select the confidence level for the interval (e.g., 95%).

In Appendix 6.E, look down the leftmost column of Table 6.E for the expected proportion with the variable of interest. Next, read across the table to the chosen width and confidence level, yielding the required sample size.

When studying the specificity of a diagnostic test, the investigator must estimate the sample size of subjects who do not have the disease in question. There are also techniques for estimating the sample size for studies that use receiver operating characteristic (ROC) curves (26), likelihood ratios (27), and reliability (28) as outcomes (Chapter 12).

**Example 6.5. Calculating Sample Size for a Descriptive Study of a Dichotomous Variable**

*Problem:* The investigator wishes to determine the sensitivity of a new diagnostic test for pancreatic cancer. Based on a pilot study, she expects that 80% of patients with pancreatic cancer will have positive tests. How many such patients will be required to estimate a 95% confidence interval for the test's sensitivity of 0.80 ± 0.05?

*Solution:* The ingredients for the sample size calculation are as follows:

1. Expected proportion = 0.20. (Because 0.80 is more than half, sample size is estimated from the proportion expected to have negative result, that is, 0.20.)
2. Total width = 0.10 (0.05 below and 0.05 above).
3. Confidence level = 95%.

Reading across from 0.20 in the leftmost column of Table 6.E and down from a total width of 0.10, the middle number (representing a 95% confidence level) yields the required sample size of 246 patients with pancreatic cancer.

# ■ WHAT TO DO WHEN SAMPLE SIZE IS FIXED

Especially when doing secondary data analysis, the sample size may have been determined before the study was planned. In this situation, or if the number of participants who are available or affordable for study is limited, the investigator must work backward from the sample size. She estimates the effect size that can be detected at a given power (usually 80%) or, less commonly, the power to detect a given effect. The investigator can use the sample size tables in the chapter appendixes, interpolating when necessary, or use the sample size formulas in the appendixes for estimating the effect size.

A good general rule is that a study should have a power of 80% or greater to detect a reasonable effect size. It is often tempting to pursue research hypotheses that have lower levels of power if the cost of doing so is small. The investigator should keep in mind, however, that she might face the dilemma of deciding whether to report a study that may have found no effect as a result of insufficient power.

**Example 6.6. Calculating the Detectable Effect Size When Sample Size Is Fixed**

*Problem:* There are 100 patients with systemic lupus erythematosus (SLE) who might be willing to participate in a study of whether a 6-week meditation program affects disease activity, as compared with a control group that receives a pamphlet describing relaxation. If the standard deviation of the change in a validated SLE disease activity scale score is expected to be five points in both the control and the treatment groups, what size difference will the investigator be able to detect between the two groups, at $\alpha$ (two-sided) = 0.05 and $\beta$ = 0.20?

*Solution:* In Table 6.A, reading down from $\alpha$ (two-sided) = 0.05 and $\beta$ = 0.20 (the rightmost column), 44 patients per group are required to detect a standardized effect size of 0.6, which is equal to three points (0.6 × 5 points). Thus the investigator (who will have about 50 patients per group) will be able to detect a difference of a little less than three points between the two groups.

# ■ STRATEGIES FOR MINIMIZING SAMPLE SIZE AND MAXIMIZING POWER

When the estimated sample size is greater than the number of subjects that can be studied realistically, the investigator should proceed through several steps. First, the calculations should be checked, as it is easy to make mistakes. Next, the "ingredients" should be reviewed. Is the effect size unreasonably small or the variability unreasonably large? Could $\alpha$ or $\beta$, or both, be increased without harm? Would a one-sided alternative hypothesis be adequate? Is the confidence level too high or the interval unnecessarily narrow?

These technical adjustments can be useful, but it is important to realize that statistical tests ultimately depend on the information contained in the data. Minor changes in the ingredients, such as switching from a two-sided to a one-sided alternative hypothesis, do not change the quantity or quality of the data that will be collected. There are, however, several strategies for reducing the required sample size or for increasing power for a given sample size that actually increase the information content of the collected data. Many of these strategies involve modifications of the research hypothesis; the investigator should carefully consider whether the new hypothesis still answers the research question that she wished to study.

## Use Continuous Variables

When continuous variables are an option, they usually permit smaller sample sizes than dichotomous variables. Blood pressure, for example, can be expressed either as millimeters of mercury (continuous) or as the presence or absence of hypertension (dichotomous). The former permits a smaller sample size for a given power or a greater power for a given sample size.

In the example, the continuous outcome addresses the effect of nutrition supplements on the mean birth weight in the entire sample. The dichotomous outcome is concerned with its effects on the proportion of babies who have a categorically low birth weight, which may be a more valid surrogate for neonatal morbidity and developmental abnormalities.

## Use Paired Measurements

In some experiments or cohort studies with continuous outcome variables, paired measurements—one at baseline, another at the conclusion of the study—can be made in each subject. The outcome variable is the change between these two measurements. In this situation, a $t$ test on the paired measurements can be used to compare the mean value of this change in the two groups. This technique often permits a smaller sample size because, by comparing each subject with herself, it removes the between-subject part of the variability of the outcome variable. For example, the change in weight on a diet has less variability than the final weight, because final weight is highly correlated with initial weight. Sample size for this type of $t$ test is estimated in the usual way, except that the standardized effect size ($E/S$ in Table 6.A) is the anticipated difference in the change in the variable divided by the standard deviation of that change.

**Example 6.7. Use of Continuous versus Dichotomous Variables**

*Problem:* Consider a placebo-controlled trial to determine the effect of prenatal nutrition supplements on birth weight in a population at risk for low-birth-weight infants (<2,500 g). Suppose that previous studies have established that birth weight is approximately normally distributed, with a mean of 3,500 g and a standard deviation of 770 g, and that about 10% of infants have low birth weight. The placebo is anticipated to have no effect; nutrition supplements are anticipated to increase the mean birth weight by 300 g. This change in mean birth weight can be estimated, based on the distribution of newborn birth weights, to correspond to a reduction in the proportion of low-birth-weight infants to 5%.

One design might treat birth weight as a dichotomous variable: low birth weight versus not low birth weight. Another might use all the information contained in the measurement and treat birth weight as a continuous variable. How many live births would each design require at $\alpha$ (two-sided) = 0.05 and $\beta$ = 0.20? How does the change in design affect the research question?

*Solution:* The ingredients for the sample size calculation using a *dichotomous outcome variable* (low birth weight or not low birth weight) are as follows:

1. *Null hypothesis:* The proportion of low-birth-weight babies born to mothers receiving prenatal nutrition supplements is the same as that in mothers taking placebo.
   *Alternative hypothesis:* The proportion of low-birth-weight babies born to mothers receiving prenatal nutrition supplements is different from that of mothers taking placebo.
2. $P_1$ (incidence of low birth weight in placebo group) = 0.10; $P_2$ (incidence of low birth weight in supplement group) = 0.05. The smaller of these values is 0.05, and the difference between them ($P_1 - P_2$) is 0.05.
3. $\alpha$ (two-sided) = 0.05; $\beta$ = 0.20.

Using Table 6.B.1, reading across from 0.05 in the leftmost column and down from an expected difference of 0.05, the upper number (for $\alpha$ [two-sided] = 0.05 and $\beta$ = 0.20), this design would require 434 live births in each group.

The ingredients for the sample size calculation using a continuous outcome variable (birth weight) are as follows:

1. *Null hypothesis:* Mean birth weight among babies born to mothers receiving prenatal nutrition supplements is the same as that among babies born to mothers taking placebo.
   *Alternative hypothesis:* Mean birth weight among babies born to mothers receiving prenatal nutrition supplements is different from that among babies born to mothers taking placebo.
2. Effect size = 300 g.
3. Standard deviation of birth weight = 770 g.
4. Standardized effect size = effect size ÷ standard deviation = 300 g ÷ 770 g ≈ 0.4.
5. $\alpha$ (two-sided) 0.05; $\beta$ = 0.20.

Using Table 6.A, reading across from a standardized effect size of 0.40, with $\alpha$ (two-sided) = 0.05 and $\beta$ = 0.20, this design would require about 131 live births in each group, a substantially smaller sample.

**Example 6.8. Use of the $t$ Test with Paired Measurements**

*Problem:* Recall Example 6.1, in which the investigator studying the treatment of asthma is interested in determining whether salbutamol can improve $FEV_1$ by 200 mL compared with ipratropium bromide. Sample size calculations indicated that 393 subjects per group are needed, more than are likely to be available. Fortunately, a colleague points out that asthmatic patients have great differences in their $FEV_1$ values before treatment. These between-individual differences account for much of the variability in $FEV_1$ after treatment, thus obscuring the effect of treatment. She suggests using a paired $t$ test to compare the *changes* in $FEV_1$ in the two groups. A pilot study finds that the standard deviation of the change in $FEV_1$ is only 250 mL. How many subjects would be required per group, at $\alpha$ (two-sided) = 0.05 and $\beta$ = 0.20?

*Solution:* The ingredients for the sample size calculation are as follows:

1. *Null hypothesis:* Change in mean $FEV_1$ at 1 hour after treatment is the same in asthmatic patients treated with salbutamol as it is in those treated with ipratropium bromide.
   *Alternative hypothesis:* Change in mean $FEV_1$ at 1 hour after treatment is different in asthmatic patients treated with salbutamol from what it is in those treated with ipratropium bromide.
2. Effect size = 200 mL.
3. Standard deviation of the outcome variable = 250 mL.
4. Standardized effect size = effect size ÷ standard deviation = 200 mL ÷ 250 mL = 0.8.
5. $\alpha$ (two-sided) = 0.05; $\beta$ = 1 − 0.80 = 0.20.

Using Table 6.A, this design would require about 25 participants per group, a much more reasonable sample size than the 393 per group in Example 6.1.

*A Brief Technical Note.*    This chapter always refers to *two-sample t* tests, which are used when comparing the mean values of an outcome variable in two groups of subjects. A two-sample $t$ test can be *unpaired*, if the outcome variable itself is being compared between two groups (see Example 6.1), or *paired* if the outcome is the change in a pair of measurements, say before and after an intervention (see Example 6.8). (A *one-sample t* test would compare the mean value in a single group with the value of zero; a one-sample paired $t$ test would compare the mean change in a pair of values within a single group to zero change.)

## Use More Precise Variables

Because they reduce variability, more precise variables permit a smaller sample size in both analytic and descriptive studies. Even a modest change in precision can have a substantial effect on sample size. For example, when using the $t$ test to estimate sample size, a 20% decrease in the standard deviation of the outcome variable results in a 36% decrease in the sample size. Techniques for increasing the precision of a variable, such as making measurements in duplicate, are presented in Chapter 4.

## Use Unequal Group Sizes

Because an equal number of subjects in each of two groups usually gives the greatest power for a given total number of subjects, Tables 6.A, 6.B.1, and 6.B.2

in the appendixes assume equal sample sizes in the two groups. Sometimes, however, the distribution of subjects is not equal in the two groups, or it is easier or less expensive to recruit study subjects for one group than the other. It may turn out, for example, that an investigator wants to estimate sample size based on the 30% of the subjects in a cohort who smoke cigarettes (compared with 70% who do not smoke). Or, in a case-control study, the number of persons with the disease may be small, but it may be possible to sample a much larger number of controls. In general, the gain in power when the size of one group is increased to twice the size of the other is considerable; tripling and quadrupling one of the groups provide progressively smaller gains. Sample sizes for unequal groups can be computed from the formulas found in the text to Appendixes 6.A and 6.B or from the Web.

Here is a useful approximation for estimating sample size for case-control studies of dichotomous risk factors and outcomes using $c$ controls per case. If $n$ represents the number of cases that would have been required for one control per case (at a given $\alpha$, $\beta$, and effect size), then the approximate number of cases ($n'$) with $cn'$ controls that will be required is

$$n' = [(c + 1) \div 2c] \times n$$

For example, with $c = 2$ controls per case, then $[(2 + 1) \div (2 \times 2)] \times n = 3/4 \times n$; thus only 75% as many cases are needed. As $c$ gets larger, $n'$ approaches 50% of $n$ (when $c = 10$, for example, $n' = 11/20 \times n$).

---

**Example 6.9. Use of Multiple Controls per Case in a Case-Control Study**

*Problem:* An investigator is studying whether exposure to household insecticide is a risk factor for aplastic anemia. The original sample size calculation indicated that 25 cases would be required, using one control per case. Suppose that the investigator has access to only 18 cases. How should the investigator proceed?

*Solution:* The investigator should consider using multiple controls per case (after all, she can find lots of patients who do not have aplastic anemia). By using three controls per case, for example, the approximate number of cases that will be required is $[(3 + 1) \div (2 \times 3)] \times 25 = 17$.

---

## Use a More Common Outcome

When the outcome is dichotomous, using a more frequent outcome, up to a frequency of about 0.5, is usually one of the best ways to increase power: If an outcome occurs more often, there is more of a chance to detect its predictors. Power actually depends more on the number of subjects with a specified outcome than it does on the total number of subjects in the study. Studies with rare outcomes, like the occurrence of cervical cancer in healthy women, require very large sample sizes to have adequate power.

One of the best ways to make an outcome more common is to enroll subjects at greater risk of developing that outcome (such as women with a family history of breast cancer). Others are to extend the follow-up period, so that there is more time to accumulate outcomes, or to loosen the definition of what constitutes an outcome (e.g., by including ductal carcinoma *in situ*). All these techniques, however, may change the research question, so they should be used with caution.

---

**Example 6.10. Use of a More Common Outcome**

*Problem:* Suppose an investigator is comparing the efficacy of an antiseptic gargle versus a placebo gargle in preventing upper respiratory infections. Her initial calculations indicated that her anticipated sample of 200 volunteer college students was inadequate, in part because she expected that only about 20% of her subjects would have an upper respiratory infection during the 3-month follow-up period. Suggest a few changes in the study plan.

*Solution:* Here are two possible solutions: (a) Study a sample of pediatric residents, who are likely to experience a much greater incidence of upper respiratory infections than college students; or (b) follow the sample for a longer period of time, say 6 or 12 months. Both of these solutions involve modification of the research hypothesis, but neither change seems sufficiently large to affect the overall research question about the efficacy of antiseptic gargle.

---

# ■ HOW TO ESTIMATE SAMPLE SIZE WHEN THERE IS INSUFFICIENT INFORMATION

Often the investigator finds that she is missing one or more of the ingredients for the sample size calculation and becomes frustrated in her attempts to plan the study. This is an especially frequent problem when the investigator is using an instrument of her design (such as a new questionnaire on quality of life in patients with urinary incontinence), or enrolling a sample that has not previously been studied (such as subjects taking a new drug). How should she go about deciding what effect size or standard deviation to use?

The first strategy is an **extensive search** for previous findings on the topic, thoroughly reviewing the relevant literature, sometimes going beyond the medical journals listed in MEDLINE. Roughly comparable situations and mediocre or dated findings may be good enough. (The sample size calculation is just an estimate.) If the literature review is unproductive, she should contact other investigators about their judgment on what to expect, and whether they are aware of any unpublished results that may be relevant. If there is still no information available, she may consider doing a small **pilot study** or obtaining a data set for a secondary analysis, to obtain the missing ingredients, before embarking on the main study. This may be especially useful for estimating the standard deviation of a measurement, or the proportion of subjects with a particular characteristic. For continuous variables that have a roughly bell-shaped distribution, the standard deviation can be estimated as one-quarter of the difference between the high and low ends of the range of values that occur commonly, ignoring extreme values. For example, if most subjects are likely to have a serum sodium level between 135 and 143 meq/L, the standard deviation of serum sodium is about 2 meq/L ($1/4 \times 8$ meq/L).

Another strategy, when the mean and standard deviation of a continuous or categorical variable are in doubt, is to **dichotomize** that variable. Categories can be lumped into two groups, and continuous variables can be split at their mean or median. The chi-squared statistic can then be used to make a reasonable estimate of the sample size. Dividing the quality of life into "better than the median" or "the median or less" avoids having to estimate its standard deviation in the sample at the cost of underestimating the actual power of the study.

If all this fails, the investigator should just make an **educated guess** about the likely values of the missing ingredients. The process of thinking through the problem and imagining the findings will usually result in a reasonable estimate, and that is what sample size planning is about.

# ■ COMMON ERRORS TO AVOID

Many inexperienced investigators (and some experienced ones!) make mistakes when planning sample size. A few of the more common ones follow:

1. Dichotomous variables can appear to be continuous when they are expressed as a percentage or rate. For example, vital status (alive or dead) might be misinterpreted as continuous when expressed as percent alive, or as number of deaths per year. Similarly, in survival analysis a dichotomous outcome can appear to be continuous (e.g., mean survival duration in months). For all of these, the outcome is actually dichotomous and the appropriate simple approach in planning sample size would be the chi-squared test.
2. The sample size estimates the number of subjects who need to be followed, not the number who need to be enrolled. The investigator should always plan for dropouts and for subjects with missing data.
3. The tables at the end of the chapter assume that the two groups being studied have equal sample sizes. Often that is not the case; for example, a cohort study of whether use of vitamin supplements reduces the risk of sunburn would probably not enroll equal numbers of subjects who used, or did not use, vitamins. If the sample sizes are not equal, then the formulas that follow the tables should be used.
4. When using the *t* test to estimate the sample size, what matters is the standard deviation (SD) of the outcome variable. Thus if the outcome is *change* in a continuous variable, the investigator should use the SD of that change rather than the SD of the variable itself.
5. The most common error is estimating the sample size late during the design of the study. Do it early in the process, when fundamental changes can still be made.
6. Be aware of clustered data. If there appear to be two "levels" of sample size (e.g., one for physicians and another for patients), clustering is a likely problem.

# ■ SUMMARY

1. When estimating sample size for an **analytic study,** the following steps need to be taken: (a) state the **null** and **alternative hypotheses,** specifying the number of **sides**; (b) select a **statistical test** that could be used to analyze the data, based on the types of predictor and outcome variables; (c) estimate the **effect size** and its **variability** from the results of previous studies or a pilot study; and (d) specify appropriate values for $\alpha$ and $\beta$, based on the importance of avoiding Type I and Type II errors.
2. Other considerations in calculating sample size for analytic studies include adjusting for potential **dropouts,** and strategies for dealing with **categorical variables, survival analysis, clustered samples, matching, multivariate adjustment,** and **equivalence studies.**

3. The steps for estimating sample size for **descriptive studies,** which do not have hypotheses, are to (a) estimate the **proportion** of subjects with a dichotomous outcome or the **standard deviation** of a continuous outcome; (b) specify the desired **precision** (width of the confidence interval); and (c) specify the **confidence level** (e.g., 95%).

4. When sample size is predetermined, the investigator can work backward to estimate the detectable **effect size** or, less commonly, the **power.**

5. Strategies **to minimize** the required sample size include using **continuous** variables, more **precise** measurements, **paired** measurements, **unequal group sizes,** and more **common outcomes.**

6. When there seems not to be enough information to estimate the sample size, the investigator should **review the literature** in related areas, think about doing a small **pilot study** or secondary data analysis, or consider **dichotomizing** a variable at its median. If none of these is feasible, an educated guess can give a useful ballpark estimate.

# EXERCISES

1. Review the exercise at the end of Chapter 5. Determine how many cases of stomach cancer would be required for the study. What if the investigator wanted a power of 0.90? Or a level of statistical significance of 0.01?

2. Muscle strength declines with advancing age. Preliminary evidence suggests that part of this loss of muscle strength might be due to progressive deficiency of dehydroepiandrosterone (DHEA). Investigators plan a randomized trial to administer DHEA or identical placebo for 6 months to elderly subjects, and then measure muscle strength. Previous studies have reported a mean grip strength in elderly persons of 20 kg with a standard deviation of 5 kg. Assuming $\alpha$ (two-sided) = 0.05 and $\beta$ = 0.10, how many subjects would be required to demonstrate a 10% or greater difference between strength in the treated and placebo groups? How many subjects would be required if a one-sided test is justified? How many subjects would be needed if $\beta$ = 0.20?

3. In exercise 2, sample size calculations indicated that 131 subjects per group were needed, more than can be enrolled. A colleague points out that elderly people have great differences in grip strength. This accounts for much of the variability in the strength measured after treatment and might be obscuring the treatment effect. She suggests that you measure strength at baseline and again after treatment, using the change in strength as the outcome variable. A small pilot study shows that the standard deviation of the change in strength during a 6-month period is only 2 kg. How many subjects would be required per group using this design, assuming $\alpha$ (two-sided) = 0.05 and $\beta$ = 0.10?

4. An investigator suspects that left-handedness is more common in dyslexic than in nondyslexic third graders. Previous studies indicated that about 10% of people are left-handed and that dyslexia is uncommon. A case-control study is planned that will select all the dyslexic students in a school district as cases, with an equal number of nondyslexic students randomly selected as controls. What sample size would be required to show that the odds ratio for dyslexia is 2.0 among left-handed students compared with right-handed students? Assume $\alpha$ = 0.05 (two-sided) and $\beta$ = 0.20.

**5.** An investigator seeks to determine the mean priority score of R0-1 NIH grant applications, with a 99% confidence interval of +20 points. Priority scores range from 100 to 500, with the lowest score the best. A previous study found that the standard deviation of priority scores was about 100. What sample size is needed?

# References

1. Lehr R. Sixteen S-squared over D-squared: a relation for crude sample size estimates. *Stat Med* 1992;11:1099–102.
2. Lakatos E, Lan KK. A comparison of sample size methods for the logrank statistic. *Stat Med* 1992;11:179–91.
3. Shih JH. Sample size calculation for complex clinical trials with survival endpoints. *Control Clin Trials* 1995;16:395–407.
4. Donner A. Sample size requirements for stratified cluster randomization designs [published erratum appears in *Stat Med* 1997;30;16:2927]. *Stat Med* 1992;11:743–50.
5. Liu G, Liang KY. Sample size calculations for studies with correlated observations. *Biometrics* 1997;53:937–47.
6. Kerry SM, Bland JM. Trials which randomize practices II: sample size. *Fam Pract* 1998;15:84–7.
7. Hayes RJ, Bennett S. Simple sample size calculation for cluster-randomized trials. *Int J Epidemiol* 1999;28:319–26.
8. Schlesselman JJ. *Case-control studies: design, conduct, analysis.* New York: Oxford University Press, 1982.
9. Drescher K, Timm J, Jöckel KH. The design of case-control studies: the effect of confounding on sample size requirements. *Stat Med* 1990;9:765–76.
10. Lui KJ. Sample size determination for case-control studies: the influence of the joint distribution of exposure and confounder. *Stat Med* 1990;9:1485–93.
11. Bull SB. Sample size and power determination for a binary outcome and an ordinal exposure when logistic regression analysis is planned. *Am J Epidemiol* 1993;137:676–84.
12. Dupont WD, Plummer WD, Jr. Power and sample size calculations for studies involving linear regression. *Control Clin Trials* 1998;19:589–601.
13. Hsieh FY, Bloch DA, Larsen MD. A simple method of sample size calculation for linear and logistic regression. *Stat Med* 1998;17:1623–34.
14. Sasieni PD. From genotypes to genes: Doubling the sample size. *Biometrics* 1997;53:1253–61.
15. Elston RC, Idury RM, Cardon LR, Lichter JB. The study of candidate genes in drug trials: sample size considerations. *Stat Med* 1999;18:741–51.
16. García-Closas M, Lubin JH. Power and sample size calculations in case-control studies of gene-environment interactions: comments on different approaches. *Am J Epidemiol* 1999;149:689–92.
17. Torgerson DJ, Ryan M, Ratcliffe J. Economics in sample size determination for clinical trials. *QJM* 1995;88:517–21.
18. Laska EM, Meisner M, Siegel C. Power and sample size in cost-effectiveness analysis. *Med Decis Making* 1999;19:339–43.
19. Willan AR, O'Brien BJ. Sample size and power issues in estimating incremental cost-effectiveness ratios from clinical trials data. *Health Econ* 1999;8:203–11.
20. Patel HI. Sample size for a dose-response study [published erratum appears in *J Biopharm Stat* 1994;4:127]. *J Biopharm Stat* 1992;2:1–8.
21. Day SJ, Graham DF. Sample size estimation for comparing two or more treatment groups in clinical trials. *Stat Med* 1991;10:33–43.
22. Nam JM. Sample size determination in stratified trials to establish the equivalence of two treatments. *Stat Med* 1995;14:2037–49.

23. Bristol DR. Determining equivalence and the impact of sample size in anti-infective studies: a point to consider. *J Biopharm Stat* 1996;6:319–26.

24. Tai BC, Lee J. Sample size and power calculations for comparing two independent proportions in a "negative" trial. *Psychiatry Res* 1998;80:197–200.

25. Hauschke D, Kieser M, Diletti E, Burke M. Sample size determination for proving equivalence based on the ratio of two means for normally distributed data. *Stat Med* 1999;18:93–105.

26. Obuchowski NA. Computing sample size for receiver operating characteristic studies. *Invest Radiol* 1994;29:238–43.

27. Simel DL, Samsa GP, Matchar DB. Likelihood ratios with confidence: sample size estimation for diagnostic test studies. *J Clin Epidemiol* 1991;44:763–70.

28. Walter SD, Eliasziw M, Donner A. Sample size and optimal designs for reliability studies. *Stat Med* 1998;17:101–10.

## ■ APPENDIX 6.A

### Sample Size Required per Group When Using the *t* Test to Compare Means of Continuous Variables

#### ■ TABLE 6.A

Sample Size *per Group* for Comparing Two Means

| E/S* | β = | One-sided α = 0.005 Two-sided α = 0.01 | | | One-sided α = 0.025 Two-sided α = 0.05 | | | One-sided α = 0.05 Two-sided α = 0.10 | | |
|------|-----|-------|-------|-------|-------|-------|-------|-------|-------|-------|
| | | 0.05 | 0.10 | 0.20 | 0.05 | 0.10 | 0.20 | 0.05 | 0.10 | 0.20 |
| 0.10 | | 3,565 | 2,978 | 2,338 | 2,600 | 2,103 | 1,571 | 2,166 | 1,714 | 1,238 |
| 0.15 | | 1,586 | 1,325 | 1,040 | 1,157 | 935 | 699 | 963 | 762 | 551 |
| 0.20 | | 893 | 746 | 586 | 651 | 527 | 394 | 542 | 429 | 310 |
| 0.25 | | 572 | 478 | 376 | 417 | 338 | 253 | 347 | 275 | 199 |
| 0.30 | | 398 | 333 | 262 | 290 | 235 | 176 | 242 | 191 | 139 |
| 0.40 | | 225 | 188 | 148 | 164 | 133 | 100 | 136 | 108 | 78 |
| 0.50 | | 145 | 121 | 96 | 105 | 86 | 64 | 88 | 70 | 51 |
| 0.60 | | 101 | 85 | 67 | 74 | 60 | 45 | 61 | 49 | 36 |
| 0.70 | | 75 | 63 | 50 | 55 | 44 | 34 | 45 | 36 | 26 |
| 0.80 | | 58 | 49 | 39 | 42 | 34 | 26 | 35 | 28 | 21 |
| 0.90 | | 46 | 39 | 21 | 34 | 27 | 21 | 28 | 22 | 16 |
| 1.00 | | 38 | 32 | 26 | 27 | 23 | 17 | 23 | 18 | 14 |

*E/S is the standardized effect size, computed as E (expected effect size) divided by S (standard deviation of the outcome variable). To estimate the sample size, read across from the *standardized effect size,* and down from the specified values of α and β for the required sample size in each group.

### Calculating Variability

Variability is usually reported as either the standard deviation (SD) or the standard error of the mean (SEM). For the purposes of sample size calculation, the standard deviation of the variable is most useful. Fortunately, it is easy to convert from one measure to another: the standard deviation is simply the standard error times the square root of N, where N is the number of subjects that make up the mean. Suppose a study reported that the weight loss in 25 persons on a low-fiber diet was 10 ± 2 kg (mean ± SEM). The standard deviation would be $2 \times \sqrt{25} = 10$ kg.

### General Formula for Other Values

The general formula for other values of $E$, $S$, $\alpha$, and $\beta$, or for unequal group sizes, where $E$ and $S$ are defined above, follows. Let:

$z_\alpha$ = the standard normal deviate for $\alpha$ (If the alternative hypothesis is two-sided, $z_\alpha$ = 2.58 when $\alpha$ = 0.01, $z_\alpha$ − 1.96 when $\alpha$ = 0.05, and $z_\alpha$ = 1.645 when $\alpha$ = 0.10. If the alternative hypothesis is one-sided, $z_\alpha$ = 1.645 when $\alpha$ = 0.05.)

$z_\beta$ = the standard normal deviate for $\beta$ ($z_\beta$ = 0.84 when $\beta$ = 0.20, and $z_\beta$ = 1.282 when $\beta$ = 0.10)

$q_1$ = proportion of subjects in group 1
$q_2$ = proportion of subjects in group 2
$N$ = **total** number of subjects required

Then:

$$N = [(1/q_1 + 1/q_2)S^2(z_\alpha + z_\beta)^2] \div E^2.$$

(Because this formula is based on approximating the $t$ statistic with a z statistic, it will slightly underestimate the sample size when N is less than about 30. Table 6.A uses the $t$ statistic to estimate sample size.)

# ■ APPENDIX 6.B

## Sample Size Required per Group When Using the Chi-Squared Statistic to Compare Proportions of Dichotomous Variables

### ■ TABLE 6.B.1
Sample Size *per Group* for Comparing Two Proportions

**Upper number:** $\alpha = 0.05$ (one-sided) or $\alpha = 0.10$ (two-sided); $\beta = 0.02$
**Middle number:** $\alpha = 0.025$ (one-sided) or $\alpha = 0.05$ (two-sided); $\beta = 0.02$
**Lower number:** $\alpha = 0.025$ (one-sided) or $\alpha = 0.05$ (two-sided); $\beta = 0.10$

| Smaller of P1 and P2* | Difference Between $P_1$ and $P_2$ | | | | | | | | | |
|---|---|---|---|---|---|---|---|---|---|---|
| | 0.05 | 0.10 | 0.15 | 0.20 | 0.25 | 0.30 | 0.35 | 0.40 | 0.45 | 0.50 |
| 0.05 | 381 | 129 | 72 | 47 | 35 | 27 | 22 | 18 | 15 | 13 |
| | 473 | 159 | 88 | 59 | 43 | 33 | 26 | 22 | 18 | 16 |
| | 620 | 207 | 113 | 75 | 54 | 41 | 33 | 27 | 23 | 19 |
| 0.10 | 578 | 175 | 91 | 58 | 41 | 31 | 24 | 20 | 16 | 14 |
| | 724 | 219 | 112 | 72 | 51 | 37 | 29 | 24 | 20 | 17 |
| | 958 | 286 | 146 | 92 | 65 | 48 | 37 | 30 | 25 | 21 |
| 0.15 | 751 | 217 | 108 | 67 | 46 | 34 | 26 | 21 | 17 | 15 |
| | 944 | 270 | 133 | 82 | 57 | 41 | 32 | 26 | 21 | 18 |
| | 1,252 | 354 | 174 | 106 | 73 | 53 | 42 | 33 | 26 | 22 |
| 0.20 | 900 | 251 | 121 | 74 | 50 | 36 | 28 | 22 | 18 | 15 |
| | 1,133 | 313 | 151 | 91 | 62 | 44 | 34 | 27 | 22 | 18 |
| | 1,504 | 412 | 197 | 118 | 80 | 57 | 44 | 34 | 27 | 23 |
| 0.25 | 1,024 | 278 | 132 | 79 | 53 | 38 | 29 | 23 | 18 | 15 |
| | 1,289 | 348 | 165 | 98 | 66 | 47 | 35 | 28 | 22 | 18 |
| | 1,714 | 459 | 216 | 127 | 85 | 60 | 46 | 35 | 28 | 23 |
| 0.30 | 1,123 | 300 | 141 | 83 | 55 | 39 | 29 | 23 | 18 | 15 |
| | 1,415 | 376 | 175 | 103 | 68 | 48 | 36 | 28 | 22 | 18 |
| | 1,883 | 496 | 230 | 134 | 88 | 62 | 47 | 36 | 28 | 23 |
| 0.35 | 1,197 | 315 | 146 | 85 | 56 | 39 | 29 | 23 | 18 | 15 |
| | 1,509 | 395 | 182 | 106 | 69 | 48 | 36 | 28 | 22 | 18 |
| | 2,009 | 522 | 239 | 138 | 90 | 62 | 47 | 35 | 27 | 22 |
| 0.40 | 1,246 | 325 | 149 | 86 | 56 | 39 | 29 | 22 | 17 | 14 |
| | 1,572 | 407 | 186 | 107 | 69 | 48 | 35 | 27 | 21 | 17 |
| | 2,093 | 538 | 244 | 139 | 90 | 62 | 46 | 34 | 26 | 21 |
| 0.45 | 1,271 | 328 | 149 | 85 | 55 | 38 | 28 | 21 | 16 | 13 |
| | 1,603 | 411 | 186 | 106 | 68 | 47 | 34 | 26 | 20 | 16 |
| | 2,135 | 543 | 244 | 138 | 88 | 60 | 44 | 33 | 25 | 19 |
| 0.50 | 1,271 | 325 | 146 | 83 | 53 | 36 | 26 | 20 | 15 | — |
| | 1,603 | 407 | 182 | 103 | 66 | 44 | 32 | 24 | 18 | — |
| | 2,135 | 538 | 239 | 134 | 85 | 57 | 42 | 30 | 23 | — |
| 0.55 | 1,246 | 315 | 141 | 79 | 50 | 34 | 24 | 18 | — | — |
| | 1,572 | 395 | 175 | 98 | 62 | 41 | 29 | 22 | — | — |
| | 2,093 | 522 | 230 | 127 | 80 | 53 | 37 | 27 | — | — |
| 0.60 | 1,197 | 300 | 132 | 74 | 46 | 31 | 22 | — | — | — |
| | 1,509 | 376 | 165 | 91 | 57 | 37 | 26 | — | — | — |
| | 2,009 | 496 | 216 | 118 | 73 | 48 | 33 | — | — | — |

*continued*

■ **TABLE 6.B.1** *continued*

**Upper number:** $\alpha = 0.05$ (one-sided) or $\alpha = 0.10$ (two-sided); $\beta = 0.02$
**Middle number:** $\alpha = 0.025$ (one-sided) or $\alpha = 0.05$ (two-sided); $\beta = 0.02$
**Lower number:** $\alpha = 0.025$ (one-sided) or $\alpha = 0.05$ (two-sided); $\beta = 0.10$

| Smaller of P1 and P2* | Difference Between $P_1$ and $P_2$ | | | | | | | | | |
|---|---|---|---|---|---|---|---|---|---|---|
| | 0.05 | 0.10 | 0.15 | 0.20 | 0.25 | 0.30 | 0.35 | 0.40 | 0.45 | 0.50 |
| 0.65 | 1,123 | 278 | 121 | 67 | 41 | 27 | — | — | — | — |
| | 1,415 | 348 | 151 | 82 | 51 | 33 | — | — | — | — |
| | 1,883 | 459 | 197 | 106 | 65 | 41 | — | — | — | — |
| 0.70 | 1,024 | 251 | 108 | 58 | 35 | — | — | — | — | — |
| | 1,289 | 313 | 133 | 72 | 43 | — | — | — | — | — |
| | 1,714 | 412 | 174 | 92 | 54 | — | — | — | — | — |
| 0.75 | 900 | 217 | 91 | 47 | — | — | — | — | — | — |
| | 1,133 | 270 | 112 | 59 | — | — | — | — | — | — |
| | 1,504 | 354 | 146 | 75 | — | — | — | — | — | — |
| 0.80 | 751 | 175 | 72 | — | — | — | — | — | — | — |
| | 944 | 219 | 88 | — | — | — | — | — | — | — |
| | 1,252 | 286 | 113 | — | — | — | — | — | — | — |
| 0.85 | 578 | 129 | — | — | — | — | — | — | — | — |
| | 724 | 159 | — | — | — | — | — | — | — | — |
| | 958 | 207 | — | — | — | — | — | — | — | — |
| 0.90 | 381 | — | — | — | — | — | — | — | — | — |
| | 473 | — | — | — | — | — | — | — | — | — |
| | 620 | — | — | — | — | — | — | — | — | — |

The one-sided estimates use the z statistic.

*$P_1$ represents the proportion of subjects expected to have the outcome in one group; $P_2$ in the other group. (In a case-control study, $P_1$ represents the proportion of cases with the predictor variable; $P_2$ the proportion of controls with the predictor variable.) To estimate the sample size, read across from the *smaller* of $P_1$ and $P_2$, and down the *expected difference* between $P_1$ and $P_2$. The three numbers represent the sample size required in each group for the specified values of $\alpha$ and $\beta$.

Additional detail for $P_1$ and $P_2$ between 0.01 and 0.10 is given in Table 6.B.2.

## General Formula for Total Sample Size

The general formula for calculating the *total* sample size (N) required for a study using the z statistic, where $P_1$ and $P_2$ are defined above, is as follows (see Appendix 6.A for definitions of $z_\alpha$ and $z_\beta$). Let

$$q_1 = \text{proportion of subjects in group 1}$$
$$q_2 = \text{proportion of subjects in group 2}$$
$$N = total \text{ number of subjects}$$
$$P = q_1 P_1 + q_2 P_2$$

Then

$$N = \frac{[z_\alpha \sqrt{P(1-P)(1/q_1 + 1/q_2)} + z_\beta \sqrt{P_1(1-P_1)(1/q_1) + P_2(1-P_2)(1/q_2)}]^2}{(P_1 - P_2)^2}.$$

(This formula does not include the Fleiss-Tytun-Ury continuity correction and thus underestimate the required sample size by up to about 10%. Tables 6.B.1 and 6.B.2 do include this continuity correction.)

■ **TABLE 6.B.2**

Sample Size *per Group* for Comparing Two Proportions, the Smaller of Which Is Between 0.01 and 0.10

**Upper number:** $\alpha = 0.05$ (one-sided) or $\alpha = 0.10$ (two-sided); $\beta = 0.02$
**Middle number:** $\alpha = 0.025$ (one-sided) or $\alpha = 0.05$ (two-sided); $\beta = 0.02$
**Lower number:** $\alpha = 0.025$ (one-sided) or $\alpha = 0.05$ (two-sided); $\beta = 0.10$

| Smaller of $P_1$ and $P_2$ | Expected Difference Between $P_1$ and $P_2$ | | | | | | | | | |
|---|---|---|---|---|---|---|---|---|---|---|
| | 0.01 | 0.02 | 0.03 | 0.04 | 0.05 | 0.06 | 0.07 | 0.08 | 0.09 | 0.10 |
| 0.01 | 2,019 | 700 | 396 | 271 | 204 | 162 | 134 | 114 | 98 | 87 |
| | 2,512 | 864 | 487 | 332 | 249 | 197 | 163 | 138 | 120 | 106 |
| | 3,300 | 1,125 | 631 | 428 | 320 | 254 | 209 | 178 | 154 | 135 |
| 0.02 | 3,205 | 994 | 526 | 343 | 249 | 193 | 157 | 131 | 113 | 97 |
| | 4,018 | 1,237 | 651 | 423 | 306 | 238 | 192 | 161 | 137 | 120 |
| | 5,320 | 1,625 | 852 | 550 | 397 | 307 | 248 | 207 | 177 | 154 |
| 0.03 | 4,367 | 1,283 | 653 | 414 | 294 | 224 | 179 | 148 | 126 | 109 |
| | 5,493 | 1,602 | 813 | 512 | 363 | 276 | 220 | 182 | 154 | 133 |
| | 7,296 | 2,114 | 1,067 | 671 | 474 | 359 | 286 | 236 | 199 | 172 |
| 0.04 | 5,505 | 1,564 | 777 | 482 | 337 | 254 | 201 | 165 | 139 | 119 |
| | 6,935 | 1,959 | 969 | 600 | 419 | 314 | 248 | 203 | 170 | 146 |
| | 9,230 | 2,593 | 1,277 | 788 | 548 | 410 | 323 | 264 | 221 | 189 |
| 0.05 | 6,616 | 1,838 | 898 | 549 | 380 | 283 | 222 | 181 | 151 | 129 |
| | 8,347 | 2,308 | 1,123 | 686 | 473 | 351 | 275 | 223 | 186 | 159 |
| | 11,123 | 3,061 | 1,482 | 902 | 620 | 460 | 360 | 291 | 242 | 206 |
| 0.06 | 7,703 | 2,107 | 1,016 | 615 | 422 | 312 | 243 | 197 | 163 | 139 |
| | 9,726 | 2,650 | 1,272 | 769 | 526 | 388 | 301 | 243 | 202 | 171 |
| | 12,973 | 3,518 | 1,684 | 1,014 | 691 | 508 | 395 | 318 | 263 | 223 |
| 0.07 | 8,765 | 2,369 | 1,131 | 680 | 463 | 340 | 263 | 212 | 175 | 148 |
| | 11,076 | 2,983 | 1,419 | 850 | 577 | 423 | 327 | 263 | 217 | 183 |
| | 14,780 | 3,965 | 1,880 | 1,123 | 760 | 555 | 429 | 343 | 283 | 239 |
| 0.08 | 9,803 | 2,627 | 1,244 | 743 | 502 | 367 | 282 | 227 | 187 | 158 |
| | 12,393 | 3,308 | 1,562 | 930 | 627 | 457 | 352 | 282 | 232 | 195 |
| | 16,546 | 4,401 | 2,072 | 1,229 | 827 | 602 | 463 | 369 | 303 | 255 |
| 0.09 | 10,816 | 2,877 | 1,354 | 804 | 541 | 393 | 302 | 241 | 198 | 167 |
| | 13,679 | 3,626 | 1,702 | 1,007 | 676 | 491 | 377 | 300 | 246 | 207 |
| | 18,270 | 4,827 | 2,259 | 1,333 | 893 | 647 | 495 | 393 | 322 | 270 |
| 0.10 | 11,804 | 3,121 | 1,461 | 863 | 578 | 419 | 320 | 255 | 209 | 175 |
| | 14,933 | 3,936 | 1,838 | 1,083 | 724 | 523 | 401 | 318 | 260 | 218 |
| | 19,952 | 5,242 | 2,441 | 1,434 | 957 | 690 | 527 | 417 | 341 | 285 |

The one-sided estimates use the *z* statistic.

## ■ APPENDIX 6.C

### Total Sample Size Required When Using the Correlation Coefficient ($r$)

■ **TABLE 6.C**

Sample Size for Determining Whether a Correlation Coefficient Differs from Zero

| One-sided $\alpha$ =<br>Two-sided $\alpha$ =<br><br>$\beta$ =<br>$r$ * | 0.005<br>0.01 | | | 0.025<br>0.05 | | | 0.05<br>0.010 | | |
|---|---|---|---|---|---|---|---|---|---|
| | **0.05** | **0.10** | **0.20** | **0.05** | **0.10** | **0.20** | **0.05** | **0.10** | **0.20** |
| 0.05 | 7,118 | 5,947 | 4,663 | 5,193 | 4,200 | 3,134 | 4,325 | 3,424 | 2,469 |
| 0.10 | 1,773 | 1,481 | 1,162 | 1,294 | 1,047 | 782 | 1,078 | 854 | 616 |
| 0.15 | 783 | 655 | 514 | 572 | 463 | 346 | 477 | 378 | 273 |
| 0.20 | 436 | 365 | 287 | 319 | 259 | 194 | 266 | 211 | 153 |
| 0.25 | 276 | 231 | 182 | 202 | 164 | 123 | 169 | 134 | 98 |
| 0.30 | 189 | 158 | 125 | 139 | 113 | 85 | 116 | 92 | 67 |
| 0.35 | 136 | 114 | 90 | 100 | 82 | 62 | 84 | 67 | 49 |
| 0.40 | 102 | 86 | 68 | 75 | 62 | 47 | 63 | 51 | 37 |
| 0.45 | 79 | 66 | 53 | 58 | 48 | 36 | 49 | 39 | 29 |
| 0.50 | 62 | 52 | 42 | 46 | 38 | 29 | 39 | 31 | 23 |
| 0.60 | 40 | 34 | 27 | 30 | 25 | 19 | 26 | 21 | 16 |
| 0.70 | 27 | 23 | 19 | 20 | 17 | 13 | 17 | 14 | 11 |
| 0.80 | 18 | 15 | 13 | 14 | 12 | 9 | 12 | 10 | 8 |

*To estimate the total sample size, read across from $r$ (the expected correlation coefficient) and down from the specified values of $\alpha$ and $\beta$.

### General Formula for Other Values

The general formula for other values of $r$, $\alpha$, and $\beta$ is as follows (see Appendix 6.A for definitions of $z_\alpha$ and $z_\beta$). Let

$$r = \text{expected correlation coefficient}$$
$$C = 0.5 \times \ln\left[(1 + r)/(1 - r)\right]$$
$$N = \text{Total number of subjects required}$$

Then

$$N = [(z_\alpha + z_\beta) \div C]^2 + 3.$$

### Estimating Sample Size for Difference Between Two Correlations

If testing whether a correlation, $r_1$, is different from $r_2$ (i.e., the null hypothesis is that $r_1 = r_2$; the alternative hypothesis is that $r_1 \neq r_2$), let

$$C_1 = 0.5 \times \ln\left[(1 + r_1)/(1 - r_1)\right]$$
$$C_2 = 0.5 \times \ln\left[(1 + r_2)/(1 - r_2)\right]$$

Then

$$N = [(z_\alpha + z_\beta) \div (C_1 - C_2)]^2 + 3.$$

# ■ APPENDIX 6.D

## Sample Size for a Descriptive Study of a Continuous Variable

### ■ TABLE 6.D
Sample Size for Common Values of W/S*

| W/S | Confidence Level | | |
|-----|------|------|------|
|      | **90%** | **95%** | **99%** |
| 0.10 | 1,083 | 1,537 | 2,665 |
| 0.15 | 482 | 683 | 1,180 |
| 0.20 | 271 | 385 | 664 |
| 0.25 | 174 | 246 | 425 |
| 0.30 | 121 | 171 | 295 |
| 0.35 | 89 | 126 | 217 |
| 0.40 | 68 | 97 | 166 |
| 0.50 | 44 | 62 | 107 |
| 0.60 | 31 | 43 | 74 |
| 0.70 | 23 | 32 | 55 |
| 0.80 | 17 | 25 | 42 |
| 0.90 | 14 | 19 | 33 |
| 1.00 | 11 | 16 | 27 |

*$W/S$ is the standardized width of the confidence interval, computed as $W$ (desired total width) divided by $S$ (standard deviation of the variable). To estimate the total sample size, read across from the *standardized width* and down from the specified confidence level.

## General Formula for Other Values

For other values of $W$, $S$, and a confidence level of $(1 - \alpha)$, the total number of subjects required ($N$) is

$$N = 4z_\alpha^2 S^2 \div W^2$$

(see Appendix 6.A for the definition of $z_\alpha$).

## ■ APPENDIX 6.E

### Sample Size for a Descriptive Study of a Dichotomous Variable

■ **TABLE 6.E**
Sample Size for Proportions

**Upper number: 90% confidence level**
**Middle number: 95% confidence level**
**Lower number: 99% confidence level**

| Expected Proportion (P)* | Total Width of Confidence Interval (W) | | | | | | |
|---|---|---|---|---|---|---|---|
| | **0.10** | **0.15** | **0.20** | **0.25** | **0.30** | **0.35** | **0.40** |
| 0.10 | 98 | 44 | — | — | — | — | — |
| | 138 | 61 | — | — | — | — | — |
| | 239 | 106 | — | — | — | — | — |
| 0.15 | 139 | 62 | 35 | 22 | — | — | — |
| | 196 | 87 | 49 | 31 | — | — | — |
| | 339 | 151 | 85 | 54 | — | — | — |
| 0.20 | 174 | 77 | 44 | 28 | 19 | 14 | — |
| | 246 | 109 | 61 | 39 | 27 | 20 | — |
| | 426 | 189 | 107 | 68 | 47 | 35 | — |
| 0.25 | 204 | 91 | 51 | 33 | 23 | 17 | 13 |
| | 288 | 128 | 72 | 46 | 32 | 24 | 18 |
| | 499 | 222 | 125 | 80 | 55 | 41 | 31 |
| 0.30 | 229 | 102 | 57 | 37 | 25 | 19 | 14 |
| | 323 | 143 | 81 | 52 | 36 | 26 | 20 |
| | 559 | 249 | 140 | 89 | 62 | 46 | 35 |
| 0.40 | 261 | 116 | 65 | 42 | 29 | 21 | 16 |
| | 369 | 164 | 92 | 59 | 41 | 30 | 23 |
| | 639 | 284 | 160 | 102 | 71 | 52 | 40 |
| 0.50 | 272 | 121 | 68 | 44 | 30 | 22 | 17 |
| | 384 | 171 | 96 | 61 | 43 | 31 | 24 |
| | 666 | 296 | 166 | 107 | 74 | 54 | 42 |

*To estimate the sample size, read across the *expected proportion* (P) who have the variable of interest and down from the desired *total width* (W) of the confidence interval. The three numbers represent the sample size required for 90%, 95%, and 99% confidence levels.

## General Formula for Other Values

The general formula for other values of P, W, and a confidence level of $(1 - \alpha)$, where P and W are defined above, is as follows. Let

$z_\alpha$ = the standard normal deviate for a two-sided $\alpha$, where $(1 - \alpha)$ is the confidence level (e.g., since $\alpha = 0.05$ for a 95% confidence level, $z_\alpha = 1.96$; thus, for a 90% confidence level $z_\alpha = 1.65$, and for a 99% confidence level $z_\alpha = 2.58$).

Then the total number of subjects required is:

$$N = 4z_\alpha^2 P(1 - P) \div W^2$$

# Section II
# Study Designs

# 7

# Designing an Observational Study: Cohort Studies

## Steven R. Cummings, Thomas B. Newman, and Stephen B. Hulley

**C**ohort studies involve following groups of subjects over time. There are two primary purposes: **descriptive,** typically to describe the incidence of certain outcomes over time; and **analytic,** to analyze associations between predictors and those outcomes. Two basic variations of this design are possible: **prospective** studies, in which the investigator defines the sample and measures predictor variables before any outcomes have occurred; and **retrospective** studies, in which the investigator defines the sample and collects data about predictor variables after the outcomes have occurred.

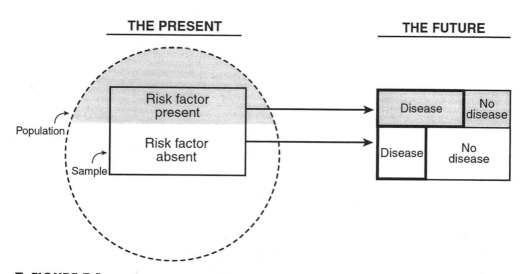

**■ FIGURE 7.1**

In a prospective cohort study, the investigator: (a) Selects a sample from the population (the dotted line signifies its large and undefined size); (b) measures the predictor variables (in this case whether a dichotomous risk factor is present (shaded)); (c) measures the outcome during follow-up (in this case a disease (outlined in bold) that developed in a higher proportion of subjects who had the risk factor).

# ■ PROSPECTIVE COHORT STUDIES

## Structure

**Cohort** was the Roman term for a group of soldiers that marched together. In clinical research, a cohort is a group of subjects followed over time. In a prospective cohort study, the investigator chooses or defines a sample of subjects. She measures characteristics in each subject, such as exercise habits, that might predict the subsequent outcomes. She follows these subjects with periodic measurements of the outcomes of interest (Fig. 7.1).

---

**Example 7.1. Prospective Cohort Study**

The Nurses' Health Study examines incidence and risk factors for common diseases in women (1). The basic steps in performing the study were to

1. *Assemble the cohort.* In 1976 the investigators obtained lists of registered nurses ages 25 to 42 in the 11 most populous states and mailed them an invitation to participate in the study.
2. *Measure predictor variables and potential confounders.* They mailed a questionnaire about diet and other potential risk factors and obtained completed questionnaires from 121,700 nurses. They sent questionnaires every 2 years for the next two decades that asked about additional risk factors and updated the status of some risk factors that had been measured at baseline.
3. *Follow up the cohort and measure outcomes.* The periodic questionnaires also included questions about the occurrence of a variety of disease outcomes, which were then confirmed by review of medical records.

The prospective approach allowed investigators to design the set of measurements made at baseline, and the cohort design allowed them to collect data on subsequent outcomes. The large size of the cohort and extended period of follow-up have provided an unparalleled opportunity to study risk factors for various forms of heart disease, cancer, and other common diseases. For example, the investigators examined the hypothesis that high intake of dietary fiber is associated with a decreased risk of colorectal cancer. Fiber intake was assessed in 1980, and 787 cases of colon cancer were confirmed between 1980 and 1994. The rate of colon cancer among women in the lowest decile of dietary fiber intake was similar to the rate in women in the highest decile of fiber intake (relative risk = 1.0; 95% confidence interval, 0.7 to 1.4). The investigators also adjusted the analysis for potential confounding factors, and this did not change the result. The large number of cases of colon cancer and the quality of the methods support the conclusion that high intake of dietary fiber does not prevent colon cancer.

---

## Strengths

The prospective cohort design is a powerful strategy for defining the incidence and investigating the potential causes of a condition. Because potential causative factors are measured before the outcome occurs, a cohort study can establish that they preceded the outcome. This time sequence strengthens the inference that the factor may be a cause of the outcome.

A prospective study gives the investigator an opportunity to measure important variables completely and accurately. This may be particularly important for studies of certain types of predictors, such as dietary habits, that are difficult for a subject to remember accurately. Measuring current levels of the predictor variable before the outcome occurs will generally produce more accurate data than attempts to reconstruct past exposures after the outcome has already happened. This also prevents measurements from being biased by knowledge or biologic effects of the outcome of interest.

Prospective cohort studies are uniquely valuable for studying the antecedents of fatal diseases. When fatal diseases are studied retrospectively, the set of the cases that comes to the attention of the investigator may not be representative of all such deaths, and it is necessary to reconstruct past predictor variables from medical records or friends and relatives of the deceased.

## Weaknesses

The prospective cohort design is an expensive and inefficient way to study rare outcomes. Even diseases we think of as relatively common, such as colon cancer, in fact, happen so infrequently in any given year that large numbers of people must be followed for long periods of time to observe enough outcomes to produce meaningful results.

Prospective cohort designs become more efficient as the outcomes become more common. Therefore a prospective cohort study of risk factors for progression after treatment of patients with colon cancer will be smaller and less time-consuming than a prospective cohort study of risk factors for the occurrence of colon cancer in a healthy population.

When a cohort is assembled to study mainly one disease, investigators often exclude people who already have any history of the disease. (This is called an "inception cohort.") By excluding subjects who are known to have the outcomes of interest, the investigator assumes that the predictor variables that are measured at the beginning of the study have not been influenced by the outcomes. However, some conditions can be present and producing symptoms before the diagnosis is made. The potential problem that a predictor variable such as eating habits can then be influenced by the outcome can be minimized in two ways: First, sensitive tests can be used to screen and exclude potential subjects who have "subclinical" forms of the disease of interest. Second, the investigator can extend the time frame, asking at baseline about former eating habits or increasing the duration of follow-up, so that the period from measurement of predictor occurrence of outcome is longer than the preclinical phase of the disease.

## ■ RETROSPECTIVE COHORT STUDIES

### Structure

The design of a **retrospective cohort study** is essentially the same as that of a prospective cohort study: A group of subjects is followed over time with measurements of potential predictor variables at the beginning and then ascertainment of subsequent outcomes (Fig. 7.2). The difference is that the assembly of the cohort, baseline measurements, follow-up, and outcomes have all happened in the past. This type of study is only possible if adequate data about the risk factors and outcomes are available on a cohort of subjects that has been assembled for other purposes.

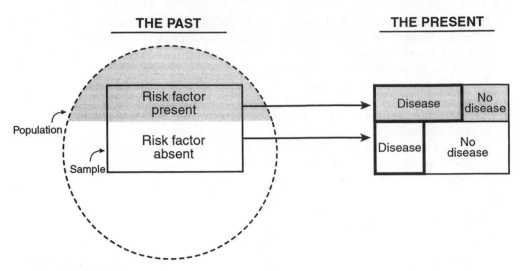

THE PAST

THE PRESENT

**■ FIGURE 7.2**

In a retrospective cohort study, the investigator (a) identifies a cohort that has been assembled in the past, (b) collects data on predictor variables (measured in the past), (c) collects data on outcome variables (measured in the past or present).

---

**Example 7.2. Retrospective Cohort Study**

To describe the natural history of thoracic aortic aneurysms and risk factors for rupture of these aneurysms, Clouse and colleagues analyzed data from the medical records of 133 patients who had aneurysms (2). The basic steps in performing the study were to

1. *Identify a suitable cohort.* The investigators used the residents of Olmstead County, Minnesota. They searched a database of diagnoses made between 1980 and 1995 and found 133 residents who had a diagnosis of aortic aneurysm.
2. *Collect data about predictor variables.* They reviewed patients' records to collect gender, age, size of aneurysm, and risk factors for cardiovascular disease at the time of diagnosis.
3. *Collect data about subsequent outcomes that occurred at a later time.* They collected data from the medical records of the 133 patients to determine whether the aneurysm ruptured or was surgically repaired.

The investigators found that the 5-year risk of rupture was 20% and that women were 6.8 times more likely to suffer a rupture than men (95% confidence interval, 2.3 to 20). They also found that 31% of aneurysms with diameters of more than 6 cm, and none with diameters of less than 4 cm, ruptured.

---

## Strengths

Retrospective cohort studies have the same strengths as prospective cohort studies. They can establish that predictor variables precede outcomes, and because measurements are collected before the outcomes are known, the measurement of predictor variables cannot be biased by knowledge of which subjects have the outcome of interest.

Retrospective cohort studies have the advantage over prospective ones of being much less costly and time-consuming. In retrospective studies, the subjects are already assembled, baseline measurements have already been made, and the follow-up period has already taken place.

## Weaknesses

The main disadvantages of a retrospective cohort study are the limited control the investigator has over the design of the approach to sampling the population, and over the nature and the quality of the predictor variables. The existing data may not include the subjects and information that are important to answering the research question. Even if the existing data include information about key variables, they may be incomplete, inaccurate, or measured in ways that are not ideal for answering the research question.

# ■ NESTED CASE-CONTROL AND CASE-COHORT STUDIES*

## Structure

A **nested case-control** design has a case-control study "nested" within a prospective or retrospective cohort study. It is an excellent design for predictor variables that are expensive to measure and that can be assessed at the end of the study.

The investigator begins with a suitable cohort of subjects with enough cases to provide adequate statistical power to answer the research question. The investigator describes the criteria that define the outcome of interest and then identifies all the individuals in the cohort who have developed the outcome (the cases). Next, she selects a sample of the subjects who were also part of the cohort but who have not developed the outcome of interest (the controls). The investigator then retrieves samples, images, or records that were taken before the outcomes had occurred, measures the predictor variables for cases and controls, and compares levels of the risk factor in cases to the levels in the sample of controls (Fig. 7.3).

Controls selected for nested case-control studies should be a probability sample of all members of the cohort who did not develop the outcome. However, if subjects have been followed for different lengths of time, it may be best, for each case, to select a control that entered the study at approximately the same time or had the same length of follow-up. In certain situations, matching controls to selected characteristics of cases (most commonly age, sex, or race) might also improve the statistical power of this design, but the decision to match should be considered cautiously, and often an unmatched design with statistical adjustment after the study is preferable (Chapter 9).

A **nested case-cohort** design is similar to the case-control strategy except that, instead of selecting controls who have not developed the outcome of interest, the investigator selects a random sample of all the members of the cohort, regardless of outcomes. A few subjects who are part of the random sample will have developed the outcome (the number is very small when the outcome is uncommon): These can be classified as "cases" when the data are analyzed. An advantage of the case-cohort design is that a single random sample of the cohort can provide the controls for several case-control studies of different outcomes. In addition, the random sample of the cohort can provide information on the prevalence of risk factors.

---

*These terms are used inconsistently in the literature; the definitions provided here are the simplest. For a detailed discussion, see Szklo and Nieto (3).

**MEASUREMENTS IN THE PRESENT OF SPECIMENS FROM THE PAST**

**THE PRESENT**

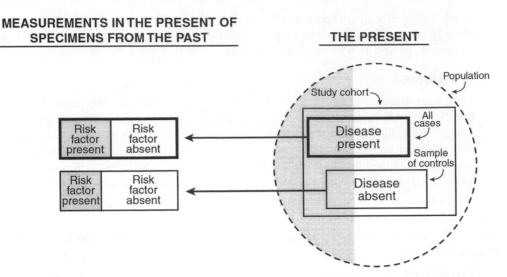

■ **FIGURE 7.3**

In a nested case-control study, the investigator (a) identifies a cohort with banked specimens or information, (b) identifies those participants who developed the outcome during follow-up (the cases), (c) selects a sample from the rest of the cohort (the controls), (d) measures predictor variables in cases and controls.

---

**Example 7.3. Nested Case-Control Design**

To determine whether higher levels of sex hormones increased the risk of breast cancer, Cauley and colleagues conducted a nested case-control study (4). The basic steps in performing this study were to

1. *Identify a cohort with banked samples.* The investigators used serum and data from the Study of Osteoporotic Fractures. Because this case-control study was conceived years after the cohort study began, this would be considered a case-control study nested in a retrospective cohort. (However, serum samples had been drawn by the same investigators during the baseline examination and put into frozen storage at $-190°C$ with the expectation that just such a study would be designed, so in a sense it was a prospective design.)
2. *Identify cases at the end of follow-up.* Based on responses to follow-up questionnaires and review of death certificates, the investigators identified 97 subjects who had developed a first occurrence of breast cancer during 3.2 years of follow-up.
3. *Select controls.* The investigators selected a random sample of 244 women in the cohort who did not develop breast cancer during that follow-up period.
4. *Measure predictors on baseline samples from cases and controls.* Levels of sex hormones, including estradiol and testosterone, were measured in the samples of frozen serum from the baseline examination of cases and controls. The laboratory was blinded to whether the samples came from cases or controls.

Women who had high levels of either estradiol or testosterone had a threefold increase in the risk of a subsequent diagnosis of breast cancer compared with women who had very low levels of these hormones.

## Strengths

Nested case-control and case-cohort studies are especially useful for costly measurements on serum and other specimens that have been archived at the beginning of the study and preserved for later analysis. Making expensive measurements on all the cases and a sample of the controls is much less costly than making the measurements on the entire cohort. When data are available for the entire cohort at no additional cost, as is the case for measurements made before the outcome occurred, nothing is gained by studying only a sample of controls and the whole cohort should be used.

This design preserves all the advantages of cohort studies that result from collecting predictor variables before the outcomes have happened. In addition, it avoids the potential biases of conventional case-control studies that cannot make measurements on fatal cases and that draw cases and controls from different populations.

## Weaknesses

The design shares certain disadvantages of other cohort designs: the possibilities that observed associations are due to the effect of confounding variables and that baseline measurements may be affected by silent preclinical disease.

## Other Considerations

Nested case-control and case-cohort designs have been used less often than they should be. An investigator planning large prospective studies should consider preserving biologic samples (e.g., banks of frozen sera) or storing images or records that are expensive to analyze, for subsequent nested case-control analyses. She should ensure that the conditions of storage will preserve substances of interest for many years, setting aside specimens for periodic measurements to confirm that the concentrations have remained stable. It may also be useful to collect new samples or information during the follow-up period, which can be used in the case-control comparisons.

# ■ MULTIPLE-COHORT STUDIES AND EXTERNAL CONTROLS

## Structure

Several cohorts can be followed and compared. For example, double-cohort studies begin with two separate samples of subjects: typically, one group with exposure to a potential risk factor and a second control group with no exposure or a lower level of exposure (Fig. 7.4). After defining suitable cohorts that have an adequate number of subjects or outcomes and are likely to have different levels of exposure to the predictor of interest, the investigator proceeds to measure predictor variables and to assess outcomes as in any other type of cohort study.

The multiple-cohort design is common in occupational and environmental medicine. For example, two separate groups may have different levels of exposure to a certain factor, and differences in subsequent outcomes are used to assess the effect of the exposure. Although the double-cohort design uses two different samples of subjects, it should not be confused with the case-control design (Chapter 8). The samples in a double-cohort study are chosen based on the level of a

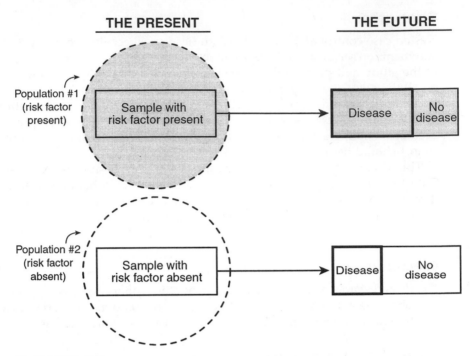

**■ FIGURE 7.4**

In a prospective double-cohort study, the investigator (a) selects samples from populations with different levels of the predictor, (b) measures outcome variables during follow-up. (Double-cohort studies can also be conducted retrospectively.)

---

**Example 7.4. Multiple Cohort Design**

To determine whether physicians who were exposed to radiation had higher mortality rates, Matanoski and colleagues (5) undertook a retrospective triple cohort study. The basic steps in performing the study were to

1. *Identify cohorts with different exposures.* The investigators obtained the membership lists for the Radiological Society of North America, the American College of Physicians, and the American Academy of Ophthalmology and Otolaryngology; the lists included all who had joined since 1920.
2. *Determine outcomes.* The investigators determined the vital status for all members of these societies, including year and cause of death for those who had died.

Radiologists had a higher mortality rate from cancer than the members of the other two societies, supporting the hypothesis that exposure to radiation increased cancer mortality rates.

---

predictor variable. In contrast, in a case-control study the samples are chosen based on the presence or absence of the outcome.

A variant of the multiple-cohort design is to compare the outcomes of members of a study cohort with data from a census or registry, which take the place of a second cohort. For example, to determine whether uranium miners had an increased incidence of lung cancer, Wagoner and colleagues (6) compared the incidence of respiratory cancer in 3,415 uranium miners with that of white men who lived in the same states. The increased incidence of lung cancer observed in the miners helped establish occupational exposure to ionizing radiation as an important cause of lung cancer.

## Strengths

The multiple-cohort design may be the only feasible approach for studying rare exposures, and exposures to potential occupational and environmental hazards. Using data from a census or registry as the external control group has the additional advantage of being population based and economical. Otherwise, the strengths of this design are similar to those of other cohort studies.

## Weaknesses

The problem of confounding is accentuated in a multiple-cohort study. The cohorts often differ in important ways (besides exposure to the predictor variable) that could influence the outcomes. Although some of these differences, such as age and race, can be measured and used to adjust the findings statistically, other important characteristics of the control population may not be available.

Multiple-cohort studies that are done retrospectively share a shortcoming common to other retrospective cohort studies. Important data may be imprecisely recorded, incomplete, or nonexistent.

# ■ PLANNING A COHORT STUDY

The hallmark of a cohort study is the definition of a group of subjects at the beginning of a period of follow-up (Fig. 7.1). The subjects should be appropriate to the research question and available for follow-up. They should sufficiently resemble the population to which the results will be generalized. The number of subjects should provide adequate precision and power.

The quality of the study will depend on the precision and accuracy of the measurements of predictor and outcome variables. The ability to draw inferences about cause and effect will also depend on how completely the investigator has measured potential confounders (Chapter 9). Predictor variables may change during the study; whether and how frequently measurements should be repeated depends on practical considerations like cost, and on the importance to the research question of observing these changes. Outcomes should be assessed using standardized criteria and blindly, without knowing the values of the predictor variables.

The ability to **follow the entire cohort** is an important goal. Loss of subjects can be minimized in several ways (Table 7.1). Subjects who plan to move out of reach during the study or who will be difficult to follow for other reasons should be excluded. At entry to the study, the investigator should collect information that will allow the subjects to be found if they move or die, such as the names, addresses, and telephone numbers of their personal physician and of one or two close friends or relatives who do not live with them. It is important to obtain the subjects' Social Security and (for those over 65) Medicare numbers. This information will allow the investigator to determine the vital status of subjects who are lost to follow-up using the National Death Index and to obtain hospital discharge information from the Social Security Administration for subjects who receive Medicare. Periodic contact with the subjects once or twice a year helps keep track

■ **TABLE 7.1**
Strategies for Minimizing Losses During Follow-up

*During enrollment*

1. Exclude those likely to be lost
   a. Planning to move
   b. Unwilling to return
2. Obtain information to allow future tracking
   a. Address, telephone number(s), and e-mail address of subject
   b. Social Security/Medicare numbers
   c. Name, address, and telephone number, and e-mail address for one or two close friends or relatives who do not live with the subject
   d. Name, e-mail, address, and telephone number of primary physician

*During follow-up*

1. Periodic contact with subjects
   a. By telephone: may require calls during weekends and evenings
   b. By mail: repeated mailings by e-mail or with stamped, self-addressed return cards
   c. Other: newsletters, token gifts with study logo
2. For those who are not reached by phone or mail:
   a. Contact friends, relatives, or physicians
   b. Request forwarding addresses from postal service
   c. Seek address through other sources, such as telephone directories, the Internet, and ultimately a credit bureau search
   d. (for subjects receiving Medicare) Collect data about hospital discharges from Social Security Administration
   e. Determine vital status from state health department or National Death Registry

of them and may improve the timeliness and accuracy of recording the outcomes of interest. Finding subjects for follow-up assessments sometimes requires persistent and repeated efforts by mail, e-mail, telephone, house calls, or professional tracking.

# ■ SUMMARY

1. In **cohort studies,** subjects are followed over time to **describe the incidence** or natural history of a condition and to **analyze predictors** (risk factors) for various outcomes. Measuring the predictor before the outcome occurs establishes the sequence of events and helps control bias in that measurement.
2. **Prospective cohort** studies may require large numbers of subjects followed for long periods of time. This disadvantage can sometimes be overcome by analyzing records or samples that have already been collected, using a **retrospective** cohort design.
3. Another efficient variant is the **nested case-control** design. A bank of specimens, images, or records is collected at baseline and stored until the end of the study; measurements are made on the stored materials for all subjects who have developed a disease or other outcome, and for a subset of those who have not. In the **nested case-cohort strategy,** a single random sample of the cohort can provide controls for several case-control studies.
4. The **multiple-cohort** design, which compares the incidence of outcomes in cohorts that differ in level of a predictor variable, is useful for studying the

effects of rare and occupational exposures. A census or registry can provide an efficient external control group.

5. Inferences about **cause and effect** are strengthened by measuring all important potential confounding variables at baseline. Bias in the assessment of outcomes is prevented by **standardizing** the measurements and **blinding** them to the values of predictor variables.

6. The strengths of a cohort design can be undermined by incomplete **follow-up** of subjects. Losses can be avoided by excluding subjects who are not likely to be available for follow-up and by collecting baseline information that facilitates tracking and vigorous pursuit of all subjects.

# EXERCISES

**1.** The research question is, "Does mild vitamin D deficiency cause hip fractures in the elderly?"

    **a.** Briefly outline a study plan to address this research question with a prospective cohort study.

    **b.** An alternative approach would be to compare evidence of vitamin D deficiency in women who have had previous hip fracture with that in women who have not. Compared with this "case-control" approach, list at least one advantage and one disadvantage of your prospective cohort study. (If you like, you can come back to this question after you have read Chapter 8.)

    **c.** Could the cohort study be designed as a retrospective study, and how would this affect these advantages or disadvantages?

# References

1. Fuchs CS, Giovannucci EL, Colditz GA, et al. Dietary fiber and the risk of colorectal cancer and adenoma in women. *N Engl J Med* 1999;340:169–76.
2. Clouse WD, Hallett JW, Jr, Schaff HV, et al. Improved prognosis of thoracic aortic aneurysms: a population-based study. *JAMA* 1998;280:1926–9.
3. Szklo M, Nieto FJ. *Epidemiology: beyond the basics.* Gaithersburg, MD: Aspen, 2000:33–38.
4. Cauley JA, Lucas FL, Kuller LH, et al. Elevated serum estradiol and testosterone concentrations are associated with a high risk for breast cancer. Study of Osteoporotic Fractures Research Group. *Ann Intern Med* 1999;130:270–7.
5. Matanoski GM, Seltser R, Sartwell PE, Elliot EA. The current mortality rates of radiologists and other physician specialists: deaths from all causes and from cancer. *Am J Epidemiol* 1975;101:188–98.
6. Wagoner JK, Archer VE, Lundin FE, et al. Radiation as the cause of lung cancer among uranium miners. *N Engl J Med* 1965;273:181–7.

# 8 Designing an Observational Study: Cross-sectional and Case-control Studies

Thomas B. Newman,
Warren S. Browner,
Steven R. Cummings, and
Stephen B. Hulley

**C**hapter 7 dealt with cohort studies, in which the sequence of the measurements is the same as the chronology of cause and effect: first the predictor, then (after an interval of follow-up) the outcome. In this chapter we turn to two kinds of observational studies in which causal inference is not guided by this logical time sequence.

In a **cross-sectional** study, the investigator makes all of her measurements on a single occasion. She draws a sample from the population and looks at distributions of variables within that sample; she may then infer cause and effect from associations between variables she decides (using information from various sources) to designate as predictor and outcome. In a **case-control** study, the investigator works backward. She begins by choosing one sample from a population of patients with the outcome (the cases) and another from a population without it (the controls); then she compares the levels of the predictor variables in the two samples to see which ones are associated with the outcome.

## ■ CROSS-SECTIONAL STUDIES

### Structure

The structure of a cross-sectional study is similar to that of a cohort study except that all the measurements are made at once, with no follow-up period (Fig. 8.1). Cross-sectional designs are very well suited to the goal of describing variables and their distribution patterns. In the National Health and Nutrition Examination Survey (NHANES), for example, a sample designed to represent the U.S. population is interviewed and examined. (Search for *NHANES* on the Web.) NHANES surveys have been carried out periodically, and a NHANES follow-up (cohort) study has been added to the original cross-sectional design. But each cross-sectional study is a major source of information about the health and habits of the U.S. population in the year it is carried out, providing estimates of such things as the prevalence of smoking in various demographic groups.

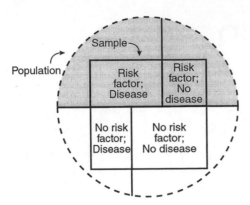

### ■ FIGURE 8.1

In a cross-sectional study, the investigator: (a) selects a sample from the population, and (b) measures predictor and outcome variables (e.g., presence or absence of a risk factor and disease).

Cross-sectional studies can also be used for examining associations, although the choice of which variables to label as predictors and which as outcomes depends on the cause-and-effect hypotheses of the investigator rather than on the study design. This choice is easy for constitutional factors such as age and race; these cannot usually be altered by other variables and therefore are predictors. For most variables, however, the choice is more difficult. For example, a cross-sectional finding in NHANES III is an association between childhood obesity and hours spent watching television (1,2). Is this because television viewing makes children obese or because obese children like to watch TV?

---

**Example 8.1. Cross-Sectional Study**

The research questions are, "What is the prevalence of chlamydia infection in women attending sexually transmitted disease (STD) clinics?" and, "Is it associated with the use of oral contraceptives?" To answer these questions in a cross-sectional study the investigator might

1. Select a sample of 100 women attending an STD clinic.
2. Measure the predictor and outcome variables by taking a history of oral contraceptive use and sending a cervical swab to the lab for chlamydia culture.

Note that there are several time elements in this study: The predictor variable addresses the use of oral contraceptives over the past year; the outcome variable is not available until several days later; and the investigator takes 6 months to examine all the women. The study is still cross-sectional, however, because the investigator makes all the measurements for each subject on a single occasion.

Suppose the findings are that 20 of the women report taking oral contraceptives and that four (20%) of these women have positive cultures, compared with eight of the 80 women (10%) not taking oral contraceptives. Then the overall prevalence of chlamydia infection in this sample of STD clinic attendees (who may not represent the general population) is 12 in 100 (12%) and there is an association between oral contraceptive use and chlamydia that has a relative prevalence of 20%/10% = 2.0. (See Appendix 8.A for the calculation.)

---

---

Statistics for Expressing Disease Frequency in Observational Studies

| Type of Study | Statistic | Definition |
|---|---|---|
| Cross-sectional | Prevalence | Number of people who *have* the disease at one point in time / Number of people at risk at that point |
| Cohort | Incidence | Number who *get* disease over a period of time / Number of people at risk during that period |

---

Example 8.1 reveals an important descriptive statistic obtained from cross-sectional studies: prevalence. **Prevalence** is the proportion of the population who *have* a disease or condition at *one point in time* and is distinguished from **incidence** (the statistic obtained from a cohort study), which is the proportion who *get it over a period of time* (Table 8.1). Prevalence and incidence can also apply to variables other than diseases, so that prevalence of smoking, recent condom use, or any other attribute can be estimated. Prevalence is useful to the health planner who wants to know how many people have certain diseases so that she can allocate enough resources to care for them, and it is useful to the clinician who must estimate the likelihood that the patient sitting in her office has a particular disease.

Example 8.1 also gives an example of an analytic statistic obtained from cross-sectional studies, the **relative prevalence.** This is the ratio of the prevalence of an outcome in subjects classified by their level of a predictor variable, the cross-sectional analog of relative risk.

## Strengths and Weaknesses of Cross-Sectional Studies

A major strength of cross-sectional studies over cohort studies (and experiments) is that there is no waiting for the outcome to occur. This makes them fast and inexpensive, and it means that there is no loss to follow-up. A cross-sectional study can be included as the first step in a cohort study or experiment at little or no added cost. The results define the demographic and clinical characteristics of the study group at baseline and can sometimes reveal cross-sectional associations of interest. The cross-sectional design is the only one that gives the prevalence of a disease or risk factor.

Cross-sectional studies are convenient for examining **networks of causal links.** For example, the investigator in Example 8.1 could examine age as a predictor of the oral contraceptive use and then examine oral contraceptive use as a predictor of chlamydia infection.

A weakness of cross-sectional studies is the difficulty of establishing causal relationships from data collected in a cross-sectional time frame. Cross-sectional studies are also impractical for the study of rare diseases if the design involves collecting data on a sample of individuals from the general population. A cross-sectional study of stomach cancer in a general population of 45- to 59-year-old men, for example, would need about 10,000 subjects to find just one case.

Cross-sectional studies can be done on rare diseases if the sample is drawn from a population of diseased patients rather than from the general population. A case series of this sort is better suited to describing the characteristics of the disease than to analyzing differences between these patients and healthy people, although informal comparisons with prior experience can sometimes identify very strong risk factors. Of the first 1,000 patients with AIDS, for example, 727 were homosexual or bisexual males and 236 were injecting drug users (3). It did not require a formal control group to conclude that these groups were at increased risk. Furthermore, within a sample of patients with a disease there may be associations of interest (e.g., the higher risk of Kaposi's sarcoma among AIDS patients who were homosexual than among those who were injecting drug users).

The fact that cross-sectional studies can only measure prevalence and not incidence limits the information they can produce on prognosis, natural history, and disease causation. To show causation, investigators need to demonstrate that the incidence of disease differs in those exposed to a risk factor. But cross-sectional studies can only show effects on prevalence, which is the product of disease incidence and disease duration. A factor that is associated with prevalence of disease may be a cause of the disease but could also be associated with duration of the disease, by affecting the course of the disease. For example, the prevalence of severe depression is affected not just by its incidence, but by the suicide rate and the responsiveness to medication of those affected.

## Serial Surveys

A series of cross-sectional studies of a single population observed at several points in time is sometimes used to draw inferences about changing patterns over time. A good example is the use of census data to characterize changes in the age structure of the U.S. population from one decade to the next. This is not a cohort design because it does not follow a single group of people over time; there are changes in the population through birth, death, and migration into and out of the United States.

The serial survey design is also useful when the investigator wants to characterize changes in a population over time but is concerned that in a cohort design the initial examination will produce a learning effect, influencing the responses to follow-up examinations. An example is the Stanford Five-City Project, which sampled the populations of five California cities over a number of years to observe trends in the prevalence of coronary heart disease (CHD) risk factors. Two kinds of samples were drawn in each city, one a true cohort of individuals in whom the factors predicting within-individual changes could be observed, and the other a series of independent samples of new individuals who had not been contaminated by the prior examination (4).

## ■ CASE-CONTROL STUDIES

### Structure

To investigate the causes of all but the most common diseases, both cohort and cross-sectional studies of general population samples are expensive: Each would require thousands of subjects to identify risk factors for a rare disease like stomach cancer. A case series of patients with the disease can identify an obvious risk factor (such as, for AIDS, injection of illegal drugs), using prior knowledge of the prevalence of the risk factor in the general population. For most risk factors, however, it is necessary to assemble a reference group, so that the prevalence of the risk factor in subjects with the disease (cases) can be compared with the prevalence in subjects without the disease (controls).

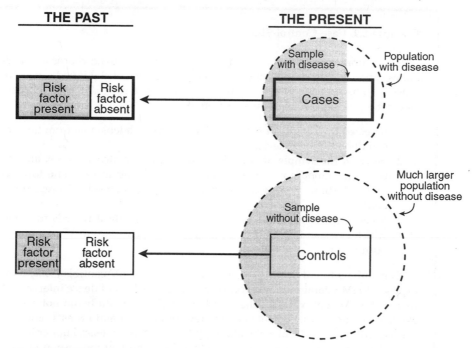

■ **FIGURE 8.2**

In a case-control study, the investigator: (a) selects a sample from a population of people with the disease (cases), (b) selects a sample from a population at risk that is free of the disease (controls), (c) measures predictor variables.

The structure of a case-control study is shown in Fig. 8.2. Whereas cohort studies begin with people at risk and follow them forward in time to see who gets the disease and cross-sectional studies look at a single point in time, case-control studies are generally retrospective. They identify one group of subjects with the disease and another without it, then look backward in time to find differences in predictor variables that may explain why the cases got the disease and the controls did not.

Case-control studies began as epidemiologic studies to try to identify risk factors for diseases. Thus the outcome traditionally used to determine case-control status has been the presence or absence of the disease. For this reason and because it makes the discussion easier to follow, we often refer to "cases" as those with the disease. However, the case-control design can also be used to look at other outcomes, such as disability among those who already have a disease. In addition, when undesired outcomes are the rule rather than the exception, the cases in a case-control study may be the rare patients with a good outcome, such as smoking cessation or recovery from a usually fatal disease.

Case-control studies are the "house red" on the research design wine list: more modest and a little riskier than the other selections but much less expensive and sometimes surprisingly good. The design of a case-control study is challenging because of the increased opportunities for bias, but there are many examples of well-designed case-control studies that have yielded important results. These include the links between maternal diethylstilbestrol use and vaginal cancer in daughters (a classic study that provided a definitive conclusion based on just seven cases!) (5), and use of short-acting calcium channel blockers and increased risk of myocardial infarction (6).

---

**Example 8.2. Case-Control Study**

Since intramuscular (IM) vitamin K is given routinely to newborns in the United States, a pair of studies reporting a doubling in the risk of childhood cancer among those who had received IM vitamin K caused quite a stir (7,8). To investigate this association further, German investigators (9)

1. **Selected the sample of cases**—107 children with leukemia from the German Childhood Cancer Registry.
2. **Selected the sample of controls**—107 children matched by sex and date of birth and randomly selected from children living in the same town as the case at the time of diagnosis (from local government residential registration records).
3. **Measured the predictor variable**—reviewed medical records to determine which cases and controls had received intramuscular vitamin K in the newborn period.

The authors found 69 of 107 cases (64%) and 63 of 107 controls (59%) had been exposed to IM vitamin K, for an odds ratio of 1.2 (95% confidence interval [CI], 0.7 to 2.3). (See Appendix 8.A for the calculation.) Thus this study did not confirm the existence of an association between the receipt of IM vitamin K as a newborn and subsequent childhood leukemia, although the point estimate and upper limit of the 95% CI leave open the possibility of a clinically important increase in leukemia.*

---

Case-control studies cannot yield estimates of the incidence or prevalence of a disease because the proportion of study subjects who have the disease is determined by how many cases and how many controls the investigator chooses to sample, rather than by their proportions in the population. What case-control studies do provide is some descriptive information on the characteristics of the cases and, more important, an estimate of the strength of the association between each predictor variable and the presence or absence of the disease. These estimates are in the form of the odds ratio, which approximates the relative risk if the prevalence of the disease is not too high (Appendix 8.B).

## Strengths of Case-Control Studies

***Efficiency for Rare Outcomes.***   One of the major strengths of case-control studies is their high yield of information from relatively few subjects. Consider a study of the effect of circumcision on subsequent carcinoma of the penis. This cancer is very rare in circumcised men but is also rare in uncircumcised men: their lifetime cumulative incidence is about 0.16% (12). To do a cohort study with a reasonable chance (80%) of detecting even a very strong risk factor (say a relative risk of 50) would require more than 6,000 men, assuming that roughly equal proportions were circumcised and uncircumcised. A randomized clinical trial of circumcision at birth would require the same sample size, but the cases would occur at a median of 67 years after entry into the study. It would take three generations of epidemiologists to follow the subjects!

---

*Although most studies have found no evidence for an association between vitamin K and childhood cancer (10,11), a problem for policymakers is that leukemia is much more common than serious bleeding from vitamin K deficiency, so that even an odds ratio of 1.1 would mean more leukemias caused than episodes of serious bleeding prevented.

Now consider a case-control study of the same question. For the same chance of detecting the same relative risk, only 16 cases and 16 controls (and not much investigator time) would be required. For diseases that are either rare or have long latent periods between exposure and disease, case-control studies are far more efficient than the other designs. In fact, they are often the only feasible option.

***Usefulness for Generating Hypotheses.*** The retrospective approach of case-control studies, and their ability to examine a large number of predictor variables makes them useful for generating hypotheses about the causes of a new outbreak of disease. For example, a case-control study of an epidemic of acute renal failure in Haitian children (13) found an odds ratio of 52.7 for ingestion of locally manufactured acetaminophen syrup. Further investigation revealed that the renal failure was due to poisoning by diethylene glycol, which was found to contaminate the glycerine solution used to make the acetaminophen syrup.

## Weaknesses of Case-Control Studies

Case-control studies have great strengths, but they also have major limitations. The information available in case-control studies is limited: There is no direct way to estimate the incidence or prevalence of the disease, nor the attributable or excess risk. There is also the problem that only one outcome can be studied (the presence or absence of the disease that was the criterion for drawing the two samples), whereas cohort and cross-sectional studies (and experiments) can study any number of outcome variables. But the biggest weakness of case-control studies is their increased susceptibility **to bias.** This bias comes chiefly from two sources: the separate sampling of the cases and controls, and the retrospective measurement of the predictor variables. These two problems and the strategies for dealing with them are the topic of the next two sections.

***Sampling Bias and How to Control It.*** The sampling in a case-control study begins with the cases. Ideally, the sample of cases would be a random sample of everyone who develops the disease under study. An immediate problem comes up, however. How do we know who has developed the disease and who has not? In cross-sectional and cohort studies the disease is systematically sought in all the study participants, but in case-control studies the cases must be sampled from patients in whom the disease has already been diagnosed and who are available for study. This sample is not representative of all patients who develop the disease because those who are undiagnosed, misdiagnosed, or dead are less likely to be included (Fig. 8.3).

In general, sampling bias is important when the sample of cases is unrepresentative with respect to the risk factor being studied. Diseases that almost always require hospitalization and are relatively easy to diagnose, such as anencephaly and traumatic amputations, can be safely sampled from diagnosed and accessible cases. On the other hand, conditions that may not come to medical attention are not well suited to retrospective studies because of the selection that precedes diagnosis. For example, women seen in a gynecologic clinic with first-trimester spontaneous abortions would probably differ from the entire population of women experiencing spontaneous abortions because those with greater access to gynecologic care or with complications would be overrepresented. If a predictor variable of interest is associated with gynecologic care in the population (such as past use of an intrauterine device), sampling from the clinic could be an important source

New cases of the disease

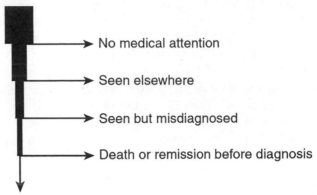

No medical attention

Seen elsewhere

Seen but misdiagnosed

Death or remission before diagnosis

Cases available for case-control study

■ **FIGURE 8.3**

Reasons that the cases in a case-control study may not be representative of all cases of the disease.

of bias. If, on the other hand, a predictor is unrelated to gynecologic care (such as blood type) there would be less likelihood of sampling bias.

Although it is important to think about these issues, in actual practice the selection of cases is often straightforward because the accessible sources of subjects are limited. The sample of cases may not be entirely representative, but it may be all that the investigator has to work with. The more difficult decisions faced by an investigator designing a case-control study often relate to the more open-ended task of selecting the controls. The general goal is to sample controls from a population at risk for the disease that is otherwise similar to the cases. Four strategies for sampling controls follow:

1. *Hospital- or clinic-based controls.* One strategy to compensate for the possible selection bias caused by obtaining cases from a hospital or clinic is to select controls from the same facilities. For example, in a study of past use of an intrauterine device (IUD) as a risk factor for spontaneous abortion, controls could be sampled from a population of women seeking care for vaginitis at the same gynecologic clinic. Compared with a random sample of women from the same area, these controls would presumably better represent the population of women who, had they developed a spontaneous abortion, would have come to the clinic and become a case.

However, selection of an unrepresentative sample of controls to compensate for an unrepresentative sample of cases can be problematic. If the risk factor of interest also causes diseases for which the controls seek care, the prevalence of the risk factor in the control group will be falsely high, biasing the study results. If, for example, many women in the control group had vaginitis and use of an IUD increased the risk of vaginitis, there would be an excess of IUD users among the controls, masking a possible real association between IUD use and spontaneous abortion.

Because hospital-based and clinic-based control subjects are usually unwell and because their diseases may be positively or negatively associated with the risk factors being studied, the use of hospital- or clinic-based controls is not always successful in compensating for an unrepresentative sample of cases. Such control groups are often used, however, because of another consideration in selecting controls: **convenience.** Clinical investigators work in clinics and hospitals, and the populations of control subjects most readily accessible to them are those that are in the hospital or clinic for other reasons. What the investigator must decide is whether the added convenience of hospital- or clinic-based controls is worth the possible threat to the validity of the study.

2. *Matching.* Matching is a simple method of ensuring that cases and controls are comparable with respect to major factors that are related to the disease but not of interest to the investigator. So many risk factors and diseases are related to age and sex, for example, that the study results may be meaningless unless the cases and controls are comparable with regard to these two variables. One approach to avoiding this problem is to choose controls that match the cases on these constitutional predictor variables. Matching does have its adverse consequences, however, particularly when modifiable predictors such as income or serum cholesterol level are matched. The reasons for this and the alternatives to matching are discussed in Chapter 9.

3. *Using a population-based sample.* Population-based case-control studies are now possible for many diseases, because of a rapid increase in the use of disease registries. In the San Francisco Bay Area, for example, there are registries of all new cases of cancer, birth defects, AIDS, and sudden infant death. Because cases obtained from such registries are generally representative of the general population of patients in the area with the disease, the choice of a control group is simplified: It should be a representative sample from the population living in the area covered by the registry. In Example 8.2, all residents of the town were registered with the local government, making such a sample straightforward. An alternative technique for generating a random sample is **random-digit dialing.**

Random-digit dialing can include a matching strategy by repeatedly dialing the same prefix as the case (thereby matching roughly on city district) until an age- and sex-matched individual is reached. There are some problems with random-digit dialing, however. First, because it requires that all controls live in a household with a telephone, cases with no telephones need to be excluded, potentially reducing the sample size and generalizability of the study. Second, a large and nonrandom portion of the controls might not consent to be in a study after being randomly dialed. Finally, as the number of telephone numbers per household proliferates, there is the problem that households with multiple telephone lines (which are not representative of all households) will be overrepresented.

When registries are available, population-based case-control studies are clearly the most desirable. As the disease registry approaches completeness and the population it covers approaches stability (i.e., no migration in or out), the population-based case-control study approaches a case-control study that is nested within a cohort study or clinical trial (Chapter 7). This design has the potential for eliminating sampling bias, because both cases and controls are selected from the same population. When designing the sampling approach for a case-control study, the **nested case-control** design is useful to keep in mind as the model to emulate.

4. *Using two or more control groups.* Because selection of a control group can be so tricky, particularly when the cases are not a representative sample of those with disease, it is sometimes advisable to use two or more control groups selected in different ways. The Public Health Service study of Reye's syndrome and medications (14), for example, used four types of controls: emergency room controls (seen in the same emergency room as the case), inpatient controls (admitted to

the same hospital as the case), school controls (attending the same school or day care center as the case), and community controls (identified by random-digit dialing). The odds ratios for salicylate use in cases compared with each of these control groups (in the order listed earlier) were 39, 66, 33 and 44, and each was statistically significant. The consistent finding of a strong association using control groups that would have a variety of sampling biases makes a convincing case for the inference that there is a real association in the population.

What happens if the control groups give conflicting results? Luckily, this happens less often than one might expect, and when it does it may be helpful, revealing inherent fragility to the case-control method for the research question at hand. If possible, the investigator should seek additional information to try to determine the magnitude of potential biases from each of the control groups. In any case, it is better to have inconsistent results and conclude that the answer is not known than to have just one control group and draw the wrong conclusion.

***Differential Measurement Bias and How to Control It.*** The second particular problem of case-control studies is bias that affects one group more than the other caused by the retrospective approach to measuring the predictor variables. Case-control studies of birth defects, for example, are hampered by differential recall bias: Parents of babies with birth defects may be more likely to recall drug exposures than parents of normal babies, because they will already have been worrying about what caused the defect. Differential recall bias cannot occur in a cohort study because the parents are asked about exposures before the baby is born.

In addition to the strategies set out in Chapter 4 for controlling biased measurements (standardizing the operational definitions of variables, choosing objective approaches, supplementing key variables with data from several sources, etc.), there are two specific strategies for avoiding bias in measuring risk factors in case-control studies:

1. **Use data recorded before the outcome occurred.** It may be possible, for example, to examine the prenatal records in a case-control study of birth defects. This excellent strategy is limited to the extent that recorded information about the risk factor of interest is available and of satisfactory reliability. Bias can still occur, however, if the investigator searches the medical records for evidence of past habits more vigorously in the cases than in the controls.
2. **Use blinding.** The general approach to blinding was discussed in Chapter 4, but there are some issues that are specific to designing interviews in case-control studies. Because both observers and study subjects could be blinded both to the case-control status of each subject and to the risk factor being studied, four types of blinding are possible (Table 8.2)

Ideally, neither the study subjects nor the investigators should know which subjects are cases and which are controls. If this can be done successfully, differential bias in measuring the predictor variable is eliminated. In practice, this is often difficult. The subjects know whether they are sick or well, so they can be blinded to case-control status only if controls are drawn from patients who are also ill with diseases that they believe might be related to the risk factors being studied. (Of course, if the disease of any of the controls is related to the risk factor being studied, it will cause sampling bias.) Efforts to blind interviewers are hampered

■ **TABLE 8.2**
Approaches to Blinding Interview Questions in a Case-Control Study

| Person Blinded | Blinding Case-control Status | Blinding Risk Factor Measurement |
|---|---|---|
| Subject | Possible if both cases and controls have diseases that could plausibly be related to the risk factor. | Include ''dummy'' risk factors and be suspicious if they differ between cases and controls. May not work if the risk factor for the disease has already been publicized. |
| Observer | Possible if cases are not externally distinguishable from controls, but subtle signs and statements volunteered by the subjects make it difficult. | Possible if interviewer is not the investigator, but may be difficult to maintain. |

by the obvious nature of some diseases (an interviewer can hardly help noticing if the patient is jaundiced or has had a laryngectomy), and by the clues that interviewers may discern in the patient's responses.

Blinding to the specific risk factor being studied is usually easier than blinding as to case-control status. Both the study subjects and the interviewer can be kept in the dark about the study hypotheses by including "dummy" questions about plausible risk factors not associated with the disease. For example, if the specific hypothesis to be tested is whether honey intake is associated with increased risk of infant botulism, equally detailed questions about jelly, yogurt, and bananas could be included in the interview. This type of blinding does not actually prevent differential bias, but it allows an estimate of whether it is a problem: If the cases report more exposure to honey but no increase in the other foods, then differential measurement bias is less likely. This strategy would not work if the association between infant botulism and honey had previously been widely publicized or if some of the dummy risk factors turned out to be real risk factors.

Blinding the observer to the case-control status of the study subject is a particularly good strategy for laboratory measurements such as blood tests and x-rays. Blinding under these circumstances is easy and should always be done: Someone other than the individual who will make the measurement simply applies coded identification labels to each specimen. Its importance is illustrated by 15 case-control studies comparing measurements of bone mass between hip fracture patients and controls; much larger differences were formed in the studies that used unblinded measurements than in the blinded studies (15).

## ■ CHOOSING AMONG OBSERVATIONAL DESIGNS

The pros and cons of the main observational designs presented in the last two chapters are summarized in Table 8.3. We have already described these issues in detail and will make only one final point here. Among all these designs, none is best and none is worst; each has its place and purpose, depending on the research question and the circumstances.

■ **TABLE 8.3**
Advantages and Disadvantages of the Major Observational Designs

| Design | Advantages | Disadvantages* |
|---|---|---|
| **Cohort** | | |
| All | Establishes sequence of events<br>Can study several outcomes<br>Number of outcome events grows over time<br>Yields incidence, relative risk, excess risk | Often requires large sample sizes<br>Less feasible for rare outcomes |
| Prospective | More control over selection of subjects<br>More control over measurements<br>Avoids bias in measuring predictors | More expensive<br>Longer duration |
| Retrospective | Less expensive<br>Shorter duration | Less control over selection of subjects<br>Less control over measurements |
| Multiple cohort | Useful when distinct cohorts have different or rare exposures | Potential for bias and confounding from sampling several populations |
| **Cross-Sectional** | May study several outcomes<br>Relatively short duration<br>A good first step for a cohort study<br>Yields prevalence, relative prevalence | Does not establish sequence of events<br>Not feasible for rare predictors or rare outcomes<br>Does not yield incidence or true relative risk |
| **Case-Control** | Useful for studying rare conditions<br>Short duration<br>Relatively inexpensive<br>Relatively small<br>Yields odds ratio (usually a good approximation of relative risk unless the outcome is common) | Potential for bias and confounding from sampling two populations<br>Does not establish sequence of events<br>Potential survivor bias<br>Limited to one outcome variable<br>Does not yield prevalence, incidence, or excess risk |
| **Combination Designs** | | |
| Nested case-control | Advantages of a retrospective cohort design, only much more efficient | Sometimes requires banked samples stored until outcomes occur |
| Nested case-cohort | Can use a single control group for multiple studies | |

*All these observational designs have the disadvantage (compared with experiments) of being susceptible to the influence of confounding variables.

## ■ SUMMARY

1. In a **cross-sectional** study, the variables are all measured at a single point in time, with no structural distinction between predictors and outcomes. Cross-sectional studies are valuable for providing **descriptive** information about **prevalence**; they also have the advantage of avoiding the time, expense, and dropout problems of a follow-up design.

2. Cross-sectional studies yield **weaker evidence for causality** than cohort studies, however, because the predictor variable is not shown to precede the outcome. A further weakness is the need for a large sample size (compared with that of a case-control study) when studying the prevalence of uncommon diseases and variables in the general population. The cross-sectional design can be used for an uncommon disease in a **case series** of patients with that disease, and it often serves as the first step of a cohort study or experiment.

3. In a **case-control study,** the prevalence of risk factors in a sample of subjects who have a disease or other outcome of interest (the cases) is compared with that in a sample who do not (the controls). This design, in which people with and without the disease are sampled separately, is relatively **inexpensive** and uniquely **efficient** for studying **rare diseases.**

4. One problem with case-control studies is their susceptibility to **sampling bias.** The likelihood of sampling bias depends on both the disease and risk factor in question. Four approaches to reducing sampling bias are (a) to sample controls and cases in the same (admittedly unrepresentative) way; (b) to **match** the cases and controls; (c) to do a population-based study; and (d) to use **several** control groups, sampled in different ways.

5. The other major problem with case-control studies is their retrospective design, which makes them susceptible to **differential measurement bias** (between cases and controls). Such bias can be reduced by obtaining **past measurements** of the predictor variable and by **blinding** the subjects and observers.

## EXERCISES

1. The research question is, ``How much does a family history of ovarian cancer increase the risk for ovarian cancer?'' You plan a case-control study to answer this question.
   **a.** How would you pick the cases?
   **b.** How would you pick the controls?
   **c.** Comment on potential sources of bias in the sampling of cases and controls.
   **d.** How would you measure ``family history of ovarian cancer'' as the predictor variable of interest? Comment on the sources of bias in this measurement.
   **e.** What measure of association would you use, and what test of statistical significance?
   **f.** Do you think the case-control method is an appropriate approach to this research question? Discuss the advantages and disadvantages of the case-control design relative to other possibilities for this research question.

2. The research question is, ``Does maternal height or weight predict infant

birth weight?'' During a 12-month period an investigator assembles data on consecutive newborns in a large maternity hospital. The study is limited to term newborns as defined by delivery 38 to 42 weeks after the mother's last menstrual period. In the maternity ward, the investigator measures each infant's birth weight and the mother's height and weight. Based on the data obtained, the investigator concludes that birth weight is strongly dependent on both maternal height and weight.

**a.** What kind of study is this?

**b.** Explain why you agree or disagree with the investigator's conclusions?

# References

1. Andersen RE, Crespo CJ, Bartlett SJ, Cheskin LJ, Pratt M. Relationship of physical activity and television watching with body weight and level of fatness among children: results from the Third National Health and Nutrition Examination Survey. *JAMA* 1998;279:938–42.
2. Robinson TN. Does television cause childhood obesity? *JAMA* 1998;279:959–60.
3. Jaffe HW, Bregman DJ, Selik RM. Acquired immune deficiency in the U.S.: the first 1000 cases. *J Infect Dis* 1983;148:339–45.
4. Farquhar JW, Fortmann SP, Maccoby N, et al. The Stanford Five-City Project: design and methods. *Am J Epidemiol* 1985;122:323–34.
5. Herbst AL, Ulfelder H, Poskanzer DC. Adenocarcinoma of the vagina: association of maternal stilbestrol therapy with tumor appearance in young women. *N Engl J Med* 1971;284:878–81.
6. Psaty BM, Heckbert SR, Koepsell TD, et al. The risk of myocardial infarction associated with antihypertensive drug therapies. *JAMA* 1995;274:620–5.
7. Golding J, Paterson M, Kinlen LJ. Factors associated with childhood cancer in a national cohort study. *Br J Cancer* 1990;62:304–8.
8. Golding J, Greenwood R, Birmingham K, Mott M. Childhood cancer, intramuscular vitamin K, and pethidine given during labour. *BMJ* 1992;305:341–6.
9. Von Kries R, Gobel U, Hachmeister A, Kaletsch U, Michaelis J. Vitamin K and childhood cancer: a population based case-control study in Lower Saxony, Germany. *BMJ* 1996;313:199–203.
10. Klebanoff MA, Read JS, Mills JL, Shiono PH. The risk of childhood cancer after neonatal exposure to vitamin K. *N Engl J Med* 1993;329:905–8.
11. McKinney PA, Juszczak E, Findlay E, Smith K. Case-control study of childhood leukaemia and cancer in Scotland: findings for neonatal intramuscular vitamin K. *BMJ* 1998;316:173–7.
12. Kochen M, McCurdy S. Circumcision and the risk of cancer of the penis: a life-table analysis. *Am J Dis Child* 1980;134:484–6.
13. O'Brien KL, Selanikio JD, Hecdivert C, et al. Epidemic of pediatric deaths from acute renal failure caused by diethylene glycol poisoning. Acute Renal Failure Investigation Team. *JAMA* 1998;279:1175–80.
14. Hurwitz ES, Barrett MJ, Bregman D, et al. Public Health Service study of Reye's syndrome and medications. Report of the main study. *JAMA* 1987;257:1905–11.
15. Cummings SR. Are patients with hip fractures more osteoporotic? Review of the evidence. *Am J Med* 1985;78:487–94.

## ■ APPENDIX 8.A

### Calculating Measures of Association

***Cross-Sectional Studies.*** The research questions for Example 8.1 were, "What is the prevalence of chlamydia infection in women attending STD clinics." and "Is it associated with the use of oral contraceptives?" The hypothetical findings are that 20 of the women report taking oral contraceptives and that four of these women have positive cultures, compared with eight of the 80 women not taking oral contraceptives. A two-by-two table of these findings is as follows:

| | Outcome Variable: Cervical Culture Results | | |
|---|---|---|---|
| **Predictor Variable: Contraceptive History** | **Chlamydia Present** | **Chlamydia Absent** | **Total** |
| Users of oral contraceptives (OCs) | 4(*a*) | 16(*b*) | 20(*a* + *b*) |
| Nonusers of OCs | 8(*c*) | 72(*d*) | 80(*c* + *d*) |
| Total | 12(*a* + *c*) | 88(*b* + *d*) | 100 (*a* + *b* + *c* + *d*) |

Prevalence of chlamydia infection in users = $a/(a + b)$ = 4/20 = 20%.
Prevalence of chlamydia infection in nonusers = $c/(c + d)$ = 8/80 = 10%.
Prevalence of chlamydia infection overall = $(a + c)/(a + b + c + d)$ = 12/100 = 12%.

$$\textbf{Relative prevalence*} = \frac{\text{Prevalence of chlamydia in OC users}}{\text{Prevalence of chlamydia in nonusers}} = \frac{a/(a + b)}{c/(c + d)}$$
$$= \frac{4/20}{8/80} = 2.0$$
$$\textbf{Excess prevalence*} = \frac{a}{a + b} - \frac{c}{c + d} = \frac{4}{20} - \frac{8}{80} = 10\%$$

Thus the prevalence of chlamydia infection in this population of STD clinic patients is 20% among oral contraceptive users, 10% among nonusers, and 12% overall. There is an association between oral contraceptive use and chlamydia infection that is characterized by a relative prevalence of 2.0 and by an excess prevalence of 10%.

***Case-Control Studies.*** The research question for Example 8.2 was whether there is an association between intramuscular vitamin K and risk of childhood leukemia. The findings were that 69/107 leukemia cases and 63/107 controls had received intramuscular vitamin K. A two-by-two table of these findings is as follows:

| | Outcome Variable: Diagnosis | |
|---|---|---|
| **Predictor Variable: Medication History** | **Childhood Leukemia** | **Control** |
| IM vitamin K | 69(*a*) | 63(*b*) |
| No IM vitamin K | 48(*c*) | 54(*d*) |
| Total | 107 | 107 |

$$\text{Relative risk} \approx odds\ ratio = \frac{ad}{bc} = \frac{69 \times 54}{63 \times 48} = 1.2$$

Because the disease (leukemia in this instance) is rare, the odds ratio provides a good estimate of the relative risk.

---

*Relative prevalence and excess prevalence are the cross-sectional analogs of relative risk and excess risk.

# ■ APPENDIX 8.B

## Why the Odds Ratio Can Be Used as an Estimate for Relative Risk in a Case-Control Study

The data in a case-control study represent two samples: The cases are drawn from a population of people who have the disease and the controls from a population of people who do not have the disease. The predictor variable is measured, and the following two-by-two table produced:

|                     | Disease | No Disease |
|---------------------|---------|------------|
| Risk factor present | $a$     | $b$        |
| Risk factor absent  | $c$     | $d$        |

If this two-by-two table represented data from a cohort study, then the incidence of the disease in those with the risk factor would be $a/(a + b)$ and the relative risk would be simply $[a/(a + b)]/[c/(c + d)]$. However, it is not appropriate to compute either incidence or relative risk in this way because the two samples are not drawn from the population in the same proportions. Usually, there are roughly equal numbers of cases and controls in the study samples but many fewer cases than controls in the population. Instead, relative risk in a case-control study can be approximated by the odds ratio, computed as the cross-product of the two-by-two table, $ad/cb$.

The basis for this extremely useful fact cannot be understood intuitively, but is relatively easy to demonstrate algebraically. Consider the situation for the full population, represented by $a'$, $b'$, $c'$, and $d'$.

|                     | Disease | No Disease |
|---------------------|---------|------------|
| Risk factor present | $a'$    | $b'$       |
| Risk factor absent  | $c'$    | $d'$       |

Here it is appropriate to calculate the risk of disease among people with the risk factor as $a'/(a' + b')$, the risk among those without the risk factor as $c'/(c' + d')$, and the relative risk as $[a'/(a' + b')]/[c'/(c' + d')]$. We have already discussed the fact that $a'/(a' + b')$ is not equal to $a/(a + b)$. However, if the disease is relatively uncommon (as most are), then $a'$ is much smaller than $b'$, and $c'$ is much smaller than $d'$. This means that $a'/(a' + b')$ is closely approximated by $a'/b'$ and that $c'/(c' + d')$ is closely approximated by $c'/d'$. Thus the relative risk of the population can be approximated as follows:

$$\frac{a'/(a' + b')}{c'/(c' + d')} \approx \frac{a'/b'}{c'/d'}$$

The latter term is the odds ratio of the population (literally, the ratio of the odds of disease in those with the risk factor, $a'/b'$, to the odds of disease in those without the risk factor, $c'/d'$). This can be rearranged as the cross-product:

$$\left(\frac{a'}{b'}\right)\left(\frac{d'}{c'}\right) = \left(\frac{a'}{c'}\right)\left(\frac{d'}{b'}\right)$$

However, $a'/c'$ in the population equals $a/c$ in the sample if the cases are representative of all cases in the population (i.e., have the same prevalence of the risk factor). Similarly, $b'/d'$ equals $b/d$ if the controls are representative.

Thus the population parameters in this last term can be replaced by the sample parameters, and we are left with the fact that the odds ratio observed in the sample, $ad/bc$, is a close approximation of the relative risk in the population, $[a'/(a' + b')]/[c'/(c' + d')]$, provided that the disease is rare and sampling error (systematic as well as random) is small.

# 9 Enhancing Causal Inference in Observational Studies

## Thomas B. Newman, Warren S. Browner, and Stephen B. Hulley

**O**ne of the most important aspects of clinical research is the inference that an association represents a **cause-effect** relation. In this chapter we discuss ways to strengthen causal inferences based on associations in observational studies. We begin with a discussion of how to avoid **spurious associations** and then concentrate on ruling out **real associations** that do not represent cause-effect, especially those due to confounding.

Suppose that a study reveals an association between coffee drinking and myocardial infarction (MI). One possibility is that coffee drinking is a cause of MI. Before reaching this conclusion, however, four rival explanations must be considered (Table 9.1). The first two of these, **chance** (random error) and **bias** (systematic error), represent spurious associations: Coffee drinking and MI are not really associated in the population, only in the study findings.

Even if the association is real, however, it may not represent a cause-effect relation. Two rival explanations must be considered. One is the possibility of an **effect-cause** relation—that having an MI makes people drink more coffee. (This is just cause and effect in reverse.) The other is the possibility of **confounding**—that some third factor (such as cigarette smoking) is a cause of MI and is also associated with coffee drinking.

## ■ SPURIOUS ASSOCIATIONS
### Ruling Out Spurious Associations Due to Chance

Imagine that there is no association between coffee drinking and MI in the population, and that 60% of the entire population drinks coffee, whether or not they have had an MI. If we were to select a random sample of 20 MI patients, we would expect about 12 of them to drink coffee. But by chance alone we might happen to get 19 coffee drinkers in a sample of 20 MI patients. In that case, unless we were lucky enough to get a similar chance excess of coffee drinkers among the controls, a spurious association between coffee consumption and MI would be observed. Such an association due to **random error** (chance) is called a Type I error (Chapter 5).

Strategies for minimizing random errors are available in both the design and analysis phases of research (Table 9.2). The design strategies of increasing the

■ **TABLE 9.1**

The Five Explanations When an Association Between Coffee Drinking and Myocardial Infarction (MI) Is Observed in a Sample

| Explanation | Type of Association | What's Really Going on in the Population? | Causal Model |
|---|---|---|---|
| 1. Chance (random error) | Spurious | Coffee drinking and MI are not related | |
| 2. Bias (systematic error) | Spurious | Coffee drinking and MI are not related | |
| 3. Effect-Cause | Real | MI is a cause of coffee drinking | Coffee drinking ← MI |
| 4. Confounding | Real | Coffee drinking is associated with a third, extrinsic factor that is a cause of MI | Factor X ↗ ↘ Coffee drinking    MI |
| 5. Cause-Effect | Real | Coffee drinking is a cause of MI | Coffee drinking → MI |

precision of measurements and increasing the sample size are important ways to reduce random error that are discussed in Chapters 4 and 6. The analysis strategy of calculating $P$ values and confidence intervals helps the investigator quantify the magnitude of the observed association in comparison with what might have occurred by chance alone. For example, a $P$ value of 0.10 indicates that the observed difference between the two groups was as large a difference as would occur by chance alone about one time in 10.

## Ruling Out Spurious Associations Due to Bias

Associations that are spurious because of bias are trickier. To understand bias it is important to distinguish between the research question and the question actually answered by the study (Chapter 1). The research question is the uncertainty in the universe the investigator really wishes to settle, and the question answered

■ **TABLE 9.2**

Strengthening the Inference That an Association Has a Cause-Effect Basis: Ruling Out Spurious Associations

| Type of Spurious Association | Design Phase (How to prevent the rival explanation) | Analysis Phase (How to evaluate the rival explanation) |
|---|---|---|
| Chance (due to random error) | Increase sample size and other strategies (Chapters 4 and 6). | Interpret $P$ value in context of prior evidence (Chapter 5). |
| Bias (due to systematic error) | Carefully consider the potential consequences of each difference between the research question and the study plan: Subjects Predictor Outcome | Obtain additional data to see if potential biases have actually occurred. Check consistency with other studies (especially those using different methods). |

by the study reflects the compromises the investigator needed to make for the study to be feasible. Bias can be thought of as a systematic difference between the research question and the actual question answered by the study that may cause the study to give the wrong answer to the research question. Strategies for minimizing these **systematic errors** are available in both the design and analysis phases of research (Table 9.2).

***Design Phase.***    Many kinds of bias have been identified, and dealing with some of them has been a major topic of this book. To the specific strategies noted in Chapters 3, 4, 7, and 8 we now add a general approach to minimizing sources of bias. Write down the research question and the study plan side by side, as in Fig. 9.1. Then carefully think through the following three concerns:

1. Do the **samples** of study subjects (e.g., cases and controls) sufficiently represent the population(s) of interest?
2. Does the **measurement of the predictor variable** sufficiently represent the predictor of interest?
3. Does the **measurement of the outcome variable** sufficiently represent the outcome of interest?

For each question answered "No" or "Maybe not," consider whether the bias is large enough that the study could give the wrong answer to the research question.

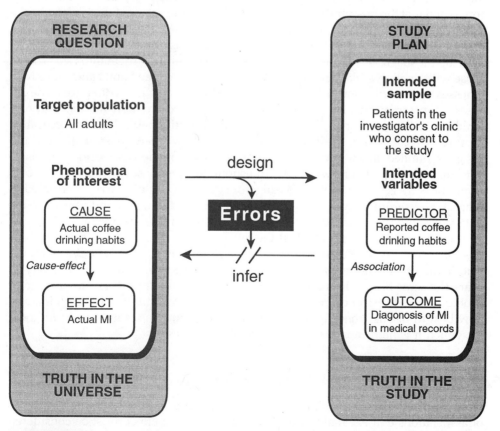

■ **FIGURE 9.1**

Minimizing bias by comparing the research question and the study plan.

To illustrate this with our coffee and MI example, consider the implications of drawing the sample of control subjects from a population of hospitalized patients. If many of these patients have chronic illnesses that have caused them to reduce their coffee intake, the sample of controls will not represent the target population from which the MI patients arose; there will be a shortage of coffee drinkers. Furthermore, if coffee drinking is measured by questionnaire, the answers on the questionnaire may not accurately represent actual coffee drinking, the predictor of interest. And if esophageal spasm, which can be exacerbated by coffee, is misdiagnosed as MI, a spurious association between coffee and MI could be found because the measured outcome (diagnosis of MI) did not accurately represent the outcome of interest (actual MI).

The next step is to think about possible strategies for preventing each potential bias. If the bias is easily preventable, revise the study plan and ask the three questions again. If the bias is not easily preventable, decide whether the study is still worth doing by making a judgment on the likelihood of the potential bias and the degree to which it will compromise the conclusions.

***Analysis Phase.*** The investigator is often faced with one or more potential biases after the data have been collected. Some may have been anticipated but too difficult to prevent, and others may not have been suspected until it was too late to avoid them.

In either situation, one approach is to obtain additional information to estimate the magnitude of the potential bias. Suppose, for example, the investigator is concerned that the hospitalized control subjects do not represent the target population of people free of MI because they have decreased their coffee intake due to chronic illness. The magnitude of this sampling bias could be estimated by reviewing the diagnoses of the control subjects and separating them into two groups: those with an illness like peptic ulcer that might alter coffee habits and those with illnesses that would not. If both types of controls drank less coffee than the MI cases, then sampling bias would be a less likely explanation for the findings. Similarly, if the investigator is concerned that a questionnaire does not accurately capture coffee drinking (perhaps because of poorly worded questions), she could assign a blinded interviewer to question a subset of the cases and controls to determine the agreement with their questionnaire responses. Finally, if the outcome measure is in doubt, the investigator could specify objective electrocardiographic and serum enzyme changes needed for the diagnosis, and reanalyze the data excluding the subset of cases that do not meet these criteria.

The investigator can also look at the results of other studies. If the conclusions are consistent, the association is less likely to be due to bias. This is especially true if the other studies have used different methods and are thus unlikely to share the same biases. In many cases, potential biases turn out not to be a major problem. The decision on how vigorously to pursue additional information and how best to discuss these issues in reporting the study are matters of judgment for which it is helpful to seek advice from colleagues.

# ■ REAL ASSOCIATIONS OTHER THAN CAUSE-EFFECT

Once spurious associations have been determined to be unlikely, the two types of associations that are real but do not represent cause-effect must be considered (Table 9.3).

■ **TABLE 9.3**

Strengthening the Inference That an Association Has a Cause-Effect Basis: Ruling Out Other Real Associations

| Type of Real Association | Design Phase (How to prevent the rival explanation) | Analysis Phase (How to evaluate the rival explanation) |
| --- | --- | --- |
| Effect-Cause (the outcome is actually the cause of the predictor) | Do a longitudinal study | Consider biologic plausibility |
| | Obtain data on the historic sequence of the variables | Consider findings of other studies with different designs |
| Confounding (another variable is associated with the predictor and a cause of the outcome) | See Table 9.4 | See Table 9.5 |

## Effect-Cause

One possibility is that the cart has come before the horse—the outcome has caused the predictor. Effect-cause is often a problem in cross-sectional and case-control studies, especially when the predictor variable is a laboratory test for which no previous values are available. Suppose, for example, that a study finds high serum C-reactive protein levels (a marker for inflammation) in men recovering from myocardial infarction. The MI may have caused the high C-reactive protein levels rather than vice versa.

Effect-cause is less commonly a problem in cohort studies because risk factor measurements can be made in a group of patients who do not yet have the disease. Even in cohort studies, however, effect-cause is possible if the disease has a long latent period and those with subclinical disease cannot be identified at baseline. A good example is the association between low serum cholesterol levels and excess cancer mortality that has been observed in many cohort studies (1). Excess cancer mortality risk associated with low serum cholesterol decreases over time (whereas the excess heart disease mortality in those with high cholesterol continues undiminished) (2). This suggests that preexisting but hidden cancer caused low cholesterol levels at baseline in some subjects. Effect-cause is further supported by the observation that cancer death is associated with *falling* cholesteral levels (3).

This example illustrates a general approach to ruling out effect-cause: drawing inferences from assessments of the variables at different points in time. In addition, effect-cause is often unlikely on the grounds of biologic implausibility. For example, it is unlikely that predisposition to lung cancer causes cigarette smoking.

## Confounding

The other rival explanation in Table 9.3 is confounding, which occurs when there is an extrinsic factor involved in the association that is the real cause of the outcome. The general connotation of confounding is something that confuses interpretation, but in epidemiologic research the term has a more specific statistical meaning. A **confounding variable** is one that is **associated with the predictor variable and is a cause of the outcome variable.**

Cigarette smoking is a likely confounder in the coffee and MI example because smoking is associated with coffee drinking and is a cause of MI. If this is the actual explanation, then the association between coffee and MI does not represent cause-effect even though it is perfectly real; the coffee is an innocent bystander. Appendix 9.A gives a numeric example of how cigarette smoking could cause an apparent association between coffee drinking and MI.

Aside from bias, confounding is often the only likely alternative explanation to cause-effect and the most important one to try to rule out. It is also the most challenging; the rest of this chapter is devoted to strategies for coping with confounders.

## ■ COPING WITH CONFOUNDERS IN THE DESIGN PHASE

In observational studies, most strategies for coping with confounding variables require that an investigator be aware of and able to measure them. (This is not true of experiments, which can control unmeasured confounders by randomization. See Chapter 10.) The first step is to list the variables (like age and sex) that may be associated with the predictor variable of interest and that may also be a cause of the outcome. The investigator must then choose between the design and analysis strategies for controlling the influence of these potential confounding variables.

The two design-phase strategies (Table 9.4), specification and matching, involve changes in the sampling scheme. Cases and controls (in a case-control study) or exposed and unexposed subjects (in a cohort study) are sampled in such a way

## ■ TABLE 9.4
Design Phase Strategies for Coping with Confounders

| Strategy | Advantages | Disadvantages |
|---|---|---|
| **Specification** | Easily understood | Limits generalizability |
| | Focuses the sample of subjects for the research question at hand | May make it difficult to acquire an adequate sample size |
| **Matching** | Can eliminate influence of strong constitutional confounders like age and sex | May be time-consuming and expensive, less efficient than increasing the number of subjects (e.g., the number of controls per case) |
| | Can eliminate influence of confounders that are difficult to measure | Decision to match must be made at outset of study and can have irreversible adverse effect on analysis and conclusions |
| | Can increase precision (power) by balancing the number of cases and controls in each stratum | Requires early decision about which variables are predictors and which are confounders |
| | May be a sampling convenience, making it easier to select the controls in a case-control study | Removes the option of studying matched variables as predictors or as intervening variables |
| | | Requires matched analysis |
| | | Creates the danger of overmatching (i.e., matching on a factor that is not a confounder, thereby reducing power) |

that they have comparable values of the confounding variable. This removes the confounder as an explanation for any association that is observed between predictor and outcome.

## Specification

The simplest strategy is to design inclusion criteria that specify a value of the potential confounding variable and exclude everyone with a different value. For example, the investigator studying coffee and MI could specify that only nonsmokers would be included in the study. If an association were then observed between coffee and MI, it obviously could not be due to smoking.

Specification is an effective strategy, but, as with all restrictions in the sampling scheme (Chapter 3), it has disadvantages. First, even if coffee does not cause MI in nonsmokers, it may cause them in smokers. (This phenomenon—an effect of coffee on MI that is different in smokers from that in nonsmokers—is called **effect modification** or **interaction.**) Thus specification limits the generalizability of information available from a study, in this instance compromising our ability to generalize to smokers. Second, if smoking is highly prevalent among the patients available for the study, the investigator may not be able to recruit a large enough sample of nonsmokers.

These problems can become serious if specification is used to control too many confounders or to control them too narrowly. Sample size and generalizability would be major problems if a study were restricted to lower-income, nonsmoking, 70- to 75-year-old men.

## Matching

In a case-control study, matching involves selecting cases and controls with matching values of the confounding variable(s). Matching and specification are both sampling strategies that prevent confounding by allowing comparison only of cases and controls that share comparable levels of the confounder. Matching differs from specification, however, in preserving generalizability because subjects at all levels of the confounder can be studied.

Matching is usually done individually (**pairwise matching**). In the study of coffee drinking as a predictor of MI, for example, each case (a patient with an MI) could be individually matched to one or more controls that smoked roughly the same amount as the case (e.g., 10 to 20 cigarettes per day). The coffee drinking of each case then would be compared with the coffee drinking of the matched control(s) of that case.

An alternative approach to matching is to do it in groups (**frequency matching**). For each level of smoking, the number of cases with that amount of smoking could be counted, and an appropriate number of controls with the same level of smoking could be selected. If the study called for two controls per case and there were 20 cases that had smoked 10 to 20 cigarettes per day, the investigators would select 40 controls that smoked this amount, matched as a group to the 20 cases.

Matching is most commonly used in case-control studies, but it can also be used with other designs. For example, to investigate the effects of acute respiratory distress syndrome (ARDS) on subsequent quality of life, 73 survivors of ARDS were matched with controls with comparable severity of underlying illness or injury but no ARDS (4). The matched pairs were then interviewed 2 years after their initial hospitalization about their current quality of life. The subjects who had survived ARDS were faring worse than their paired controls in most domains. This illustrates the use of matching in a double cohort design.

***Advantages to Matching.***    There are four main advantages to matching (Table 9.4). The first three relate to the control of confounding variables; the last is a matter of logistics.

- Matching is an effective way to prevent confounding by **constitutional factors** like age and sex that are strong determinants of outcome, are not susceptible to intervention, and are unlikely to be an intermediary in a causal pathway.
- Matching can be used to control confounders that **cannot be measured** and controlled in any other way. For example, matching siblings (or, better yet, twins) with one another can control for a whole range of genetic and familial factors that would be impossible to measure, and matching for clinical center in a multicenter study can control for unspecified differences among the populations seen at the centers.
- Matching may increase the **precision** of comparisons between groups (and thus the power of the study to find a real association) by balancing the number of cases and controls at each level of the confounder. This may be important if the available number of cases is limited or if the cost of studying the subjects is high. However, the effect of matching on precision is modest and not always favorable. In general, the desire to enhance precision is a less important reason to match than the need to control confounding.
- Finally, matching may be used primarily as a **sampling convenience,** to narrow down an otherwise impossibly large number of potential controls. For example, in a nationwide study of toxic shock syndrome, victims were asked to identify friends to serve as controls (5). This convenience, however, runs the risk of "overmatching" (discussed later).

***Disadvantages to Matching.***    There are a number of disadvantages to matching (Table 9.4).

- Matching sometimes requires additional **time and expense** to identify a match for each subject. In case-control studies, for example, the more matching criteria there are, the larger the pool of controls that must be searched to match each case. Cases for which no match can be found will need to be discarded. The possible increase in statistical power from matching must thus be weighed against the potential loss of otherwise eligible cases or controls.
- Because matching is a sampling strategy, the decision to match must be made at the beginning of the study and is **irreversible.** This precludes further analysis of the effect of the matched variables on the outcome. It also can create a serious error if the matching variable is not a fixed (constitutional) variable like age or sex, but a variable intermediate in the causal pathway between the predictor and outcome. For example, if an investigator wishing to investigate the effects of alcohol intake on risk of MI matched on serum high-density lipoprotein (HDL) levels, she would miss beneficial effects of alcohol mediated through an increase in HDL. Although the same error can occur with the analysis phase strategies discussed later, matching builds the error into the study in a way that cannot be undone; with the analysis phase strategies the error can be avoided simply by appropriately altering the analysis.
- Correct analysis of matched data requires **special analytic techniques** that compare each subject only with the individual(s) with whom she has been matched, and not with subjects who have differing levels of confounders. The use of

ordinary statistical analysis techniques on matched data can lead to incorrect results (generally biased toward no effect) because the assumption that the groups are sampled independently is violated. This sometimes creates a problem because the appropriate matched analyses, especially multivariate techniques, are less familiar to most investigators and less readily available in packaged statistical programs than are the usual unmatched techniques.

A final disadvantage of matching is the possibility of **overmatching,** which occurs when the matching variable is not a confounder because it is not associated with the outcome. Overmatching can reduce the power of a case-control study, making it more difficult to find an association that really exists in the population. In the study of toxic shock syndrome that used friends for controls, for example, matching may have inappropriately controlled for regional differences in tampon marketing, making it more probable that cases and controls would use the same brand of tampon. It is important to note, however, that overmatching will not distort the estimated relative risk (provided that a matched analysis is used); it will only reduce its statistical significance.* Thus when the findings of the study are statistically significant (as was the case in the toxic shock example), overmatching is not a problem.

## ■ COPING WITH CONFOUNDERS IN THE ANALYSIS PHASE

Both design-phase strategies (Table 9.5) require deciding at the outset of the study which variables are predictors and which are confounders. **Stratification** and **adjustment,** two analysis-phase strategies, allow the investigator to defer that decision until she has looked at the data and seen which variables may be confounders.

Sometimes there are several predictor variables, each of which may act as a confounder to the others. For example, although coffee drinking, smoking, sex, and personality type are associated with MI, they are also associated with each other. The goal may be to determine which of these predictor variables are independently associated with MI and which are associated with MI only because they are associated with other (causal) risk factors. In this section, we discuss analytic methods for assessing the independent contribution of predictor variables in observational studies.

### Stratification

Like specification and matching, stratification ensures that only cases and controls (or exposed and unexposed subjects) with similar levels of a potential confounding variable are compared. It involves segregating the subjects into strata (subgroups)

---

*The reason that overmatching reduces power can be seen with a matched pairs analysis of a case-control study. In the matched analysis, only case-control pairs that are discordant for exposure to the risk factor are analyzed. Matching on a variable associated with the risk factor will lead to fewer discordant pairs, and hence smaller effective sample size and less power. Of course, this happens to some extent any time matching is used, not just with overmatching. The difference with overmatching is that this cost comes with no benefit, because the matching was not necessary to control confounding. If a matched analysis is not used, then the estimate of the effect size will be distorted, because the matching causes the cases and controls to be more likely to have the same value of the risk factor.

■ **TABLE 9.5**
Analysis Phase Strategies for Coping with Confounders

| Strategy | Advantages | Disadvantages |
|---|---|---|
| **Stratification** | Easily understood | Number of strata limited by sample size needed for each stratum: |
| | Flexible and reversible; can choose which variables to stratify upon after data collection | Few covariables can be considered |
| | | Few strata per covariable leads to less complete control of confounding |
| | | Relevant covariables must have been measured |
| **Statistical adjustment** | Multiple confounders can be controlled simultaneously | Model may not fit: |
| | Information in continuous variables can be fully used | Incomplete control of confounding (if model does not fit confounder-outcome relationship) |
| | Flexible and reversible | Inaccurate estimates of strength of effect (if model does not fit predictor-outcome relationship) |
| | | Results may be hard to understand |
| | | Relevant covariables must have been measured |

according to the level of the potential confounder and then examining the relation between the predictor and outcome separately in each stratum. Stratification is illustrated in Appendix 9.A. By considering smokers and nonsmokers separately ("stratifying on smoking"), the confounding effects of smoking can be removed.

Like matching, stratification is easily understood. An advantage of stratification is its flexibility: by performing several stratified analyses, the investigators can decide which variables appear to be confounders and ignore the remainder. (This may be done by determining whether the results of stratified analyses substantially differ from those of unstratified analyses; see Appendix 9.A.) No choices need be made at the beginning of the study that might later be regretted.

The principal disadvantage of stratified analysis is the limited number of variables that can be controlled simultaneously. For example, possible confounders in the coffee and MI study might include age, systolic blood pressure, serum cholesterol, cigarette smoking, and alcohol intake. To stratify on these five variables, even if there were only three strata for each, would require $3^5$ (= 243) strata! With this many strata there will be some that have zeroes in the margins (e.g., strata with cases but no controls), and data in these strata cannot be used.

To maintain a sufficient number of subjects in each stratum, a variable is often divided into just two strata. When the strata are too broad, however, the confounder may not be adequately controlled. For example, if the preceding study stratified using only two age strata (e.g., age $< 50$ and age $> 50$), confounding would still be possible if within each stratum the subjects drinking the most coffee were also the oldest and thus at highest risk of MI.

## Adjustment

Several statistical techniques are available to **adjust** for confounders. These techniques **model** the nature of the associations among the variables to isolate the effects of predictor variables and confounders. For example, a study of the effect of lead ingestion on IQ in children might examine parental education as a potential confounder. Statistical adjustment might model the relation between parents' years of schooling and the child's IQ as a straight line. The IQs of children with different lead levels could then be adjusted to remove the effect of parental education using the approach described in Appendix 9.B. Similar adjustments can be made for several confounders simultaneously, using software for multivariate analysis.

One of the **great advantages of multivariate adjustment** techniques is the capacity to control the influence of many confounders simultaneously. Another advantage is their use of all the information in continuous variables. It is easy, for example, to adjust for a parent's education level in 1-year intervals, rather than stratifying into just two or three categories.

There are, however, two **disadvantages of multivariate adjustment.** First, the model may not fit. Computerized statistical packages have made these models so accessible that the investigator may not stop to consider whether their use is appropriate to the particular study. Taking the example in Appendix 9.B, the investigator should examine the data to see whether the relation between the parents' years of schooling and the child's IQ is actually linear. If the pattern is very different (e.g., quadratic), then attempts to adjust IQ for parental education using a linear model will be imperfect and the estimate of the independent effect of lead will be incorrect.

Second, the resulting highly derived statistics are difficult to understand intuitively. This is particularly a problem if a simple model does not fit and transformations (e.g., parental education squared) or interaction terms (e.g., child sex times parental education) are needed.

## ■ CHOOSING A STRATEGY

What general guidelines can be offered for when to use each of these strategies? The use of specification to control confounding is most appropriate for situations in which the investigator is chiefly interested in specific subgroups of the population; this is really just a special form of the general process in every study of establishing criteria for selecting the study subjects (Chapter 3).

An important decision to make in the design phase of the study is whether to match. Matching is most appropriate for fixed constitutional factors such as age, race, and sex. Matching may also be helpful when the sample size is small compared with the number of strata necessary to control for known confounders, and when the confounders are more easily matched than measured. However, because matching can permanently compromise the investigator's ability to observe real associations, it should be used sparingly, and in situations where it is clear that analysis-phase strategies are not as good.

The decision to stratify or adjust can wait until after the data are collected and the investigator can analyze the data to see which factors are potential confounders (i.e., associated with both the predictor of interest and the outcome). However, it is important to consider which factors may be used for adjustment at the time the study is designed, in order to know which variables to measure. Also, since strategies for controlling the influence of a specific confounding variable can only succeed to the degree that the confounder is well measured, it is important to design measurement approaches that have adequate precision and accuracy (Chapter 4).

## Evidence Favoring Causality

The approach to enhancing causal inference has largely been a negative one thus far—how to rule out the four rival explanations in Table 9.1. A complementary strategy is to seek characteristics of associations that provide positive evidence for causality, of which the most important are the consistency and strength of the association, the presence of a dose-response relation, and biologic plausibility.

When the results are **consistent** in studies of various designs, it is less likely that chance or bias is the cause of an association. Real associations that represent effect-cause or confounding, however, will also be consistently observed. For example, if cigarette smokers drink more coffee and have more MIs in the population, studies will consistently observe an association between coffee drinking and MI.

The **strength** of the association is also important. For one thing, stronger associations give more significant $P$ values, making chance a less likely explanation. Stronger associations also provide better evidence for causality by reducing the likelihood of confounding. Associations due to confounding are indirect (i.e., via the confounder) and therefore are generally weaker than direct cause-effect associations. This is illustrated in Appendix 9.A: the very strong associations between coffee and smoking (odds ratio = 16) and between smoking and MI (odds ratio = 4) led to a much weaker association between coffee and MI (odds ratio = 2.25).

A **dose-response** relation provides positive evidence for causality. The association between cigarette smoking and lung cancer is an example: Moderate smokers have higher rates of cancer than nonsmokers, and heavy smokers have even higher rates. Whenever possible, predictor variables should be measured continuously or in several categories, so that any dose-response relation that is present can be observed. Once again, however, a dose-response relation can be observed with effect-cause associations or with confounding. For example, if heavier coffee drinkers also were heavier smokers, their MI risk would be greater than that of moderate coffee drinkers.

Finally, **biologic plausibility** is an important consideration for drawing causal inference—if a causal mechanism that makes sense biologically can be proposed, evidence for causality is enhanced, whereas associations that do not make sense given our current understanding of biology are less likely to represent cause-effect. It is important not to overemphasize biologic plausibility, however. Investigators can come up with a suggested mechanism for virtually any association.

## ■ SUMMARY

1. The design of observational studies should anticipate the need to interpret **associations.** The inference that the association represents a **cause-effect** relation is strengthened by strategies that reduce the likelihood of the **four rival explanations—chance, bias, effect-cause,** and **confounding.**

2. The role of **chance** can be minimized by designing a study with **adequate sample size and precision** to assure a low Type I error rate. Once the study is completed, the likelihood that chance is the basis of the association can be

judged from the $P$ value and the consistency of the results with previous evidence.

3. **Bias** arises from differences between the population and phenomena addressed by the research question and the actual subjects and measurements in the study. Bias can be avoided by basing design decisions on a judgment as to whether these differences will lead to a wrong answer to the research question.

4. **Effect-cause** is made less likely by designing a study that permits assessment of **temporal sequence**, and by considering biologic plausibility.

5. **Confounding** is made less likely by the following strategies:
   a. **Specification** or **matching** in the design phase, which alters the sampling strategy to ensure that only groups with similar levels of the confounder are compared. These strategies should be used sparingly because they can irreversibly limit the information available from the study.
   b. **Stratification** or **adjustment** in the analysis phase, which accomplishes the same goal statistically and preserves more options for coping with confounders. Adjustment permits many factors to be controlled simultaneously, but the data may not fit the statistical model and the resulting measures of association may not be easy to grasp intuitively.

6. Causal inference is further enhanced by positive evidence: the **consistency and strength of the association,** the presence of a **dose-response** relation, and **biologic plausibility.**

# EXERCISES

> **1.** You are planning a case-control study to address the research question, "Does eating more fruits and vegetables reduce the risk of coronary heart disease (CHD) in the elderly?" Suppose that your study shows that people in the control group report a higher intake of fruits and vegetables than people with CHD.
>
> What are the possible explanations for this inverse association between intake of fruits and vegetables and CHD? How could each of these possibilities be altered in the design phase of the study? How could they be addressed in the analysis phase?
>
> Give special attention to the possibility that the association between eating fruits and vegetables and CHD may be confounded by exercise (if people who eat more fruits and vegetables also exercise more, and this is the cause of their lower CHD rates). What approaches could you use to cope with exercise as a possible confounder, and what are the advantages and disadvantages of each plan?

# References

1. Jacobs D, Blackburn H, Higgins M, et al. Report of the Conference on Low Blood Cholesterol: mortality associations. *Circulation* 1992;86:1046–60.
2. Pekkanen J, Nissinen A, Punsar S, Karvonen MJ. Short- and long-term association of serum cholesterol with mortality: the 25-year follow-up of the Finnish cohorts of the seven countries study. *Am J Epidemiol* 1992;135:1251–8.
3. Sharp SJ, Pocock SJ. Time trends in serum cholesterol before cancer death. *Epidemiology* 1997;8:132–6.

4. Davidson T, Caldwell E, Curtis J, et al. Reduced quality of life in survivors of acute respiratory distress syndrome compared with critically ill control patients. *JAMA* 1999;281:354–60.

5. Shands KN, Schmid GP, Dan BB, et al. Toxic-shock syndrome in menstruating women: association with tampon use and *Staphylococcus aureus* and clinical features in 52 cases. *N Engl J Med* 1980;303:1436–42.

# ■ APPENDIX 9.A

## Hypothetical Example of Confounding

Confounding by cigarette smoking can be the cause of an apparent association between coffee drinking and MI. The entries in these tables are numbers of subjects. Thus the top left entry of Panel 1 means that, among the smokers, 80 MI cases drank coffee (out of $80 + 20 = 100$ total MI cases).

1. Both in smokers and in nonsmokers, coffee drinking is not associated with MI.

|  | Smokers | | Nonsmokers | |
| --- | --- | --- | --- | --- |
|  | MI | No MI | MI | No MI |
| Coffee | 80 | 40 | 10 | 20 |
| No Coffee | 20 | 10 | 40 | 80 |

Odds ratio for MI associated with coffee:

$$\text{in smokers} = \frac{80 \times 10}{20 \times 40} = 1$$

$$\text{in nonsmokers} = \frac{10 \times 80}{40 \times 20} = 1$$

2. However, if we did not stratify on smoking (i.e., if we did not consider smokers or nonsmokers separately), coffee drinking and MI would appear to be related. Combining the two preceding tables gives

| | Smokers and Nonsmokers Combined | |
| --- | --- | --- |
|  | MI | No MI |
| Coffee | 90 | 60 |
| No Coffee | 60 | 90 |

Odds ratio for MI associated with coffee:

$$\text{in smokers and non} \atop \text{smokers combined} = \frac{90 \times 90}{60 \times 60} = 2.25$$

3. Smoking is a confounder because it is strongly associated with coffee drinking (below, left) and with MI (below, right):*

| | MI and No MI Combined | | | Coffee and No Coffee Combined | |
| --- | --- | --- | --- | --- | --- |
|  | Coffee | No Coffee | | MI | No MI |
| Smokers | 120 | 30 | Smokers | 100 | 50 |
| Nonsmokers | 30 | 120 | Nonsmokers | 50 | 100 |

$$\text{Odds ratio for} \atop \text{coffee drinking} \atop \text{associated with smoking} = \frac{120 \times 120}{30 \times 30} = 16 \qquad \text{Odds ratio for MI} \atop \text{associated with smoking} = \frac{100 \times 100}{50 \times 50} = 4$$

*These tables were obtained by rearranging numbers in Panel 1 and then combining tables.

# ■ APPENDIX 9.B

## A Simplified Example of Adjustment

Suppose that a study finds two major predictors of the IQ of children: the parental education level and the child's blood lead level. Consider the following hypothetical data on children with normal and high lead levels:

|  | Average Years of Parental Education | Average IQ of Child |
|---|---|---|
| High lead level | 10.0 | 95 |
| Normal lead level | 12.0 | 110 |

Note that the parental education level is also associated with the child's blood lead level. The question is, "Is the difference in IQ more than can be accounted for on the basis of the difference in parental education?" To answer this question we look at how much difference in IQ the difference in parental education levels would be expected to produce. We do this by plotting parental educational level versus IQ in the children with normal lead levels (Fig. 9.2).*

The dotted line in Fig. 9.2 shows the relationship between the child's IQ and parental education in children with normal lead levels; there is an increase in the child's IQ of five points for each 2 years of parental education. Thus, we can adjust the IQ of the normal lead group to account for the difference in mean parental education by sliding down the line from point $A$ to point $A'$. (Because

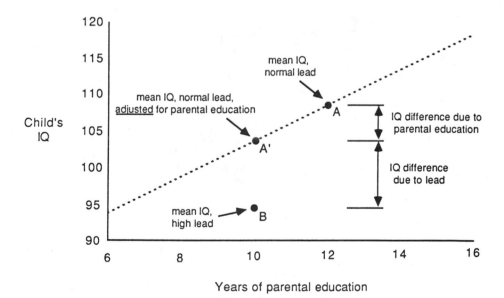

## ■ FIGURE 9.2

Hypothetical graph of child's IQ as a linear function (*dotted line*) of years of parental education.

---

*This description of analysis of covariance (ANCOVA) is simplified. Actually, parental education is plotted against the child's IQ in both the normal and high lead groups, and the single slope that fits both plots the best is used. The model for this form of adjustment thus assumes linear relationships between education and IQ in both groups, and that the slopes of the lines in the two groups are the same.

the group with normal lead levels had 2 more years of parental education on the average, we adjust their IQs downward by five points to make them comparable in mean parental education to the high-lead group.) This still leaves a 10-point difference in IQ between points $A'$ and $B$, suggesting that lead has an independent effect on IQ of this magnitude. Thus of the 15-point difference in IQ of children with low and high lead levels, five points can be accounted for by their parents' different education levels and the remaining 10 are attributable to the lead exposure.

# 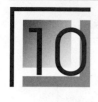 Designing an Experiment: Clinical Trials I

## Steven R. Cummings, Deborah Grady, and Stephen B. Hulley

In clinical trials, the investigator applies a treatment (termed **intervention**) and observes the effect on an outcome. The major advantage of a trial over an observational study is the ability to demonstrate causality. In particular, **randomly assigning** the intervention can eliminate the influence of confounding variables, and **blinding** its administration can eliminate the possibility that the observed effects of the intervention are due to other treatments or to biased ascertainment.

However, clinical trials are generally expensive, are time-consuming, address a narrow clinical question, and sometimes expose participants to potential harm. For these reasons, trials are best reserved for relatively mature research questions, when observational studies and other lines of evidence suggest that an intervention might be effective but stronger evidence is required as the basis for practice guidelines. Not every research question is amenable to the clinical trial design. For example, it is not feasible to study whether drug treatment of high-LDL cholesterol in children will prevent heart attacks many decades later. But the principles of evidence-based medicine require clinical trial evidence whenever possible.

This chapter focuses on the classic **randomized blinded trial** (Fig. 10.1), addressing the selection of participants, measurement of baseline variables, randomization, and choice of intervention and control. In the next chapter we will come to outcomes, analysis, and other trial designs.

## ■ SELECTING THE PARTICIPANTS

Selection of the participants begins with deciding what kind of participants to study and how to go about recruiting them. Chapter 3 discussed how to specify entry criteria defining a target population that is appropriate to the research question and an accessible population that is practical to study, how to design an efficient and scientific approach to selecting participants, and how to recruit them. Here are some further points that are especially relevant to clinical trials.

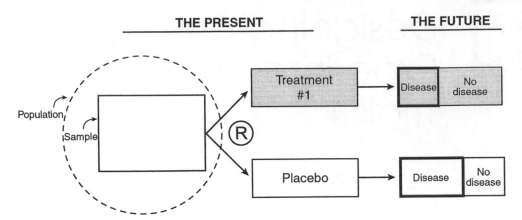

**THE PRESENT**                                    **THE FUTURE**

■ **FIGURE 10.1**

In a randomized trial, the investigator (a) selects a sample from the population, (b) measures baseline variables, (c) randomizes the participants, (d) applies interventions (one should be a blinded placebo, if possible), (e) follows up the cohort, (f) measures outcome variables (blindly, if possible) and analyzes the results.

## Define Entry Criteria

In a clinical trial, inclusion and exclusion criteria have the joint goal of identifying an important population for whom a statistically significant impact of the intervention on the outcome is feasible and likely. This means that the entry criteria should optimize the rate of the primary outcome, the expected effectiveness of the active treatment, the generalizability of findings from the trial, the ease of recruitment, and the likelihood of compliance with treatment and follow-up.

If the outcome of interest is a rare event, such as breast cancer, it is usually necessary to recruit participants who have a high risk of the outcome to reduce the sample size and follow-up time to feasible levels. On the other hand, narrowing the inclusion criteria to higher-risk people limits the generalizability of the results and makes it more difficult to recruit participants into the trial.

The investigator must have reliable estimates of the rate of the primary outcome in people who might be included. These estimates can be based on data from vital statistics, longitudinal observational studies, or rates observed in the untreated group of trials with outcomes similar to those in the planned trial. For example, expected rates of breast cancer in 60-year-old women can be estimated from cancer registry data, from large observational studies such as the Nurses Health Study (1), or from rates of breast cancer observed in large trials of mammographic screening.

Including participants with a high risk of the outcome can decrease the number of subjects needed for the trial. If risk factors for the outcome have been established, then the selection criteria can be designed to include participants who have a minimum estimated risk of the outcome of interest. The Breast Cancer Prevention Trial of tamoxifen for prevention of breast cancer, for example, applied combinations of risk factors for breast cancer in an algorithm designed to include women who had a 5-year risk of breast cancer of at least 1.7% (2). Another way to increase the rate of events is to limit enrollment to people who already have the disease. The Heart and Estrogen/Progestin Replacement Study (HERS) included 2,763 women who already had coronary heart disease (CHD) to test whether estrogen plus progestin reduced the risk of new CHD events (3). This approach was much more feasible and less costly than a study of women without CHD, which would require about 25,000 participants (4).

Additionally, a trial can be smaller and shorter if it includes people who are likely to have the greatest effect from the treatment. For example, tamoxifen appears to decrease the risk of breast cancer that is estrogen receptor positive but not that of cancer that is estrogen receptor negative. Thus a trial testing the effect of tamoxifen on the risk of breast cancer would be smaller and shorter if participants are at high risk of estrogen receptor positive breast cancer (5,6).

Limiting inclusion to participants at high risk of the disease has two disadvantages. The results of the trial may not be generalizable to lower-risk populations. For example, because the HERS study included only women with CHD, it left uncertainty about whether the findings could be generalized to women without CHD. Furthermore, documenting the basis of the increased risk, such as a history of CHD, may require collecting data or making measurements that make recruitment of participants more complicated, difficult, and expensive.

Although probability samples of general populations confer advantages in observational studies, this type of sampling is generally not feasible and has limited value for most randomized trials. Inclusion of participants with diverse characteristics will increase the confidence that the result of a trial applies broadly. However, setting aside issues of adherence to randomized treatment, it is generally true that results of a trial done in a convenience sample (e.g., women with CHD who respond to advertisements) will be similar to results obtained in probability samples of eligible people (all women with CHD).

Exclusion criteria should be parsimonious because unnecessary exclusions may diminish the generalizability of the results, make it more difficult to recruit the necessary number of participants, and increase the complexity and cost of recruitment. There are five reasons for excluding people from a clinical trial (Table 10.1).

The treatment may be unsafe in people who are susceptible to known or suspected adverse effects of the active treatment. For example, tamoxifen increases the risk of venous thrombosis so that women who have a history of thromboembolic disease should not take the drug and should be excluded. Conversely, the treatment may be known to be so beneficial for some people, such as women with recently diagnosed estrogen receptor positive breast cancer, that it would be unacceptable to assign them to the placebo group. Persons in whom the active treatment is unlikely to be effective should be excluded, as well as those who are unlikely to be adherent to the intervention or unlikely to complete follow-up. It is wise to exclude people who are not likely to contribute a primary outcome to the study (e.g., because they will move during the period of follow-up). Occasionally, practical problems, such as impaired mental status that makes it difficult to follow instructions, justify exclusion. Investigators should carefully weigh potential exclusion criteria that apply to many people (e.g., diabetes or upper age limits) as these have a large impact on the feasibility and costs of recruitment and generalizability of results.

## Design an Adequate Sample Size and Plan the Recruitment Accordingly

Trials with too few participants to detect substantial effects are wasteful, unethical, and may produce misleading conclusions (7). Estimating the sample size is one of the most important early parts of planning a trial (Chapters 5 and 6). Recruitment for a trial is usually more difficult than recruitment for an observational study because participants must be willing to be randomly assigned and to take

■ **TABLE 10.1**
Reasons for Excluding People from a Clinical Trial

| Reason | Example (A trial of tamoxifen vs. placebo to prevent breast cancer) |
|---|---|
| 1. A study treatment would be harmful | |
|     Unacceptable risk of adverse reaction to active treatment | Prior venous thromboembolic event (tamoxifen increases risk of venous thromboembolic events) |
|     Unacceptable risk of assignment to placebo | Recent estrogen receptor–positive breast cancer (treatment with tamoxifen is an effective standard of care) |
| 2. Active treatment cannot or is unlikely to be effective | |
|     Not at risk for the outcome | Bilateral mastectomy |
|     Has a type of disease that is not likely to respond to treatment | Has a breast cancer susceptibility gene that causes estrogen receptor negative cancer |
|     Taking a treatment that is likely to interfere with the intervention | Taking estrogen (which competes with tamoxifen) |
| 3. Unlikely to adhere to the intervention | Poor adherence during run-in |
| 4. Unlikely to complete follow-up | Plans to move before trial ends<br>Short life expectancy because of a serious illness<br>Unreliable participation in visits before randomization |
| 5. Practical problems with participating in the protocol | Impaired mental state that prevents accurate answers to questions |

a blinded therapy. For this reason, the investigator should plan a large, accessible population and enough time and money to get the desired sample size when (as usually happens) the barriers to doing so turn out to be greater than expected.

# ■ MEASURING BASELINE VARIABLES

## Collect Tracking Information

In addition to the participant's name and address, it is important to record information, such as the names, phone numbers, addresses, and email addresses of two or three friends or relatives who will always know how to reach the participant. It is also valuable to record Social Security numbers or other national I.D. numbers. These can be used to determine the vital status of participants (through the National Death Index) or to help determine the occurrence of key outcomes using health records (e.g., health insurance systems).

## Describe the Participants

Investigators should collect enough information (e.g., age, gender, and measurements of the severity of disease) to help others judge the generalizability of the findings. These measurements also provide a means for checking on the comparability of the study groups at baseline; the first table of the final report of a clinical trial typically compares the levels of baseline characteristics in the two study groups. The goal is to make sure that differences in these levels do not exceed what might be expected from the play of chance, which might suggest a technical error or bias in carrying out the randomization.

## Measure Variables that Are Risk Factors for the Outcome or that Can Be Used to Define Subgroups

Particularly in relatively small trials, it is a good idea to measure baseline variables that are likely to be strong predictors of the outcome (smoking habits of the spouse in a trial of a smoking intervention, for example). This allows the investigator to examine these predictors as secondary research questions, and it permits statistical adjustment of the primary randomized comparison to reduce the effects of chance maldistributions of baseline factors between the two study groups, increasing the efficiency of the study. It also allows the investigator to examine whether the intervention has different effects in **subgroups** classified by baseline variables, a relatively uncommon but sometimes important phenomenon termed **effect modification** or **interaction**.

## Establish Banks of Materials

Storing sera, DNA, or other biologic specimens at baseline will allow subsequent measurement of biologic predictors of the outcome, and factors such as genotypes, that might identify interactions (subgroups who respond well or poorly to the treatment). Stored specimens can also be a rich resource to study other research questions not directly related to the main outcome.

## Measure the Outcome Variable

If possible, it is generally useful to measure the outcome variable at the beginning of the study as well as at the end. In studies that have a dichotomous outcome (the incidence of CHD, for example) it may be important to demonstrate by history and electrocardiogram that the disease is not present at the outset. In studies that have a continuous-outcome variable (a study of the effects of antihypertensive drugs on blood pressure, for example) the best outcome measure is generally the degree of change over the course of the study. This approach controls for differences among the study participants in their initial blood pressure levels and may offer more power than simply comparing blood pressure values at the end of the trial. Similarly, it may also be useful to measure secondary outcomes, and outcomes of planned ancillary studies at baseline.

## Be Parsimonious

Having pointed out all these uses for baseline measurements, we should stress that the basic design of a clinical trial does not require that *any* be measured, because randomization eliminates the problem of confounding by factors that are present at the outset. Making a lot of measurements adds expense and complexity. In a randomized trial that has a limited budget, time and money are usually better spent on things that are vital to the integrity of the study, such as the sufficiency of the sample size, the success of randomization and blinding, and the completeness of follow-up. Yusuf et al. have promoted the use of large trials with very few measurements (8).

## ■ RANDOMIZING

The third step in Fig. 10.1 is to randomly assign the participants to two or more interventions. In the simplest design, one group receives an active treatment and the other receives a placebo.

The random allocation of participants to one or another of the study groups establishes the basis for testing the statistical significance of differences between these groups in the measured outcome. Random assignment provides that age, sex, and other prognostic baseline characteristics that could confound an observed association will be distributed equally, except for chance variation, among the randomized groups. The effects of any maldistributions that do occur as a result of chance are addressed in the statistical tests of the difference in outcome between the randomly assigned groups.

## Do a Good Job of Random Assignment

Because randomization is the cornerstone of a clinical trial, it is important that it be done correctly. The two most important features are the following: (a) The procedure truly allocates treatments randomly and (b) the assignments are tamperproof so that neither intentional nor unintentional factors can influence the randomization.

Ordinarily, the participant completes the baseline examinations, is found eligible for inclusion, and gives consent to enter the study before randomization. He is then randomly assigned by applying a previously established algorithm to a set of random numbers, which are typically computer-generated. For example, if the design calls for an equal probability of assignment to each of three study groups, the algorithm could specify using the random numbers 1, 2, and 3 for assignment to the three study groups. (Other numbers are ignored.)

Once a list of the random order of assignment to study groups is generated, it must be applied to participants as they enter the trial. It is essential to design the random assignment procedure so that members of the research team who have any contact with the study participants cannot influence the allocation. Random treatment assignments can be placed in advance in a set of sealed envelopes by someone who will not be involved in opening the envelopes. Each envelope must be numbered (so that all can be accounted for at the end of the study), opaque (to prevent transillumination by a strong light), and otherwise tamperproof. When a participant is randomized, his name and the number of the next envelope are first recorded; then the envelope is opened. For small studies a table of random numbers (Appendix 3.1) can be used to order the envelopes.

An effective but costly procedure for ensuring that randomization is tamperproof is to set up a separate randomization facility that the trial staff contact by telephone, fax, or email when an eligible participant is ready to be randomized. The staff member provides the name and study number of the new participant. This information is recorded and the treatment group is then randomly assigned. Treatment can also be randomly assigned by computer programs at the research site as long as these programs are tamperproof.

Rigorous precautions to prevent tampering with randomization are needed because investigators sometimes find themselves under pressure to influence the randomization process (e.g., for an individual who seems particularly suitable for an active treatment group in a placebo-controlled trial).

## Consider Special Randomization Techniques

In general, the preferred approach is to randomize equal numbers of participants to each group, but unequal allocation has been used in studies that have three or more groups, one serving as a control for each of the others (9). If no formal comparisons among the active treatment groups are planned, the larger number of comparisons that involve the control group makes the precision of its outcome measure especially important and the investigator can consider assigning a larger proportion of participants to the control group. However, there is no clear way to pick the best proportions to use, and disproportionate randomization in this and other situations can complicate the process of obtaining informed consent. Because the advantages are marginal (the effect of even a 2 : 1 disproportion on power is surprisingly modest [10]), the best decision is usually to assign equal numbers to each group.

Trials of small to moderate size will have a small gain in power if special randomization procedures are used to balance the study groups in the numbers of participants they contain (blocked randomization) and in the distribution of baseline variables known to predict the outcome (stratified blocked randomization).

**Blocked randomization** is a commonly used technique to ensure that the number of participants is equally distributed among the study groups. Randomization is done in "blocks" of predetermined size. For example, if the block size is six, randomization proceeds normally within each block until the third person is randomized to one group, after which participants are automatically assigned to the other group until the block of six is completed. This means that in a study of 30 participants exactly 15 will be assigned to each group, and in a study of 33 participants, the disproportion could be no greater than 18 : 15. Blocked randomization is less suitable for nonblinded studies because the treatment assignment of the participants at the end of each block could be predicted and manipulated. This problem can be minimized by varying the size of the blocks randomly (ranging, for example, from four to eight) according to a schedule that is not known to the investigator.

**Stratified blocked randomization** ensures that an important predictor of the outcome is more evenly distributed between the study groups than chance alone would dictate. In a trial of the effect of a drug to prevent fractures, having a vertebral fracture is such a strong predictor of outcome and response to treatment that it may be best to ensure that very similar numbers of people who have vertebral fractures are assigned to each group. This can be achieved by dividing the study cohort at baseline into participants with or without vertebral fractures, and then carrying out a blocked randomization within each of these two "strata." Stratified blocked randomization can slightly enhance the power of a small trial by reducing the variation in outcome due to chance disproportions in important baseline variables. Stratified blocked randomization is of little benefit in large trials (more than 1,000 participants) because chance assignment ensures nearly even distribution of baseline variables. An important limitation of stratified randomization is the small number of baseline variables, not more than two or three, that can be balanced by this technique.

# ■ APPLYING THE INTERVENTIONS

In a clinical trial the investigator compares the outcome in groups of participants that receive different interventions. Between-group designs always include a group that receives a treatment to be tested, and a control group that receives either no active treatment (placebo) or a standard comparison treatment. Sometimes there are also additional experimental groups that receive other treatments. There are a number of trade-offs to consider in choosing and applying these interventions.

■ **TABLE 10.2**
Randomization Eliminates Confounding by Baseline Variables and Blinding Eliminates
Confounding by Co-Interventions

| | Explanation for Association | Strategy to Rule Out Rival Explanation |
|---|---|---|
| 1. Chance | | Same as in observational studies |
| 2. Bias | | Same as in observational studies |
| 3. Effect-Cause | | (Not a possible explanation in an experiment) |
| 4. Confounding | Prerandomization confounding variables | **Randomization** |
| | Postrandomization confounding variables (unintended interventions) | **Blinding** |
| 5. Cause-Effect | | |

## Importance of Blinding

Whenever possible, the investigator should design the interventions in such a fashion that neither the study participants nor anybody who has contact with them has any knowledge of the study group assignment. In a randomized trial, *blinding is as important as randomization:* It protects the trial from treatment differences between the groups other than the randomized treatments and from biased assessment of outcomes.

Randomization only eliminates the influence of confounding variables that are present at the time of randomization; it does not eliminate confounding that occurs during follow-up (Table 10.2). In an unblinded study the investigator may give extra attention to participants he knows are receiving the active drug, and this "**co-intervention**" may be the actual cause of any difference in outcome that is observed between the groups. For example, in an unblinded trial of the effect of exercise to prevent myocardial infarction, the investigator's eagerness to find a benefit might lead him to suggest that participants in the exercise group adopt a low-fat diet and stop smoking. Co-interventions can also affect the control group if, for example, participants who discover that they are receiving placebo seek out other treatments that affect the difference in outcome between groups.

Sometimes interventions cannot be blinded. In this case, the investigator should limit and standardize other potential treatments as much as possible. For example, an investigator testing the effect of exercise for reduction in hot flashes could specify a precise regimen of exercise sessions in the treatment group. To minimize other differences in exercise, he could instruct both exercise and control participants to refrain from starting new recreational activities or hormone treatment until the trial has ended.

The second important value of blinding is to prevent **biased assessment of outcome**. In an unblinded trial, the investigator may be tempted to look more carefully for outcomes in the untreated group or to diagnose the outcome more frequently. For example, in an unblinded trial of estrogen therapy, the investigators may be more likely to ask women in the active treatment group about pain or swelling in the calf and to order ultrasound or other tests to make the diagnosis of deep vein thrombosis. Blinded assessment of outcome may not be important if the outcome of the trial is death, about which there is no uncertainty or opportunity for biased assessment. Most other outcomes, such as cause-specific death, disease diagnosis, physical measurements, questionnaire scales, and self-reported conditions, are susceptible to biased ascertainment. Blinded assessment of outcomes is most important in trials where the outcome is "soft," such as those based on participant self-report or investigator opinion. In a trial of the effect of exercise on depression, participants who receive the exercise program may report less depression due to a placebo effect, and the investigator (who wants the intervention to be effective) may be more likely to judge that participants who were assigned to exercise are less depressed. Especially when the intervention cannot be blinded, outcomes should be "hard" (i.e., based on measurements that are resistant to bias). Measurement of depression, for example, is less susceptible to bias if change in a standardized depression scale is used, rather than investigator judgment.

Blinding is more difficult to carry out successfully than randomization. Even when an intervention such as a drug can be blinded, the logistic problems can be substantial. There is the need to get the manufacturer or pharmacy to prepare the identical capsules and to develop foolproof systems for labeling and dispensing. Well before a trial starts, investigators should inspect, taste, and weigh samples of the active drug and placebo and their containers. (Investigators sometimes discover differences in the weight of bottles and taste or odor of pills only after randomization has begun—too late to change the preparations.) In addition, it may be necessary to develop a 24-hour mechanism for unblinding in the event that a participant becomes acutely ill and his personal physician needs to know what drug he is taking. Pharmacies will sometimes help to design and provide this service.

The other major difficulty in designing the system for blinding is ensuring that neither the participants nor the research team will be able to discern the effects of treatment assignment. Telltale effects of the drugs on physical symptoms or laboratory values (such as the effect of diuretics on serum potassium) may require setting up a system in which these results are reviewed by someone not involved in follow-up contacts with the participants. In the HERS trial, even though the active hormones and the placebo were provided in identical capsules, treatment with hormones caused vaginal bleeding in a substantial proportion of postmenopausal women assigned to active treatment. To address this potential unblinding, participants were instructed to report any bleeding to the gynecologic staff who did not interact with other trial staff and had no role in the ascertainment of the main outcome—coronary disease events (11).

After the study is over, it is a good idea to assess whether the participants and investigators were unblinded by asking them to guess the treatment assignments; if a higher than expected proportion guesses correctly, the published discussion of the findings can include an assessment of the potential biases the partial unblinding may have caused.

# Choice of Intervention

Investigators should consider several issues as they design their interventions, including the balance of effectiveness and safety, the feasibility of blinding, whether to treat with one or a combination of interventions, and generalizability to the way the treatment will be used in practice (e.g., whether to use a fixed treatment dose or titrate). If important decisions are uncertain, such as which dose best balances effectiveness and safety, it may be best to postpone a trial until pilot studies have been completed to help resolve the issue. However, even after gathering a lot of data about the alternatives, the best approach is often uncertain. (If the best approach were clear, there would be no need for the study.) Sometimes an investigator may hedge his bets by including two or more treatments in order to test each of several promising interventions. For example, at the time the Multiple Outcomes of Raloxifene Trial was designed, it was not clear which dose of raloxifene, 60 or 120 mg, was best, so the trial tested two doses of raloxifene for preventing fractures (9). This is sometimes a reasonable strategy, but it has its costs: a larger and more expensive trial, and the complexity of dealing with multiple hypotheses (Chapter 5). Choosing the best treatment can be especially difficult in studies that involve years of follow-up because a treatment that reflects current practice at the outset of the study may have become outmoded by the end, transforming a pragmatic test into an academic exercise.

The best balance between effectiveness and safety depends on the condition being treated. On the one hand, effectiveness is generally the paramount consideration in designing interventions to treat illnesses that cause severe symptoms and a high risk of death. Thus it may be best to choose the "highest tolerable dose." On the other hand, safety should be the primary criterion for designing interventions to reduce the risk of less severe and nonfatal conditions among healthy people: Few people will benefit from the treatment by avoiding the condition, all will be at risk of any adverse effects of the drug. In this case, it is generally best to choose the "lowest effective dose."

The development and testing of new drugs generally involves a series of relatively small randomized trials of a range of doses or combinations of treatments (called Phase II trials by the Food and Drug Administration; see Chapter 11). At this stage, it is wise to test the widest possible range of doses and regimens to guarantee that an effective and ineffective dose are included. The outcomes are often physiologic measurements on continuous scales (such as change in cholesterol level) because it is not feasible to study the effect of multiple doses on the real outcome of interest (myocardial infarction). Investigators should carefully consider the evidence that surrogate markers are likely to predict accurately the effect of treatment on the outcome of interest. When the outcome, such as myocardial infarction, depends on several processes (levels of HDL and LDL cholesterol, blood coagulability, platelet adhesiveness, endothelial cell function), the investigator should measure several surrogate markers.

Because of their limited size, it is usually not possible for Phase II studies to assess the safety of a new drug adequately. The effect of drugs on laboratory tests, such as liver function tests, is tested because these tests are easy and inexpensive. Unless the treatment has a common and severe toxicity, it may be impossible to assess the safety of a treatment until it is tested in larger trials that have adequate power to detect uncommon but important adverse effects. This reinforces the wisdom of choosing the lowest dose that appears to have adequate effectiveness.

When a choice is possible, investigators should clearly prefer interventions that can be blinded over alternatives that cannot. Creative approaches can help blind, or partially blind, many outcomes. For example, in a trial of the effect of acupuncture on pain from dysmenorrhea, the treated group can have needles placed in points thought to relieve pain, and the control group can have needles placed in other locations.

Trials to test single interventions are generally much easier to plan and implement than those testing combinations of treatments. However, many medical conditions, such as HIV infection, are treated with combinations of drugs. The most important disadvantage of testing combinations of treatments is that the result cannot provide clear conclusions about any one of the interventions. In the HERS trial, for example, postmenopausal women were treated with estrogen plus progestin therapy or placebo. The intervention did not result in a reduced risk of coronary events, but it was unclear whether estrogen alone may have had a more beneficial effect. In general, it is preferable to design trials that have only one major difference between any two study groups.

The investigator should consider how well the intervention can be incorporated in practice. Thus simple interventions are generally better than complicated ones (patients are more likely to take a pill once a day than two or three times). Complicated interventions, such as multifaceted counseling of patients about changing their behavior, may not be feasible to incorporate in general practice because they require rare expertise or are too time-consuming or costly. Such interventions are less likely to have clinical impact, even if a trial proves that they are effective.

Some treatments are generally given in doses that vary from patient to patient. In these instances, it may be best to design an intervention so that the active drug is titrated to achieve a clinical outcome such as reduction in the hepatitis C viral load. To maintain blinding, corresponding changes should be made (by someone blinded to treatment group) in the "dose" of the placebo.

## Choice of Control

The best control group receives no active treatment in a way that can be blinded, which for medications means receiving a placebo that is identical to active treatment. This strategy compensates for any placebo effect of the active intervention (i.e., through suggestion and other nonpharmacologic mechanisms) so that any outcome difference between study groups can be ascribed to a biologic effect.

Often, however, it is not possible or desirable to withhold all treatment. For example, in trials of statin drugs to reduce the risk of myocardial infarction in persons with known CHD, the investigators cannot ethically prohibit or discourage participants from taking medical treatments that are indicated for persons with known CHD, including aspirin and beta-blockers. It is important to consider such "co-interventions" for two reasons. First, if participants use medications or therapies (other than the study drug) that reduce the risk of developing the outcome of interest, the reduction in power means that the sample size will need to be larger or the trial longer. Second, the trial protocol must include plans to obtain data to allow statistical adjustment for differences between the groups in the rate of use of such "co-interventions" during the trial. However, adjusting for such postrandomization differences violates the intention-to-treat principle and should be viewed as a secondary or explanatory analysis (Chapter 11). Alternatively, the investigators may give a standard treatment, such as aspirin, to all participants in the trial. Although this approach reduces power, it minimizes the potential for differences in co-interventions between the groups and tests whether the new intervention improves outcome when given in addition to standard care.

For some medical conditions, there is already a standard treatment. In this case, new treatments should be evaluated by comparison with those already proven effective. These are known as **equivalence trials**. Ideally, the new treatment should have advantages—lower cost, less frequent administration, or greater safety—so that finding no difference in outcome would lead to the conclusion that one agent is superior. If the new treatment has no advantages, then demonstrating that it has an effectiveness that is similar to that of an older one may be valuable to the manufacturer of the new treatment, but the effort produces no advance in clinical care or public health.

In trials with active treatment as the control group, the challenge is to show convincingly that, if no significant difference is seen, the two treatments are equivalent. Statistical approaches involve testing whether the observed difference in outcomes between the two groups lies within some specified range (12). This may require larger sample sizes than trials that have placebo controls because the difference to be detected may be smaller.

As noted in Chapter 6, a basic problem with equivalence studies is that because the goal is to accept the null hypothesis rather than reject it, the normal strategies that reduce the likelihood of Type I errors do not have their usual effect in safeguarding the conclusions. The failure to find a statistically significant difference between active treatments in equivalence trials can result from designing a randomized trial that has too few participants, too few outcomes, or imprecise measurements of outcome.

## ■ SUMMARY

1. The criteria for **selecting study participants** should provide subjects at **high risk** of the outcome (if dichotomous), likely to **benefit and not be harmed** by treatment, easy to recruit, and likely to **adhere to treatment** and **follow-up** protocols.
2. **Baseline variables** should be measured parsimoniously (setting aside banks of serum, genetic material, and so on, for later analysis) to **describe** the participants, to **measure risk factors** and baseline values of the outcome, and to allow examination of **interactions** in which the intervention has different effects in different subgroups.
3. **Randomization,** which eliminates bias due to baseline **confounding** variables, should be tamperproof; in small trials **stratified blocked randomization** can reduce the impact of chance maldistributions of key predictors.
4. **Blinding the intervention** is as important as randomization and serves to control **co-intervention** and **ascertainment biases**.
5. The **choice of intervention** is a difficult decision that balances **effectiveness** and **safety**; other considerations include the need for **relevance** to clinical practice and the scientific utility of **single interventions** in preference to combinations.
6. Whenever possible, trials should include a comparison with a **placebo control**; the danger of comparing active treatments in an **equivalence trial** is the reversal of the normal safeguards of testing the null hypothesis.

# References

1. Colditz GA, Hankinson SE, Hunter DJ, et al. The use of estrogens and progestins and the risk of breast cancer in postmenopausal women. *N Engl J Med* 1995;332:1589–93.
2. Fisher B, Costantino JP, Wickerham DL, et al. Tamoxifen for prevention of breast cancer: report of the National Surgical Adjuvant Breast and Bowel Project P-1 Study. *J Natl Cancer Inst* 1998;90:1371–88.
3. Hulley S, Grady D, Bush T, et al. Randomized trial of estrogen plus progestin for secondary prevention of coronary heart disease in postmenopausal women. Heart and Estrogen/Progestin Replacement Study (HERS) Research Group. *JAMA* 1998; 280:605–13.
4. Design of the Women's Health Initiative clinical trial and observational study. The Women's Health Initiative Study Group. *Control Clin Trials* 1998;19:61–109.
5. Fisher B, Dignam J, Wolmark N, et al. Tamoxifen in treatment of intraductal breast cancer: National Surgical Adjuvant Breast and Bowel Project B-24 randomised controlled trial. *Lancet* 1999;353:1993–2000.
6. Cummings SR, Eckert S, Krueger KA, ct al. The effect of raloxifene on risk of breast cancer in postmenopausal women: results from the MORE randomized trial. Multiple outcomes of raloxifene evaluation. *JAMA* 1999;281:2189–97.
7. Freiman JA, Chalmers TC, Smith H, Jr, Kuebler RR. The importance of beta, the type II error and sample size in the design and interpretation of the randomized control trial. Survey of 71 "negative" trials. *N Engl J Med* 1978;299:690–4.
8. Yusuf S, Collins R, Peto R. Why do we need some large, simple randomized trials? *Stat Med* 1984;3:409–22.
9. Ettinger B, Black DM, Mitlak BH, et al. Reduction of vertebral fracture risk in postmenopausal women with osteoporosis treated with raloxifene: results from a 3-year randomized clinical trial. Multiple outcomes of raloxifene evaluation (MORE) investigators. *JAMA* 1999;282:637–45.
10. Friedman LM, DeMets DL, Furberg C. *Fundamentals of clinical trials*, 3rd ed. St. Louis: Mosby-Year Book, 1996.
11. Grady D, Applegate W, Bush T, et al. Heart and Estrogen/Progestin Replacement Study (HERS): design, methods, and baseline characteristics. *Control Clin Trials* 1998;19:314–35.
12. Hauck WW, Anderson S. A proposal for interpreting and reporting negative studies. *Stat Med* 1986;5:203–9.

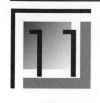

# Designing an Experiment: Clinical Trials II

## Deborah Grady, Steven R. Cummings, and Stephen B. Hulley

In the last chapter, we discussed the randomized, blinded trial: how to select participants, measure baseline variables, randomize, and apply the intervention. In this chapter, we describe how to maximize follow-up and adherence to the protocol, measure the outcome, and analyze the results. Clinical trials are very different from observational studies in that something is done to participants, and this chapter addresses the need for monitoring the results during the trial. The chapter ends by reviewing some alternatives to the classic randomized trial.

## ■ FOLLOW-UP AND ADHERENCE TO THE PROTOCOL

If a substantial number of study participants do not receive the study intervention, do not adhere to the protocol, or are lost to follow-up, the results of the trial are likely to be underpowered or biased. Strategies for **maximizing follow-up and adherence** are outlined in Table 11.1.

The effect of the intervention (and the power of the trial) is reduced to the degree that participants do not receive it. The investigator should try to choose a study drug or behavioral intervention that is easy to apply or take and is well tolerated. Adherence is likely to be poor if a behavioral intervention requires hours of practice by participants. Drugs that can be taken in a single daily dose are the easiest to remember and therefore preferable. The protocol should include provisions that will enhance adherence, such as instructing participants to take the pill at a standard point in the morning routine and giving them pill containers labeled with the day of the week.

There is also a need to consider how best to **measure adherence** to the intervention, using such approaches as self-report, pill counts, automated pill dispensers, and serum or urinary metabolite levels. This information can identify participants who are not complying, so that the investigator can help explain the finding if there is no difference between groups at the end.

Adherence to study visits and measurements can be enhanced by discussing what is involved in the study before consent is obtained, by scheduling the visits at a time that is convenient and with enough staff to prevent waiting, by calling the participant the day before each visit, and by reimbursing travel expenses and other out-of-pocket costs.

Failure to follow trial participants and measure the outcome of interest can result in biased results, diminished credibility of the findings, and decreased

■ **TABLE 11.1**

Maximizing Follow-up and Adherence to the Protocol

| Principle | Example |
|---|---|
| Choose subjects who are likely to be adherent to the intervention and protocol | Require completion of two or more comprehensive visits before randomization |
| | Exclude those who are nonadherent in a prerandomization run-in period |
| | Exclude those who are likely to move or be noncompliant |
| Make the intervention easy | Use a single tablet rather than two |
| Make study visits convenient and enjoyable | Schedule visits often enough to maintain close contact but not frequently enough to be tiresome |
| | Schedule visits at night or on weekends, or collect information by e-mail |
| | Have adequate staff to prevent waiting |
| | Provide reimbursement for travel |
| | Establish personal relationships with subjects |
| Make study measurements painless and interesting | Choose noninvasive, informative tests that are not otherwise available |
| | Provide test results of interest to participants and appropriate counseling |
| Encourage subjects to continue in the trial | Never discontinue subjects from follow-up for protocol violations, adverse events, or side effects |
| | Send participants birthday and holiday cards |
| | Send newsletters and e-mail messages |
| | Emphasize the scientific importance of adherence and follow-up |
| Find subjects who are lost to follow-up | Pursue contacts of subjects, and use a tracking service. |

statistical power. For example, a trial of nasal calcitonin spray to reduce the risk of osteoporotic fractures reported that treatment reduced fracture risk by 36% (1). However, about 60% of those randomized were lost to follow-up, and it was not known if fractures had occurred in these participants. Because the overall number of fractures was small, even a few fractures in the participants lost to follow-up could have altered the findings of the trial. This uncertainty diminished the credibility of the study findings (2).

Even if participants violate the protocol or discontinue the trial intervention, they should be followed so that their outcomes can be used in intention-to-treat analyses. In many trials, participants who violate the protocol by enrolling in another trial, discontinue the study intervention, or report adverse effects are discontinued from follow-up; this can result in biased or uninterpretable results. Consider, for example, a drug that causes a symptomatic side effect that frequently results in discontinuation of the study medication. If participants who discontinue study medication are not followed for the outcome, the rate of events in the active treatment group will be biased downward. This bias can have a serious effect on the main findings if the side effect is associated with the main outcome.

Some strategies for achieving complete **follow-up** are similar to those discussed for cohort studies (Chapter 7). At the outset of the study, participants should be informed of the importance of follow-up and investigators should record the name, address, and telephone number of one or two close acquaintances who will always know where the participant is. In addition to enhancing the investigator's ability to assess vital status, this may give him access to proxy outcome measures that can be obtained by telephone from those who absolutely refuse to come for a visit at the end. In the HERS trial, 89% of the women returned for the final clinic visit, another 8% had a final telephone contact for outcome ascertainment, and information on vital status was determined for every single participant by using phone contact, registered letters, contacts with close relatives, and a tracking service (3).

The design of the trial should make it as easy as possible for participants to adhere to the intervention and complete all follow-up visits and measurements. Long and stressful visits can deter some participants from attending. Participants are more likely to return for visits that involve noninvasive tests, such as electron beam computed tomography of the heart, than for invasive tests such as coronary angiography. Collecting follow-up information by phone or electronic means may improve adherence for participants who find visits difficult. On the other hand, participants may lose interest in a trial if there are not some social or interpersonal rewards for participation. Participants may tire of study visits that are scheduled monthly, and they may lose interest if visits only occur annually. Follow-up is also improved by making the trial experience positive and enjoyable for study participants: designing trial measurements and procedures to be painless and interesting; performing tests that would not otherwise be available; providing results of tests to participants (if the result will not influence outcomes); sending newsletters, e-mail notes of appreciation, holiday, and birthday cards; giving inexpensive gifts; and developing strong personal relationships with study staff.

Two design aspects that are specific to trials may improve adherence and follow-up: screening visits before randomization and a run-in period. Asking participants to attend one or two **screening visits** before randomization may exclude participants who find that they cannot complete such visits. The trick here is to set the hurdles for entry into the trial high enough to exclude those who will later be nonadherent, but not high enough to exclude participants who will turn out to have satisfactory adherence.

A **run-in period** may be a useful design for increasing the proportion of study participants who adhere to the intervention and follow-up procedures. During the baseline period, all participants are placed on placebo. A specified time later (usually a few weeks), those who have complied with the intervention are randomized blindly to continue taking the placebo or to begin taking the active drug. Excluding nonadherent participants before randomization in this fashion may increase the power of the study and permit a better estimate of the full effects of intervention. It is not clear, however, that a placebo run-in is more effective than the requirement that participants complete one or more screening visits before randomization.

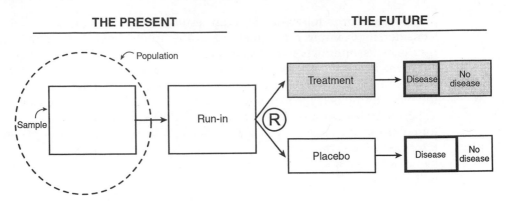

THE PRESENT                    THE FUTURE

■ **FIGURE 11.1**

In a randomized trial preceded by a run-in period to test compliance, the investigator (a) selects a sample from the population, (b) measures baseline variables, (c) randomizes the participants, (d) applies interventions, (d) follows up the cohorts, (e) measures outcome variables.

A variant of the placebo run-in design shown in Fig. 11.1 is the use of the active drug rather than the placebo for the run-in period. In addition to increasing adherence among those who enroll, an active drug run-in is designed to select participants who tolerate and respond to the intervention. The response of an intermediary variable (i.e., a surrogate that lies between the intervention and the outcome) is used as the criterion for randomization. In a trial of an antiarrhythmic drug's effect on mortality, for example, the investigator might randomize only those participants whose arrhythmias are satisfactorily suppressed without undue side effects (4). This design maximizes power by increasing the proportion of the intervention group that is responsive to the intervention. It also improves generalizability by mimicking the clinician's tendency to continue using a drug only when he sees evidence that it is working. When those who do not tolerate or do not respond to an intervention are excluded from a trial, the results may not be generalizable to those excluded.

It is also possible that the rate of adverse effects among those enrolled will underestimate the rate among all who are placed on the intervention. A trial of the effect of carvedilol on mortality in patients with congestive heart failure used a 2-week active run-in period. During the run-in, 17 people had worsening congestive heart failure and seven died (5). These people were not randomized in the trial, and these adverse effects of drug treatment were not included as outcomes.

## ■ MEASURING THE OUTCOME

In choosing the outcome measure the investigator often must balance **clinical relevance** with **feasibility** and **cost**.

### Clinical versus Surrogate Outcomes

Clinically relevant measures, such as death, myocardial infarction, hospital admission, and quality of life, are the most meaningful outcomes of trials. Surrogate markers for risk of the outcome, such as cholesterol for risk of coronary heart disease (CHD), are used when the testing of a new treatment is at a relatively early stage and when resources are too limited to permit a large study with clinical outcomes (Chapter 10). At a minimum, surrogate markers must be biologically plausible and associated with the outcome of interest; for example, bone density is commonly used as a surrogate marker for risk of fracture because the low bone density of osteoporosis has been shown to be associated with an increased risk of fracture. This does not prove, however, that treatments that cause favorable changes in the surrogate marker will produce better clinical outcomes. Distressingly, there are many instances where trials using surrogate markers for clinical outcomes have produced misleading results. For example, several studies showed that ventricular arrhythmias increase risk for death among patients with myocardial infarction. Subsequent trials also showed that certain drugs could suppress ventricular arrhythmia (the surrogate outcome). Unfortunately, the Cardiac Arrhythmia Suppression Trial (CAST) demonstrated that even though these drugs reduced the frequency of serious arrhythmia, the mortality rate was higher among treated patients (4).

## Statistical Characteristics

The outcome measure should be one that can be assessed accurately and precisely. An example of an outcome that meets these criteria is a newborn baby's weight; an example of one that does not is the presence of a congenital learning disability, a behavioral variable that represents the ill-defined end of a continuum.

Continuous outcome variables have the advantage over dichotomous ones of enhancing the power of the study, thus permitting a smaller sample size. In Chapter 6 a study with birth weight as a continuous outcome variable requires less than half the sample size needed for a study in which the outcome is the proportion of newborns who weigh less than 2,500 grams. Unfortunately, birth weight as a continuous variable is much less clinically relevant because differences in birth weight among those babies who weigh more than 2,500 grams—about 90% of all babies—may not be related to any clinical problem.

If a dichotomous outcome is unavoidable, power depends more on the number of events than on the overall number of participants (6). In the HERS trial, for example, power was not determined by the 2,763 women in the trial, but by the 348 who experienced the primary outcome—nonfatal myocardial infarction or CHD death (2). A dichotomous outcome that was more common, such as all acute coronary syndromes (nonfatal myocardial infarction, CHD death, and hospitalization for unstable angina), which occurred in 568 women, could be tested with proportionally greater power.

## Number of Outcome Variables

It is often desirable to have several outcome variables that measure different aspects of the phenomena of interest. In the HERS trial, CHD events were chosen as the primary end point. Nonfatal myocardial infarction, CHD death, revascularization, hospitalization for unstable angina and congestive heart failure, stroke and transient ischemic attack, venous thromboembolic events, and all-cause mortality were all assessed and adjudicated to provide a more detailed description of the cardiovascular effects of hormone therapy (3). However, a **single primary end point** was designated for the purpose of planning the sample size and duration of the study and to avoid the problems of interpreting tests of multiple hypotheses (Chapter 5).

## Adjudication of Outcomes

Most self-reported outcomes, such as history of stroke or a participant report of quitting smoking, are not 100% accurate. Self-reported outcomes that are important to the trial should be confirmed if possible. Occurrence of disease, such as a stroke, is generally adjudicated by (a) creating clear criteria for the outcome (new neurologic deficit with corresponding lesion on computed tomography or magnetic resonance imaging scan), (b) collecting the clinical documents needed to make the assessment (discharge summaries and radiology reports), and (c) having experts review each potential case and judge whether the criteria for the diagnosis have been met. Those who collect the information and adjudicate the cases must be blinded to the treatment assignment.

## Adverse Effects

The investigator should include outcome measures that will detect the occurrence of **adverse effects** that may result from the intervention. Revealing whether the beneficial effects of an intervention outweigh the adverse ones is a major goal of most clinical trials, even those that test apparently innocuous treatments like a health education program. Adverse effects may range from relatively minor symptoms such as rash or flulike episodes, to serious and fatal complications. The investigator should consider the problem that both the nature of the end point and the sample size requirements for detecting adverse effects may be different from those for detecting benefits. Unfortunately, rare side effects will usually be impossible to detect no matter how large the trial and are discovered (if at all) only after an intervention is in widespread clinical use.

In the early stages of testing a new treatment when potential adverse effects are unclear, investigators should ask broad, open-ended questions about all types of potential adverse effects. In large trials, assessment and coding of all potential adverse events can be very expensive and time-consuming, with a low yield of important results. Investigators should consider strategies for minimizing this burden while preserving an adequate assessment of potential harms of the intervention. For example, common events, such as respiratory infections and gastrointestinal upset, may be assessed in a subset of the participants or for a limited time. Important potential adverse events or effects that are expected because of previous research may be more accurately and efficiently assessed by specific queries. For example, since rhabdomyolysis is a reported side effect of treatment with statins, the signs and symptoms of myositis should be queried in any trial of a new statin. When data from a trial will be used to apply for approval of a new drug, the trial design must satisfy regulatory expectations for reporting adverse events. (See "Good Clinical Practices" on the U.S. FDA website.)

## ■ ANALYZING THE RESULTS

Statistical analysis of the primary hypothesis of a clinical trial is generally straightforward. If the outcome is dichotomous, the simplest approach is to compare the proportions in the study groups using a chi-squared test. When the outcome is continuous a $t$ test may be used, or a nonparametric alternative if the outcome is not normally distributed. In most clinical trials the duration of follow-up is different for each participant, necessitating the use of survival time methods. More sophisticated statistical models such as Cox proportional hazards analysis can accomplish this and at the same time adjust for chance maldistributions of baseline confounding variables. The technical details of when and how to use these methods are described elsewhere (7).

Two important issues that should be considered in the analysis of clinical trial results are the primacy of the intention-to-treat analytic approach and the ancillary role for subgroup analyses.

## Intention-to-Treat Analysis

For analysis, the investigator must decide what to do with "**cross-overs**," participants assigned to the active treatment group who do not get treatment or discontinue it and those assigned to the control group who end up getting active treatment. An analysis done by **intention-to-treat** compares outcomes between the study groups with every participant analyzed according to his randomized group assignment, regardless of whether he received the assigned intervention. Intention-to-treat analyses may underestimate the full effect of the treatment, but they guard against more important causes of biased results in clinical trials.

An alternative to intention-to-treat is to analyze only those who comply with the intervention. It is common, for example, to perform "**per protocol**" analyses that include only those participants in both groups who took more than 80% of their assigned study medication or only those who are "evaluable" (i.e., took a certain proportion of study medication, completed a certain proportion of visits, and had no other protocol violations). This seems reasonable because participants can only be affected by an intervention they actually receive. The problem arises, however, that participants who adhere to the study treatment may be different from those who drop out in ways that are related to the outcome. In the Postmenopausal Estrogen-Progestin Interventions Trial (PEPI), 875 postmenopausal women were randomly assigned to four different estrogen or estrogen plus progestin regimens and placebo (8). Among women assigned to the unopposed estrogen arm, 30% had discontinued treatment after 3 years because of endometrial hyperplasia, which is a precursor of endometrial cancer. If these women are eliminated in a per protocol analysis, an association of estrogen therapy and endometrial cancer may be missed.

The major disadvantage of the intention-to-treat approach is that participants who choose not to take the assigned intervention will nevertheless be included in the estimate of the effects of that intervention. Thus substantial discontinuation or cross-over between treatments will cause intention-to-treat analyses to underestimate the magnitude of the effect of treatment. For this reason, results of trials are often evaluated with both intention-to-treat and per protocol analyses. If both analyses produce similar results, this increases confidence in the conclusions of the trial. If they differ, results of the intention-to-treat analyses generally predominate because they preserve the value of randomization and, unlike per protocol analyses, can only bias the estimated effect in the conservative direction (favoring $H_o$). The results can only be analyzed in both ways if follow-up measures are completed regardless of whether participants adhere to treatment.

**Subgroup analyses** are defined as comparisons between randomized groups in a subset of the trial cohort. These analyses have a mixed reputation because they are easy to misuse and can lead to wrong conclusions. With proper care, however, they can provide useful ancillary information and expand the inferences that can be drawn from a clinical trial. To preserve the value of randomization, subgroups should be defined by measurements that were made before treatment was started. For example, a trial of alendronate to prevent osteoporotic fractures found that the drug decreased risk of fracture by 14% among women with low bone density. Preplanned analyses by subgroups of bone density measured at baseline revealed that the treatment was effective (36% reduction in fracture risk; $P < 0.01$) among women whose bone density was more than 2.5 standard deviations below normal. In contrast, treatment was ineffective in women with higher bone density at baseline (9). It is important to note that the value of randomization is preserved in each of the subgroups: the fracture rate among women randomized to alendronate is compared with the rate among women randomized to placebo in each subgroup—those with very low bone density (defined by measurements made before randomization) and those with higher bone density.

Subgroup analyses are prone, however, to producing misleading results for several reasons. Subgroups are, by definition, smaller than the entire trial population, and there may not be sufficient power to find important differences; investigators should avoid claiming that a drug "was ineffective" in a subgroup when the problem might reflect insufficient power to find an effect. Investigators often examine results in a large number of subgroups, increasing the likelihood of finding a different effect of the intervention in one subgroup by chance. Optimally, planned subgroup analyses should be defined before the trial begins and the number of subgroups analyzed should be reported with the results of the study. A conservative approach is to require that claims about different responses in subgroups be supported by statistical evidence that there is an interaction between treatment and the subgroup characteristic. For example, the study of alendronate found a significant interaction ($P = 0.01$) between baseline bone density and the effect of treatment on risk of fractures, supporting the conclusion that alendronate works in women with osteoporosis but not in women with higher bone density.

Subgroup analyses based on postrandomization factors do not preserve the value of randomization and often produce misleading results. Per protocol analyses limited to subjects who adhere to the randomized treatment are examples of this type of subgroup analysis.

# ■ MONITORING CLINICAL TRIALS

Why monitor a clinical trial? An important difference between clinical trials and observational studies is that in a clinical trial something is being done to the participants. For ethical reasons, investigators must assure that participants not be exposed to a harmful intervention, denied a beneficial intervention, or continued in a trial if the research question cannot possibly be answered.

The most pressing reason to monitor clinical trials is to make sure that the intervention does not turn out unexpectedly to be harmful. If the harm outweighs any benefits, the trial should be stopped. Second, if an intervention is more effective than was estimated when the trial was designed, then benefit can be observed early in the trial. When clear benefit has been proved, it may be unethical to continue the trial and delay offering the intervention to participants on placebo and to others who could benefit. Third, if there is no possibility of answering the research question, it may be unethical to continue participants in a trial that requires time and effort and that may cause some discomfort or risk. If a clinical trial is scheduled to continue for 5 years but after 4 years there is little difference in the rate of outcome events in the treated and untreated groups, then the "conditional power" (the likelihood of answering the research question given the results, thus far) becomes very small and consideration should be given to stopping the trial. In addition, because clinical trials are expensive, stopping the trial as soon as the question is answered saves money.

The research question might be answered by other trials before a given trial is finished. It is desirable to have more than one trial that provides evidence concerning a given research question, but if definitive evidence becomes available during a trial, the investigator should consider stopping.

How interim monitoring will occur should be considered in the planning of any clinical trial. Guidelines and procedures for monitoring should be detailed

---

**■ TABLE 11.2**
Monitoring a Clinical Trial

Elements to monitor
   Recruitment
   Adherence
   Randomization
   Blinding
   Follow-up
   Important variables
     Outcomes
     Adverse effects
     Potential confounders
Who will monitor
   Trial investigators if small trial with minor hazards
   Independent data monitoring board otherwise
Changes in the protocol that can result from monitoring
   Terminate the trial
   Modify the trial
     Stop one arm of the trial
     Add new measurements necessary for safety
       monitoring
     Discontinue high-risk participants
   Extend the trial in time
   Enlarge the trial sample
How often to monitor
   Often enough to meet the goals of monitoring
   Only when there is substantial new data
Statistical methods for monitoring

---

in writing before the study begins. Items to include in these guidelines are outlined in Table 11.2.

Stopping a trial should always be a carefully weighted decision that balances ethical responsibility to the participants and the advancement of scientific knowledge. Whenever a trial is stopped early, the chance to provide more conclusive results will be lost. The decision is often complex, and potential risks to participants must be weighed against possible benefits. Thus it is important that the committee that monitors the trial include physicians, participant advocates, biostatisticians, and persons experienced in conducting trials. These experts are normally outsiders who are not involved in the trial, and therefore have no personal or financial interest in its continuation.

Statistical tests of significance provide important but not conclusive information for stopping a trial. Trends over time should be evaluated for consistency, effects on related outcomes should be evaluated for consistency, and the impact of stopping the study early on the credibility of the findings should be carefully considered (Example 11.1).

There are many statistical methods for monitoring the interim results of a trial. Analyzing the results of a trial repeatedly is a form of multiple testing and thus increases the probability of a type I error. For example, if $\alpha = 0.05$ is used for each test and the results of a trial are analyzed four times during the trial and again at the end, the probability of making a type I error is increased to about 14% (14). To address this problem, statistical methods for interim monitoring generally decrease the $\alpha$ for each test ($\alpha_i$) so that the overall $\alpha = 0.05$. There are multiple approaches to deciding how to "spend $\alpha$" (Appendix 11.1).

### Example 11.1 Trials That Have Been Stopped Early

**Canadian Atrial Fibrillation Anticoagulation Study, CAFA (10):** Atrial fibrillation is a risk factor for stroke and embolic events. The CAFA study was a double-blind, randomized, placebo-controlled trial to evaluate the efficacy of warfarin in decreasing the rate of stroke, systemic embolism, or intracerebral or fatal bleeding in patients with nonrheumatic atrial fibrillation. The study was designed to enroll 660 patients and follow them on therapy for 3.5 years. During the trial (after 383 patients had been randomized and followed for a mean of 1.2 years), the results of two other randomized trials were reported showing a significant decrease in embolic events and a low rate of major bleeding events in patients with atrial fibrillation treated with warfarin. The Steering Committee of the CAFA decided that the evidence of benefit with warfarin was sufficiently compelling to stop the trial without preliminary examination of the data.

**Cardiac Arrhythmia Suppression Trial, CAST (4):** The occurrence of ventricular premature depolarizations in survivors of myocardial infarction is a risk factor for sudden death. The CAST evaluated the effect of antiarrhythmic therapy (encainide, flecainide, or moricizine) in patients with asymptomatic or mildly symptomatic ventricular arrhythmia after myocardial infarction on risk for sudden death. During an average of 10 months of follow-up, the participants treated with active drug had a higher total mortality (7.7% versus 3.0%) and a higher rate of death from arrhythmia (4.5% versus 1.5%) than those assigned to placebo. The trial was planned to continue for 5 years but was stopped after 18 months.

**Coronary Drug Project, CDP (11,12):** The CDP was a randomized, blinded trial to determine if five different cholesterol-lowering interventions (conjugated estrogen 5.0 mg/day; estrogen 2.5 mg/day; clofibrate 1.8 g/day; dextrothyroxine 6.0 mg/day; niacin 3.0 g/day) reduced the 5-year mortality rate. The CDP enrolled 8,341 men with myocardial infarction who were followed for at least 5 years. With an average of 18 months of follow-up, the high-dose estrogen arm was stopped due to an excess of nonfatal myocardial infarction (6.2% compared with 3.2%) and venous thromboembolic events (3.5% compared with 1.5%). This decision was reinforced by the fact that high-dose estrogen was also associated with testicular atrophy, gynecomastia, breast tenderness, and decreased libido. At the same time, dextrothyroxine was stopped in the subgroup of men who had demonstrated frequent premature ventricular beats on their baseline electrocardiogram because the death rate in this subgroup was 38.5% compared with 11.5% in the same subgroup receiving placebo. Dextrothyroxine therapy was stopped in all subjects shortly thereafter due to an excess mortality rate in the treated group. Two years before the planned end of the study, the 2.5-mg-dose estrogen arm was also stopped because there was no evidence of any beneficial effect and an increased risk of venous thromboembolic events among treated men.

**Physicians Health Study (13):** The Physicians Health Study was a randomized trial of the effect of aspirin (325 mg every other day) on cardiovascular mortality. The trial was stopped after 4.8 years of the planned 8-year follow-up. There was a significant reduction in myocardial infarction in the treated group (relative risk for nonfatal MI = 0.56), but the number of cardiovascular disease deaths in each group was equal. The rate of cardiovascular disease deaths observed in the study was much lower than expected (88 after 4.8 years of follow-up versus the 733 expected), and the trial was stopped because the conditional power to detect a favorable impact of aspirin therapy on cardiovascular mortality had fallen to a very low level).

# ■ ALTERNATIVES TO THE RANDOMIZED BLINDED TRIAL

## Other Randomized Designs

There are a number of variations on the classic randomized trial that may be useful when the circumstances are right.

The **factorial design** aims to answer two separate research questions in a single cohort of participants (Fig. 11.2). A good example is the Physicians' Health Study which was designed to test the effect of aspirin on myocardial infarction and of beta-carotene on cancer (15). The participants were randomly assigned to four groups, but each of the two hypotheses was tested by comparing two halves of the study cohort. First, all those on aspirin are compared with all those on aspirin placebo (disregarding the fact that half of each of these groups received beta-carotene); then all those on beta-carotene are compared with all those on beta-carotene placebo (now disregarding the fact that half of each of these groups received aspirin). The investigator has two complete trials for the price of one.

The factorial design is very efficient. The chief limitation is the possibility of interactions between the treatments and outcomes. In the example noted earlier, any influence of beta-carotene on myocardial infarction would alter the outcome for half of the participants receiving aspirin, reducing power and confusing interpretation. Factorial designs can actually be used to study such interactions, but these trials are more complicated and difficult to implement, large sample sizes are required, and the results can be hard to interpret. In clinical research, the best role for factorial designs is in studying two relatively unrelated research questions.

**Randomization of matched pairs** is a strategy for balancing baseline confounding variables that requires selecting pairs of subjects who are matched on important factors like age and sex, then randomly assigning one member of each pair to each study group. A particularly attractive version of this design can be used when the circumstances permit a contrast of treatment and control effects in two parts of the same individual at the same time. In the Diabetic Retinopathy Study, for example, each participant had one eye randomly assigned to photocoagulation treatment while the other served as a control (16).

**Group or cluster randomization** requires that the investigator randomly assign

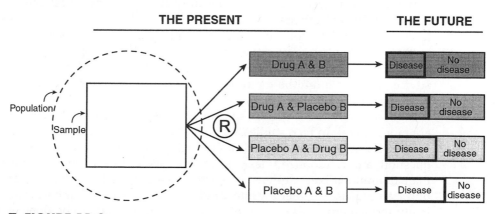

## ■ FIGURE 11.2

In a factorial randomized trial, the investigator (a) selects a sample from the population; (b) measures baseline variables; (c) randomly assigns two active interventions and their controls to four groups, as shown; (d) applies interventions; (e) follows up the cohorts; (f) measures outcome variables.

naturally occurring groups or clusters of participants to the study groups rather than assign individuals. A good example is a trial that enrolled players on 120 college baseball teams, randomly allocated half of the teams to an intervention to encourage cessation of spit-tobacco use, and observed a significantly lower rate of spit-tobacco use among players on the teams that received the intervention (17). Applying the intervention to groups of people may be more feasible and cost-effective than treating individuals one at a time, and it may better address research questions about the effects of public health programs in the population. Some interventions, such as a low-fat diet, are difficult to implement in one member of a family but not in others. Similarly, participants who receive a transferable intervention may discuss this advice with acquaintances who have been assigned to the control group. For example, a clinician in a group practice who is randomly assigned to an educational intervention is very likely to discuss this intervention with his colleagues. A disadvantage of cluster randomization is the fact that sample size estimation and analysis are more complicated (18).

## Nonrandomized Between-Group Designs

Trials that compare groups that have not been randomized are far less satisfactory than randomized trials in controlling for the influence of confounding variables. Analytic methods can adjust for baseline factors that are unequal in the two study groups, but this strategy does not deal with the problem of unmeasured confounding. Chalmers has reviewed the findings of randomized and nonrandomized studies of the same research question (19); the apparent benefits of intervention were much greater in the nonrandomized studies, even after adjusting statistically for differences in baseline variables. This and other analyses (20) indicate that the problem of confounding in nonrandomized clinical studies can be serious and that it may not be fully removed by statistical adjustment.

Sometimes subjects are allocated to the study groups by a pseudo-random mechanism. For example, every other subject (or every subject with an even hospital record number) may be assigned to the treatment group. Such designs sometimes offer logistic advantages, but the predictability of the study group assignment permits the investigator to tamper with it by manipulating the sequence or eligibility of new subjects.

Sometimes subjects are assigned to study groups by the investigator according to certain clinical criteria. For example, diabetic patients may be allocated to receive either insulin four times a day or long-acting insulin once a day according to their willingness to accept four daily injections. The problem is that those willing to take four injections per day might be more compliant with other health advice, and this might be the cause of any observed difference in the outcomes of the two treatment programs.

Nonrandomized designs are sometimes chosen in the mistaken belief that they are more ethical. In fact, studies are only ethical if they are designed well enough to have a reasonable likelihood of producing the correct answer to the research question, and randomized designs are more likely to lead to a conclusive result than nonrandomized designs. Moreover, the ethical basis for any trial is the uncertainty as to whether the intervention will be beneficial or harmful, an uncertainty termed **equipoise** that must exist if the trial needs to be done at all.

## Within-Group Designs

Designs that do not include randomization can be useful options for some types of questions (Fig. 11.3). In a **time-series design,** each participant serves as his own control to evaluate the effect of treatment. This means that innate characteris-

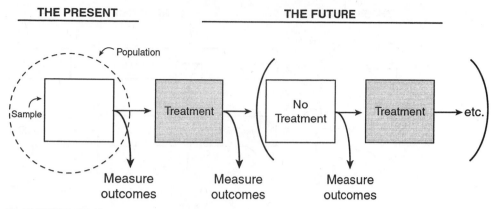

**■ FIGURE 11.3**

In a time series study, the investigator (a) selects a sample from the population, (b) measures baseline and outcome variables, (c) applies intervention to the whole cohort, (d) follows up the cohort, (e) measures outcome variables again, (f) (optional) removes intervention and measures outcome variables again.

tics such as age, sex, and genetic factors are not merely balanced (as they are in between-group studies) but actually eliminated as confounding variables.

The major disadvantage of within-group designs is the **lack of a concurrent control group.** The apparent efficacy of the intervention might be due to **learning effects** (participants do better on follow-up cognitive function tests because they learned from the baseline test), **regression to the mean** (participants who were selected for the trial because they had high blood pressure at baseline are found to have lower blood pressure at follow-up simply due to random variation in blood pressure), or **secular trends** (upper respiratory infections are less frequent at follow-up because the trial started during flu season). Within-group designs sometimes use a strategy of repeatedly starting and stopping the treatment. If repeated onset and offset of the intervention produces similar patterns in the outcome, this provides strong support that these changes are due to the treatment. This approach is only useful when the outcome variable responds rapidly and reversibly to the intervention (the effect of alcohol intake on HDL-cholesterol level, for example).

The **cross-over design** has features of both within- and between-group designs (Fig. 11.4). Half of the participants are randomly assigned to start with the control period and then switch to active treatment; the other half do the opposite. This approach (or the Latin square for more than two treatment groups) permits between-group as well as within-group analyses. The advantages of this design are substantial: It further minimizes the potential for confounding because each participant serves as his own control and substantially increases the statistical power of the trial so that it needs fewer participants. However, the disadvantages are also substantial: a doubling of the duration of the study, and the added complexity of analysis and interpretation created by the problem of **carryover effects.** A carryover effect is the residual influence of the intervention on the outcome during the period after it has been stopped. Blood pressure may not return to baseline levels for months after a course of diuretic treatment, for example. To reduce the carryover effect, the investigator can introduce an untreated **"washout"** period with the hope that the outcome variable will return to normal before starting the next intervention, but it is difficult to know whether all carryover effects have been eliminated. In general, crossover studies are only a good

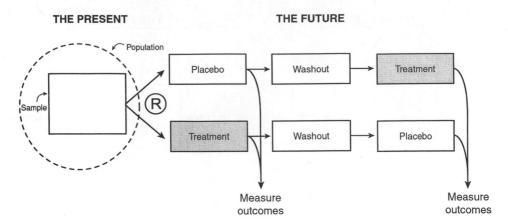

THE PRESENT                                    THE FUTURE

**■ FIGURE 11.4**

In the cross-over randomized trial, the investigator (a) selects a sample from the population, (b) measures baseline variables, (c) randomizes the participants, (d) applies interventions, (e) measures outcome variables, (f) allows washout period to reduce carryover effect, (g) applies intervention to former placebo group, (h) measures outcome variables again.

choice when the number of study subjects is limited and carryover effects are judged not to be a problem.

# ■ TRIALS FOR FDA APPROVAL OF NEW THERAPIES

Many trials are done to test the effectiveness and safety of new treatments that might be considered for approval by the U.S. Food and Drug Administration (FDA) or another national regulatory body for marketing. Trials are also done to determine whether drugs that have FDA approval for one condition might be approved for the treatment or prevention of other conditions.

The FDA publishes detailed and updated guidelines for how such trials should be conducted. (Search for "FDA" on the Web.) Guidelines also cover European and international regulations for approval (called International Committee on Harmonization [ICH] guidelines, which can be found on the Web). It is wise for investigators who conduct these trials to seek specific training in "**Good Clinical Practices**," which are guidelines available on the FDA Web site for the conduct of clinical trials by investigators and staff who enroll and treat participants.

Trials of new treatments are generally described by stage. This system refers to an orderly progression in the testing of a new treatment, from experiments in animals (**preclinical**) and initial unblinded and uncontrolled administration to a few human volunteers to test the safety of the treatment (**phase I**), to relatively small randomized blinded trials that test the effect of a range of doses on side effects and surrogate measurements of the clinical outcome that is the target of the treatment (**phase II**), to randomized trials large enough to test the hypothesis that the treatment improves the targeted condition (such as blood pressure) or reduces the risk of disease (such as stroke) with acceptable safety (**phase III**) (Table 11.3). **Phase IV** refers to large studies (which may or may not be randomized trials) conducted after a drug is approved. These studies are often conducted (and financed) by marketing departments of pharmaceutical companies with the goals

**■ TABLE 11.3**
Stages in Testing New Therapies

| Preclinical | Studies in Cell Culture and Animals |
|---|---|
| Phase I | Unblinded, uncontrolled studies in a few volunteers to test safety |
| Phase II | Relatively small randomized, controlled, blinded trials to test tolerability and different intensity or dose of the intervention on surrogate outcomes |
| Phase III | Relatively large randomized, controlled, blinded trials to test the effect of the therapy on clinical outcomes |
| Phase IV | Large trials or observational studies conducted after the therapy has been approved by the FDA to assess the rate of serious side effects and evaluate additional therapeutic uses |

of assessing the rate of serious side effects when used in very large populations and identifying additional uses of the drug that might be approved by the FDA.

# ■ DECIDING TO DO A TRIAL

In general, research questions should be answered with randomized trials if feasible. The major advantage of a randomized trial is its potential for controlling the influence of confounding variables, thus providing more conclusive answers. For some research questions, a trial may be faster and less expensive than observational studies, particularly when the outcome variable is continuous and responds rapidly to the intervention. For example, it is difficult to demonstrate the relationship between dietary fat and serum cholesterol in an observational study (because of errors in measuring in the dietary variable) but relatively easy to do so in a trial. For some research questions a trial is clearly necessary to control for confounding and to make sure that the benefit outweighs the risk. For example, observational studies have consistently found that people who take beta-carotene have a lower risk of cancer, but four large clinical trials have failed to find a benefit (21); the findings of the observational studies may be due to confounding because people who take vitamins may be more health conscious than those who do not.

However, trials are usually time-consuming and expensive, and often expose participants to discomfort or risk. Therefore they should not be performed until enough is known about the intervention to suggest that a definitive trial is possible. Such information includes definition of the *exact* intervention (therapy, counseling, surgical procedure, or drug dose, duration, and route), the likely benefit of the intervention (to allow estimation of sample size and duration of the trial), and the likely adverse effects of the intervention (to allow adequate safety protection for participants). A clinical trial should not be undertaken when, because of the absence of randomization, blinding, or sufficient numbers of participants, it is unlikely to provide a conclusive answer.

# ■ SUMMARY

1. If a substantial number of study participants **do not receive** the study intervention, **do not adhere** to the protocol, or are **lost to follow-up,** the results of the trial are likely to be underpowered, biased, or uninterpretable.

2. **Clinically relevant measures,** such as death, myocardial infarction, hospital admission, and quality of life, are the most meaningful outcomes of trials. To the extent possible, the investigator should include outcome measures that will detect the occurrence of **adverse effects** that may result from the intervention.

3. **Intention-to-treat** analyses are the primary approach to take advantage of the control over confounding provided by randomization. **Per protocol** analyses, a secondary approach that provides an estimate of the effect size in adherent subjects, should be interpreted with caution.

4. With proper care, **subgroup analyses** can provide useful ancillary information and expand the inferences that can be drawn from a clinical trial. To preserve the value of randomization, subgroups should be defined by measurements that were made before treatment was started, and analyses should compare outcomes between subsets of randomly assigned study groups.

5. An important difference between clinical trials and observational studies is that in a clinical trial, *something is being done to the participants.* **Interim monitoring** during a trial should make sure that participants are not exposed to a harmful intervention, denied a beneficial intervention, or continued in a trial if the research question cannot possibly be answered.

6. There are several variations on the randomized trial design that can substantially increase efficiency under the right circumstances:
   a. The **factorial design** allows two independent trials to be carried out for the price of one.
   b. **Matched-pair** randomization balances baseline confounding variables.
   c. **Group randomization** permits efficient studies of naturally occurring clusters.
   d. **Time-series designs** have a single (non-randomized) group with outcomes compared within each subject during periods of different interventions.
   e. **Cross-over designs** may control for confounding and minimize the required sample size if carryover effects are not a problem.

# EXERCISES

> **1. a.** Continuing with the research question, "Does mild vitamin D deficiency cause hip fractures in the elderly," briefly outline an **experiment** designed to answer the question. Contrast the advantages and disadvantages of the experimental approach compared with observational designs.
>    **b.** List some strategies for making your experiment more cost-effective.
>    **c.** There is evidence that if vitamin D has an effect on hip fractures, it may do so by improving muscle strength. What ideas does this give you for designing a more effective study?

# References

1. Chestnut CH, Silverman S, Andriano K, et al. A randomized trial of nasal spray salmon calcitonin in postmenopausal women with established osteoporosis: the PROOF study. *Am J Med*, in press.

2. Cummings S, Chapurlat R. What PROOF proves about calcitonin and clinical trials. *Am J Med*, in press.

3. Hulley S, Grady D, Bush T, et al. Randomized trial of estrogen plus progestin for secondary prevention of coronary heart disease in postmenopausal women. *JAMA* 1998;280:605–13.

4. Preliminary report: effect of encainide and flecainide on mortality in a randomized trial of arrhythmia suppression after myocardial infarction. The Cardiac Arrhythmia Suppression Trial (CAST) Investigators. *N Engl J Med* 1989;321:406–12.

5. Pfeffer M, Stevenson L. Beta-adrenergic blockers and survival in heart failure. *N Engl J Med* 1996;334:1396–7.

6. Yusuf S, Collins R, Peto R. Why do we need some large, simple randomized trials? *Stat Med* 1984;3:409–20.

7. Friedman LM, DeMets DL, Furberg C. *Fundamentals of clinical trials*, 3rd ed. St. Louis: Mosby-Year Book, 1996.

8. Writing Group for the PEPI Trial. Effects of estrogen or estrogen/progestin regimens on heart disease risk factors in postmenopausal women. *JAMA* 1995;273:199–208.

9. Cummings S, Black D, Thompson D, et al. Effect of alendronate on risk of fracture in women with low bone density but without vertebral fractures: results from the Fracture Intervention Trial. *JAMA* 1998;280:2077–82.

10. Laupacis A, Connolly SJ, Gent M, et al. How should results from completed studies influence ongoing clinical trials? The CAFA Study experience. *Ann Intern Med* 1991;115:818–22.

11. The Coronary Drug Project. Initial findings leading to modifications of its research protocol. *JAMA* 1970;214:1303–13.

12. The Coronary Drug Project. Findings leading to discontinuation of the 2.5-mg day estrogen group. The coronary Drug Project Research Group. *JAMA* 1973;226:652–7.

13. Findings from the aspirin component of the ongoing Physicians' Health Study. *N Engl J Med* 1988;318:262–4.

14. Armitage P, McPherson C, Rowe B. Repeated significance tests on accumulating data. *J R Stat Soc* 1969;132A:235–44.

15. Hennekens C, Eberlein K. A randomized trial of aspirin and beta-carotene among U.S. physicians. *Prev Med* 1985;14:165–8.

16. Diabetic Retinopathy Study Research Group. Preliminary report on effects of photocoagulation therapy. *Am J Ophthalmol* 1976;81:383–96.

17. Walsh M, Hilton J, Masouredis C, et al. Smokeless tobacco cessation intervention for college athletes: results after 1 year. *Am J Pub Health* 1999;89:228–34.

18. Donner A, Birkett N, Buck C. Randomization by cluster: sample size requirements and analysis. *Am J Epidemiol* 1981;114:906–14.

19. Chalmers T, Celano P, Sacks H, et al. Bias in treatment assignment in controlled clinical trials. *N Engl J Med* 1983;309:1358–61.

20. Pocock S. Current issues in the design and interpretation of clinical trials. *Br Med J* 1985;296:39–42.

21. Marshall J. Beta-carotene: a miss for epidemiology. *J Natl Cancer Inst* 1999;91:2068–9.

# ■ APPENDIX 11.1 Interim Monitoring of Trial Outcomes

Interim monitoring of trial results is a form of multiple testing, and thus increases the probability of a type I error. To address this problem, $\alpha$ for each test ($\alpha_i$) is generally decreased so that the overall $\alpha = 0.05$. There are multiple statistical methods for decreasing $\alpha$.

One of the easiest to understand is the Bonferroni method, where $\alpha_i = \alpha/N$ if $N$ is the total number of tests performed. For example, if the overall $\alpha$ is 0.05 and five tests will be performed, $\alpha_i$ for each test is 0.01. This method has several disadvantages, however. It requires using an equal threshold for stopping the trial at any interim analysis. Most investigators would rather use a lower threshold for stopping a trial earlier rather than later and the Bonferroni approach results in a very low $\alpha$ for the final analysis. In addition, this approach is too conservative because it assumes that each test is independent. For these reasons, Bonferroni is not generally used.

A commonly used method suggested by O'Brien and Fleming (1) uses a very small initial $\alpha_i$, then gradually increases it such that $\alpha_i$ for the final test is close to the overall $\alpha$. O'Brien-Fleming provide methods for calculating $\alpha_i$ if the investigator chooses the number of tests to be done and the overall $\alpha$. At each test, $Z_i = Z^* (N_i)^{1/2}$, where $Z_i = Z$ value for the $i$th test; $Z^*$ is determined so as to achieve the overall significance level; $N$ is the total number of tests planned and $i$ is the $i$th test. For example, for five tests and overall $\alpha = 0.05$, $Z^* = 2.04$; the initial $\alpha = 0.00001$ and the final $\alpha_5 = 0.046$. This method is unlikely to lead to stopping a trial very early unless there is a striking difference in outcome between randomized groups (as was the case in CAST [4]). In addition, this method avoids the awkward situation of getting to the end of a trial and accepting the null hypothesis even though the $P$ value is substantially less than 0.05.

A major drawback to the preceding methods is that the number of tests and the proportion of data to be tested must be decided before the trial starts. In some trials, additional interim tests are necessary when important trends occur. Lan and DeMets (2) developed a method using a specified $\alpha$-spending function that provides continuous stopping boundaries. The $\alpha_i$ at a particular time (or after a certain proportion of outcomes) is determined by the function and by the number of previous "looks." Using this method, neither the number of "looks" nor the proportion of data to be analyzed at each "look" must be specified before the trial. Of course, for each additional interim analysis conducted, the final $\alpha$ is lower.

A different set of statistical methods based on curtailed sampling techniques suggests termination of a trial if future data are unlikely to change the conclusion. The multiple testing problem is irrelevant because the decision is based only on estimation of what the data will show at the end of the trial. A common approach is to compute the conditional probability of rejecting the null hypothesis at the end of the trial, based on the accumulated data. First, conditional power is calculated assuming that $H_o$ is true (i.e., that any future outcomes in the treated and control groups will be equally distributed). Second, $H_a$ is assumed to be true (i.e., that outcomes will be distributed unequally in the treatment and control groups). The effect size is usually assumed to be the same as that used to calculate the sample size but it can be made somewhat more extreme. If the conditional power to reject the null hypothesis under either of these two assumptions is low, the null hypothesis is not likely to be rejected and the trial might be stopped.

# References

1. O'Brien P, Fleming T. A multiple testing procedure for clinical trials. *Biometrics* 1979;35:549–56.
2. DeMets D, Lan G. The alpha spending function approach to interim data analyses. *Cancer Treat Res* 1995;75:1–27.

# Designing Studies of Medical Tests

## Thomas B. Newman, Warren S. Browner, and Steven R. Cummings

**M**edical tests, such as those performed to screen for a risk factor, diagnose a disease, or estimate a patient's prognosis, are a key subject for clinical research because they are an important and costly part of health care. The study designs discussed in this chapter can be used when studying whether, or in whom, a particular test should be done.

Although clinical trials are occasionally feasible, most designs for studies of medical tests are descriptive and resemble the observational designs in Chapters 7 and 8. There are, however, some important differences. The goal of most observational studies is to identify causal relations (e.g., whether estrogen use causes breast cancer). By contrast, a study of a diagnostic test seeks to determine whether that test is useful in clinical practice. (Causality is generally irrelevant.) As a result, testing for statistical significance plays a small role in the analysis of studies of diagnostic tests, because knowing a test performs better than would be expected by chance alone is not nearly enough to determine its usefulness. Instead, **descriptive statistics** (and associated confidence intervals [CIs]) describing sensitivity, specificity, and other aspects of test performance are used. In this chapter, we review these statistics and other special issues that pertain to studies of medical tests.

## ■ DETERMINING WHETHER A TEST IS USEFUL

For a test to be useful it must pass muster on a series of increasingly difficult questions that address its reproducibility, accuracy, feasibility, and effects on clinical decisions and outcomes (Table 12.1). Favorable answers to each of these questions are necessary but insufficient criteria for a test to be worth doing. For example, if a test does not give consistent results when performed by different people or in different places, it can hardly be useful. If the test seldom supplies new information and hence seldom affects clinical decisions, it may not be worth doing. Even if it affects decisions, if these decisions do not improve the clinical outcome of patients who were tested, the test still may not be useful.

Of course, if using a test improves outcome, favorable answers to the other questions can be inferred. However, demonstrating that doing a test improves outcome is impractical for most diagnostic tests. Instead, the potential effects of a test on clinical outcomes are usually assessed indirectly, by demonstrating that the test increases the likelihood of making the correct diagnosis or is safer or less costly than existing tests. When developing a new diagnostic or prognostic test, it may be worthwhile considering what aspects of current practice are most in need

■ **TABLE 12.1**

Questions to Determine Usefulness of a Medical Test, Possible Designs to Answer Them, and Statistics for Reporting Results

| Question | Possible Designs | Statistics for Results* |
|---|---|---|
| How reproducible is the test? | Studies of intra- and interobserver and intra- and interlaboratory variability | Proportion agreement, kappa, coefficient of variation, mean and distribution of differences (avoid correlation coefficient) |
| How accurate is the test? | Cross-sectional, case control, or cohort-type designs in which test result is compared with a ``gold standard'' | Sensitivity, specificity, positive and negative predictive value, ROC curves, and likelihood ratios |
| How often do test results affect clinical decisions? | Diagnostic yield studies, studies of pre- and posttest clinical decision making | Proportion abnormal, proportion with discordant results, proportion of tests leading to changes in clinical decisions; cost per abnormal result or per decision change |
| What are the costs, risks, and acceptability of the test? | Prospective or retrospective studies | Mean costs, proportions experiencing adverse effects, proportions willing to undergo the test |
| Does doing the test improve clinical outcome or have adverse effects? | Randomized trials, cohort or case-control studies in which the predictor variable is receiving the test and the outcome includes morbidity, mortality, or costs related either to the disease or to its treatment | Risk ratios, odds ratios, hazard ratios, number needed to treat, rates and ratios of desirable and undesirable outcomes |

*Most statistics in this table should be presented with confidence intervals.

of improvement. Are current tests unreliable, expensive, dangerous, or difficult to perform?

## Common Issues for Studies of Medical Tests

***Spectrum of Disease Severity and Test Results***    Most studies of diagnostic tests are primarily descriptive rather than analytic. Since the goal is to draw inferences about populations by making measurements on samples, the way the sample is selected has a major effect on the validity of the inferences. **Spectrum bias** occurs when the spectrum of disease (or nondisease) in the sample differs from that of the population to which the investigator wishes to generalize. This can occur if the sample of patients with disease has more severe disease or the controls without the disease are healthier than those to whom the test will be applied in practice. Any test can perform well if the task is to distinguish between the very sick and the very well. It is more difficult to distinguish between one disease and another that can cause similar symptoms, or between the healthy and those with early, presymptomatic disease. The subjects in a study of a diagnostic test should have a spectrum of disease that reflects the anticipated clinical use of the test.

Spectrum bias can occur from an inappropriate spectrum of test results as well as an inappropriate spectrum of disease. For example, consider a study of interobserver agreement among radiologists reading mammograms. If they are asked to classify the films as normal or abnormal, their agreement will be much higher if most of the "positive" films that they examine are clearly abnormal and most of the "negative" films have no suspicious abnormalities.

***Sources of Variation, Generalizability, and the Sampling Scheme.***   For some research questions the main source of variation is between patients. For example, some infants with bacteremia will have an elevated white blood cell count, whereas others will not. The proportion of bacteremic infants with high white blood cell counts is not expected to vary much according to who draws the blood or what laboratory measures it. On the other hand, for many tests the results may depend on the person doing or interpreting them, or the setting in which they are done. For example, sensitivity, specificity, and interrater reliability for interpreting mammograms depend on the readers' skill and experience as well as the quality of the equipment. Sampling those who do and interpret the test can enhance the generalizability of studies of tests that require technical or interpretive skill. When accuracy or costs may vary from institution to institution, the investigators will need to sample several different institutions to obtain a generalizable result.

***Importance of Blinding.***   Many studies of diagnostic tests involve judgments, such as whether to consider a test result positive, or whether a person has a particular disease. Whenever possible, investigators should blind those interpreting test results from other information about the patient being tested. In a study of the value of ultrasonography to diagnose appendicitis, for example, those reading the sonograms should not know the results of the history and physical examination. Similarly, those making the final determination of who does and does not have appendicitis (the gold standard to which sonogram results will be compared) should not know the results of the ultrasound examination. Blinding prevents biases, preconceptions, and information from sources other than the test from affecting these judgments.

## ■ STUDIES OF TEST REPRODUCIBILITY

Sometimes the results of tests vary according to when or where they were done or who did them. **Intraobserver variability** describes the lack of reproducibility in results when the same observer or laboratory performs the test at different times. For example, if a radiologist is shown the same chest radiograph on two occasions, what proportion of the time will he agree with himself on the interpretation? **Interobserver variability** describes the lack of reproducibility among two or more observers: If another radiologist is shown the same film, how likely is he to agree with the first radiologist?

Studies of reproducibility are important for identifying tests or observers that need improvement. When reproducibility is poor—because either intra- or interobserver variability is large—a diagnostic test is unlikely to be useful. Studies of reproducibility do not require a gold standard, so they can be done for tests or diseases where none exists. Of course, both (or all) observers can agree with one another and still be wrong. Thus intra- and interobserver reproducibility address precision, not accuracy (Chapter 4).

## Designs

A cross-sectional design is used to compare test results from more than one observer or on more than one occasion from a sample of patients or specimens. Many diagnostic tests have several steps, differences in any one of which might give different results. For example, showing that several pathologists agree about the interpretation of a set of cervical cytology slides may overestimate the overall reproducibility of the test because the variability in how the sample was obtained and how the slide was prepared was not taken into account. The investigator should lay out the exact process for obtaining the test result in the operations manual (Chapters 4 and 17) and then describe it in the methods section when reporting the study results.

The extent to which an investigator needs to isolate the steps that might lead to interobserver disagreement depends partly on the goals of his study. Most studies should estimate the reproducibility of the entire testing process, since this is what determines whether the test is worth using. On the other hand, an investigator who is developing or improving a test may want to focus on the specific steps at which variability occurs, to improve the process.

## Analysis

***Categorical Variables.***     The simplest measure of interobserver agreement is the proportion of observations on which the observers agree exactly, sometimes called the **concordance rate.** However, when there are more than two categories or the observations are not evenly distributed among the categories (e.g., when the proportion "abnormal" on a dichotomous test is much different from 50%), the concordance rate can be hard to interpret, because it does not account for agreement that would be expected by chance alone. A better measure of interobserver agreement, called **kappa** ($\kappa$) (Appendix 12.1), measures the extent of agreement beyond what would be expected by chance alone. Kappa ranges from $-1$ (perfect disagreement) to 1 (perfect agreement). A kappa of 0 indicates that the amount of agreement was exactly that expected by chance.

***Continuous Variables.***     Measures of interobserver variability for continuous variables depend on the design of the study. Some studies measure the agreement between just two machines or methods (e.g., temperatures obtained from two different thermometers). The best way to describe the data from such a study is to report the mean difference between the paired measurements and the distribution of the differences, perhaps indicating the proportion of time that the difference is clinically important. For example, if a clinically important difference in temperature is thought to be 0.5° centigrade, a study comparing temperatures from tympanic and rectal thermometers could estimate the mean difference between the two (e.g., 0.1°) and how often the two measurements differed by more than 0.5°.*

---

*Although commonly used, the correlation coefficient is best avoided in studies of the reliability of laboratory tests because it is highly influenced by outlying values and does not allow readers to determine how frequently differences between the two measurements are clinically important. CIs for the mean difference should also be avoided because their dependence on sample size makes them potentially misleading. A narrow CI for the mean difference between the two measurements does not imply that they generally closely agree—only that the mean difference between them is being measured precisely. For more extensive reading on this issue, see Bland and Altman (1a).

Other studies examine interobserver or interinstrument variability of a large group of different technicians, laboratories, or machines. These results are commonly summarized using the **coefficient of variation,** which is the standard deviation of the results on a single specimen divided by their mean, expressed as a percentage. If the results are normally distributed (i.e., if a histogram with results on the same specimen would be bell shaped), then about 95% of the results on different machines will be within two standard deviations of the mean. For example, given a coefficient of variation of a serum cholesterol measurement of 2% (1), the standard deviation of multiple measurements with a mean of 200 mg/dL would be about 4 mg/dL and about 95% of laboratories would be expected to report a value between 192 and 208 mg/dL.

# ■ STUDIES OF THE ACCURACY OF TESTS

Studies in this section all address the question, "To what extent does the test give the right answer?" To be able to answer this question, there needs to be a way to tell what the right answer is. Some diseases have a gold standard, such as the results of a tissue biopsy, that is generally accepted to indicate the presence (or absence) of that disease. (Even histologic examination, however, is not perfect; there can be sampling error, inadequate preparation of the tissue, or misdiagnosis.) Other diseases have "definitional" gold standards, such as when coronary artery disease is defined as a 50% obstruction of at least one major coronary artery as seen with coronary angiography. Still others, such as rheumatologic diseases, require that a patient have a minimum number of signs, symptoms, or specific laboratory abnormalities to meet the criteria for having the disease. Of course the accuracy of any signs, symptoms, or laboratory tests used to diagnose a disease cannot be studied if they are part of the criteria for the diagnosis. Finally, as discussed later, sometimes for practical reasons the gold standard for nondisease cannot be the same as the gold standard for disease. The investigator designing a study of test accuracy must assure himself that he has chosen standards that will be acceptable to other investigators and clinicians in the field.

## Designs

***Sampling.***    Studies of diagnostic tests can have designs analogous to case-control or cross-sectional studies, whereas studies of prognostic tests usually resemble cohort studies. In the case-control design, those with and without the disease are sampled separately and the test results in the two groups are compared. Unfortunately, it is often hard to reproduce a clinically realistic spectrum of the disease and absence of the disease in the two samples. Those with the disease should not have progressed to severe stages that are relatively easy to diagnose. Controls should be patients who had symptoms consistent with a particular disease and who turned out not to have it. Case-control studies are also subject to bias in the measurement of the predictor variable, since its measurement necessarily comes after the measurement of the outcome (Chapter 8). Thus case-control sampling for diagnostic tests should be reserved for rare diseases for which no other sampling scheme is feasible.

A cross-sectional sampling scheme generally will yield more valid and interpretable results. For example, Falahati et al. (2) studied consecutive patients evaluated for acute myocardial infarction (MI) to determine the value of serum troponin-I levels for diagnosis. Because the patients were enrolled before it was known whether or not they were having an MI, the spectrum of patients in this study should be reasonably representative of patients who present to emergency rooms with a possible MI.

A variant of the cross-sectional sampling scheme that we call **tandem testing** is sometimes used to compare two (presumably imperfect) tests with one another. Both tests are done on a representative sample of patients that may or may not have the disease and the gold standard is selectively applied to the patients with discrepant or positive results on either test. This design thus allows the investigator to determine which test is more accurate without having to apply a gold standard to all the subjects with negative test results. To obtain estimates of sensitivity and specificity, however, the gold standard must also be applied to at least a random sample of patients with concordant negative results. This design has been used in studies comparing different cervical cytology methods (3).

Prognostic test studies require either prospective or retrospective cohort designs. In prospective cohort studies, the test is done at baseline, and the subjects are then followed to see who develops the outcome of interest. A retrospective cohort study may be possible if a new test becomes available, such as viral load in HIV-positive patients, and a previously defined cohort with banked blood samples is available. Then the viral load can be measured in the stored serum, to see whether it affects prognosis. The nested case-control design (Chapter 7) is particularly attractive if the outcome of interest is rare and the test is expensive.

***Predictor Variables: The Test Result.*** Although it is simplest to think of the results of a diagnostic test as being either positive or negative, many tests have categorical or continuous results. Whenever possible, investigators should use ordinal or continuous results to take advantage of all available information in the test. Most tests are more indicative of disease if they are very abnormal than if they are slightly abnormal, and most have a borderline range in which they do not provide much information.

***Outcome Variables: The Disease (or Its Outcome).*** The outcome variable in a diagnostic test study is often the presence or absence of the disease, best determined with a gold standard. Wherever possible, the assessment of outcome should not be influenced by the results of the diagnostic test being studied. This is best accomplished by blinding those applying the gold standard to the results of the test.

Sometimes uniform application of the gold standard is not ethical or feasible for studies of diagnostic tests, particularly screening tests. For example, Kerlikowske et al. studied test characteristics of mammography (4). Women with positive mammograms were referred for further tests, eventually with the "gold standard" of pathologic evaluation. However, it was not reasonable to do biopsies in women whose mammograms were negative. Instead the authors linked their data with a local tumor registry and determined whether or not breast cancer was diagnosed in the 3 years following mammography as the gold standard. This solution illustrates that some studies of tests are hybrids between diagnostic and prognostic test studies: If the test result is positive, the gold standard is applied soon, allowing one to say whether the test was truly or falsely positive. But if the test is negative, the patient is followed forward in time to see how well the test predicts something that will happen in the future.

Prognostic tests are studied in patients who already have the disease. The outcome is what happens to them, such as how long they live, what complications they develop, or what additional treatments they require. Again, blinding is important, especially for subjective outcomes. Consider a study of how well the change in oxygen saturation in the first hour predicts the need for subsequent hospital admission in patients with asthma. If those making the decision to admit are aware of this change, it may influence the admission decision, leading to a circular situation in which the true need for admission cannot be determined.

## Analysis

***Sensitivity and Specificity.***    When results of a dichotomous test are compared with a gold standard, the results can be summarized by the sensitivity and specificity of the test. The sensitivity is defined as the proportion of subjects with the disease in whom the test gives the right answer (i.e., is positive), whereas the specificity is the proportion of subjects without the disease in whom the test gives the right answer (i.e., is negative).

***ROC Curves.***    Many diagnostic tests yield ordinal or continuous results. With such tests, several values of sensitivity and specificity are possible, depending on the cutoff point chosen to define a positive test. This trade-off between sensitivity and specificity can be displayed using a graphic technique originally developed in electronics: receiver operator characteristic (ROC) curves. The investigator selects several cutoff points and determines the sensitivity and specificity at each point. He then graphs the sensitivity (or true-positive rate) on the $Y$-axis as a function of 1-specificity (the false-positive rate) on the $X$-axis. An ideal test is one that reaches the upper left corner of the graph (100% true positives and no false positives). A worthless test follows the diagonal from the lower left to the upper right corners: at any cutoff the true-positive rate is the same as the false-positive rate (Fig. 12.1). The area under the ROC curve, which thus ranges from 0.5 for a useless test to 1.0 for a perfect test, is a useful summary of the overall accuracy of a test and can be used to compare the accuracy of two or more tests.

***Likelihood Ratios.***    Although the information in a diagnostic test with continuous or ordinal results can be summarized using sensitivity and specificity or ROC curves, there is a better way. Likelihood ratios allow the investigator to take advantage of all information in a test. For each test result, the likelihood ratio is the ratio of likelihood of that result in someone with the disease to the likelihood of that result in someone who does not have it:*

$$\text{Likelihood ratio} = P\ (\text{Result}|\text{Disease})^\dagger / P\ (\text{Result}|\text{No disease})$$

The basic idea of likelihood ratios is that unless a test is perfectly accurate,

---

*For dichotomous tests the likelihood ratio for a positive test is sensitivity/(1 − specificity) and the likelihood ratio for a negative test is (1 − sensitivity/specificity). Detailed discussions of how to use likelihood ratios and prior information (the prior probability of disease) to estimate a patient's probability of disease after knowing the test result (the posterior probability) are available in standard clinical epidemiology texts (5–7). The formula is Prior odds × Likelihood Ratio = Posterior odds, where prior and posterior odds are related to their respective probabilities by odds = $P/(1 − P)$.
†The $P$ is read as "probability of" and the "|" is read as "given." Thus $P$ (Result|Disease) is the probability of result given disease, and $P$ (Result|No Disease) is the probability of that result given no disease. The likelihood ratio is a ratio of these two probabilities.

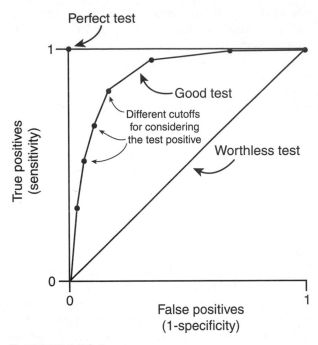

**■ FIGURE 12.1**
ROC curves for perfect, good, and worthless tests.

knowing the test result does not tell us whether or not the person tested has the disease. Instead we look at the test result and think, "How much more likely is that result to occur in someone with the disease than in someone without the disease?" If the result is one that commonly occurs in patients with the disease but is rare in those without the disease, the test has provided quite a bit of information to suggest that the patient has the disease. We combine that information with what we knew before to make our best estimate of the probability that the patient has the disease.

The higher the likelihood ratio, the better the test result for ruling in a diagnosis; a likelihood ratio greater than 100 is very high (and very unusual among tests). On the other hand, the lower a likelihood ratio (the closer it is to 0), the better the test result is for ruling out the disease. A likelihood ratio of 1 provides no information at all about the likelihood of disease.

An example of how to calculate likelihood ratios is shown in Table 12.2, results of a study that examined how well the white blood cell count predicted bacteremia or bacterial meningitis in young, febrile infants (8). A white blood cell count that is either less than 5,000 cells/mm³ or at least 15,000 cells/mm³ was more common among infants with bacteremia or meningitis than among other infants. The calculation of likelihood ratios simply quantifies this: 8% of the infants with bacteremia or bacterial meningitis had less than 5,000 cells/mm³, whereas only 4% of those without bacteremia or meningitis did. Thus the likelihood ratio is 8%/4% = 2. Similarly, the likelihood ratio for a white blood cell count between 10,000 and 14,999 cells/mm³ is 12%/36% ≃ 0.3.

***Relative Risks and Risk Differences.***    The analysis of studies of prognostic tests or risk factors for disease is similar to that of other cohort studies. If everyone

■ **TABLE 12.2**

Example of Calculation of Likelihood Ratios from a Study of Predictors of Bacterial Meningitis or Bacteremia Among Young Febrile Infants

| White Blood Cell Count (per mm³) | Meningitis or Bacteremia | | Likelihood Ratio |
|---|---|---|---|
| | Yes | No | |
| <5,000 | 5 | 96 | |
| | 8% | 4% | 2.0 |
| 5,000–9,999 | 18 | 854 | |
| | 29% | 39% | 0.7 |
| 10,000–14,999 | 8 | 790 | |
| | 12% | 36% | 0.3 |
| 15,000–19,999 | 17 | 286 | |
| | 27% | 13% | 2.1 |
| ≥20,000 | 15 | 151 | |
| | 24% | 7% | 3.4 |
| Total | 63 | 2,177 | |
| | 100% | 100% | |

in a prognostic test study is followed for a set period of time (say 3 years) with few losses to follow-up, then the results can be summarized with relative risks and risk differences. On the other hand, when the study subjects are followed for varying lengths of time, a survival-analysis technique that accounts for the length of follow-up time is preferable (9).

If follow-up is of short duration, as in survival to hospital discharge, results are sometimes summarized using sensitivity and specificity. Generally, however, sensitivity and specificity are not the best way to summarize results of prognostic test studies because they describe the test's ability to predict disease prevalence rather than incidence (Chapter 8).

# ■ STUDIES OF THE EFFECT OF TEST RESULTS ON CLINICAL DECISIONS

A test may be accurate, but if the disease is very rare, the test may be so seldom positive that it is not worth doing in most situations. Another diagnostic test may be positive more often but not affect clinical decisions because it does not provide new information beyond what was already known from the medical history, physical examination, or other tests. The study designs in this section address the yield of diagnostic tests and their effects on clinical decisions.

## Designs

***Diagnostic Yield Studies.*** Diagnostic yield studies address such questions as the following:

■ When a test is ordered for a particular indication, how often is it abnormal?

■ Can a test result be predicted from other information available at the time of testing?

■ What happens to patients with abnormal results? Do they appear to benefit?

Diagnostic yield studies estimate the proportion of positive tests among patients with a particular indication for the test. It is often reasonable to assume that (a) patients in whom a test is ordered are more likely to have a positive result than those in whom the test is not ordered and (b) those with negative results do not benefit (i.e., because their management is not changed). In these circumstances, if the observed yield of positive results on a test is sufficiently low, one can conclude that the test is unlikely to be useful in that situation.

For example, Siegel et al. (10) studied the yield of stool cultures in hospitalized patients with diarrhea. Although not all patients with diarrhea receive stool cultures, it seems reasonable to assume that those who do are, if anything, more likely to have a positive culture than those who do not. Overall, only 40 (2%) of 1,964 stool cultures were positive. Moreover, none of the positive results were in the 997 patients who had been in the hospital for more than 3 days. Since a negative stool culture is unlikely to affect management in these patients with a low likelihood of bacterial diarrhea, it is of little value in that setting. Thus the authors were able to conclude that stool cultures are unlikely to be useful in patients with diarrhea who have been in the hospital for more than 3 days.

***Before / After Studies of Clinical Decision Making.***   These designs directly address the effect of a test result on clinical decisions. The design generally involves a comparison between what clinicians do (or say they would do) before and after obtaining results of a diagnostic test. For example, Carrico et al. (11) prospectively studied the value of abdominal ultrasound in 94 children with acute lower abdominal pain. They asked the clinicians requesting the sonograms to record their diagnostic impression and what their treatment would be if a sonogram were not available. After doing the sonograms and providing the clinicians with the results, they asked again. They found that sonographic information changed the initial treatment plan in 46% of patients.

Of course (as discussed later), altering a clinical decision does not guarantee that a patient will benefit. Thus if a study with this design shows effects on decisions, it is most useful when the natural history of the disease and the efficacy of treatment are clear. In the preceding example, there is very likely a benefit from changing the decision from "discharge from hospital" to "laparotomy" in children with appendicitis, or from "laparotomy" to "observe" in children with nonspecific abdominal pain.

## Analysis

Statistical analysis and reporting of the results of these studies are generally straightforward. The proportion of positive tests and, if applicable, the proportion of tests that lead to changes in management or potentially improved outcomes should be calculated, together with the appropriate 95% CIs.

These studies can also be used to estimate the "effort/yield ratio" (12). This involves identifying the beneficial or potentially beneficial outcomes of ordering the diagnostic test and then estimating the effort that was needed to obtain those beneficial outcomes. For example, among women less than 50 years old, it takes about 500 mammograms and 48 additional diagnostic procedures per breast cancer detected (4).

# ■ STUDIES OF FEASIBILITY, COSTS, AND RISKS OF TESTS

An important area for clinical research relates to the practicalities of diagnostic testing. What proportion of patients will return a postcard with tuberculosis skin test results? What proportion of colonoscopies are complicated by hypotension? What are the medical and psychologic effects of false-positive screening tests in newborns?

## Designs

Studies of the feasibility, costs, and risks of tests are generally descriptive. The sampling scheme is important because tests often vary among the people or institutions doing them, as well as the patients receiving them.

Among studies that sample individual patients, several sampling schemes are possible. A straightforward choice is to study everyone who receives the test, as in a study of the return rate of postcards after tuberculosis skin testing. Alternatively, for some questions, the subjects in the study may be only those with results that were positive or falsely positive. For example, Bodegard et al. (13) studied families of infants who had tested falsely positive on a newborn screening test for hypothyroidism and found that fears about the baby's health persisted for at least 6 months in almost 20% of the families.

Adverse effects can occur not just from false-positive results, but also from tests in which the measurement may be correct but a patient's reaction leads to a decrement in quality of life. Rubin and Cummings (14), for example, studied women who had undergone bone densitometry to test for osteoporosis. They found that women who had been told that their bone density was abnormal were much more likely to limit their activities because of fear of falling.

## Analysis

Results of these studies can usually be summarized with simple statistics like means and standard deviations, medians, ranges, and frequency distributions. Dichotomous variables, such as the occurrence of adverse effects, can be summarized with proportions and their 95% CIs. For example, Waye et al. (15) reported that three (0.1%; 95% CI, 0.03% to 0.4%) of 2,097 ambulatory colonoscopies resulted in hypotension that required fluid resuscitation. When studying the risks of a test, there may be only a few adverse outcomes. When the number of adverse outcomes is less than five, CIs should be calculated from the binomial distribution.*

There are generally no sharp lines that divide tests into those that are or are not feasible, or those that have or do not have an unacceptably high risk of adverse effects. For this reason it is helpful in the design stage of the study to specify criteria for deciding that the test is acceptable. What rate of follow-up would be insufficient? What rate of complications would be too high?

Finally, there are several issues related to the costs of tests. Investigators wishing to focus on test expense may be tempted to report charges rather than costs because charges are more readily available and are generally much higher than costs. However, test charges vary greatly among institutions and may have little relation to what is actually paid for the test or to its actual costs. In many cases, test charges resemble the rack rate on the inside door of a hotel room—a charge much higher than most customers actually pay. On the other hand, estimating how much an institution or society must spend per test is difficult, because many of the expenses, such as laboratory space and equipment, are fixed. One approach is to use the average amount actually paid for the test; another is to multiply charges by the institution's average cost-to-charge ratio.

---

*Unfortunately, not all statistics packages do this automatically. If one end of the CI goes below zero or above 1, it is a clue that the package is using the wrong formula!

# ■ STUDIES OF THE EFFECT OF TESTING ON OUTCOMES

The best way to determine the value of a medical test is to see whether patients who are tested have a better outcome (e.g., live longer) than those who are not. Randomized trials are the ideal design for making this determination, but trials of diagnostic tests are often difficult to do. The value of tests is thus usually estimated from observational studies. The key difference between the designs described in this section and the experimental and observational designs discussed elsewhere in this book is that the predictor variable for this section is *testing*, rather than a treatment, risk factor, or test result.

## Designs

Testing itself is unlikely to have any direct benefit on the patient's health. It is only when a test result leads directly to the use of effective preventive or therapeutic interventions that the patient may benefit. Thus one important caveat about outcome studies of testing is that the predictor variable actually being studied is not just a test (e.g., a fecal occult blood test), but everything that follows (e.g., procedures for following up abnormal results, sigmoidoscopy, colonoscopy, etc.).

The outcome variable of these studies must be a measure of morbidity or mortality, not simply a diagnosis or stage of disease. For example, showing that men who are screened for prostate cancer have a greater proportion of cancers diagnosed at an early stage does not by itself establish the value of screening. It is possible that some of those cancers would not have caused any problem if they had not been detected or that treatment of the detected cancers is ineffective.

The outcome should be broad enough to include plausible adverse effects of testing and treatment, and may include psychologic as well as medical effects of testing. Thus a study of prostate-specific antigen screening for prostate cancer should include morbidity (e.g., impotence or incontinence) and mortality related to treatment. When many more people are tested than are expected to benefit (as is usually the case), less severe adverse outcomes among those without the disease may be important, because they will occur much more frequently. While negative test results may be reassuring and relieving to some patients, in others the psychologic effects of labeling or false-positive results, loss of insurance, and troublesome (but nonfatal) side effects of preventive medications may outweigh infrequent benefits.

***Observational Studies.***   Observational studies are generally quicker, easier, and less costly than experimental studies. However, they have important disadvantages as well, especially since patients who are tested tend to differ from those who were not tested in important ways that may be related to the risk of a disease or its prognosis. This is the same reason that nonexperimental studies of therapies are so difficult—a problem sometimes called **confounding by indication for treatment** (16). For example, those getting the test could be at *lower* risk of an adverse health outcome, because people who volunteer for medical tests and treatments tend to be healthier than average. On the other hand, those tested may be at *higher* risk, because patients are more likely to be tested when they or their clinicians are concerned about a disease or its sequelae.

An additional problem with observational studies of testing is the lack of standardization and documentation of any interventions or changes in management that follow positive results. If a test does not improve outcome in a particular setting, it could be because follow-up of abnormal results was poor, because patients were not compliant with the planned intervention, or because the particular intervention used in the study was not ideal.

---

**Example: An Elegant Observational Study of a Screening Test**

Selby et al. (17) did a nested case-control study in the Kaiser Permante Medical Care Program to determine whether screening sigmoidoscopy reduces the risk of death from colon cancer. They compared the rates of previous sigmoidoscopy among patients who had died of colon cancer with controls who had not. They found an adjusted odds ratio of 0.41 (95% CI, 0.25 to 0.69), suggesting that sigmoidoscopy resulted in a 60% decrease in the death rate from cancer of the rectum and distal colon.

A potential problem is that patients who undergo sigmoidoscopy may differ in important ways from those who do not, and that those differences might be associated with a difference in the expected death rate from colon cancer. To address this possible confounding, Selby et al. examined the apparent efficacy of sigmoidoscopy at preventing death from cancers of the proximal colon, above the reach of the sigmoidoscope. If patients who underwent sigmoidoscopy were less likely to die of colon cancer for other reasons, then sigmoidoscopy would appear to be protective against these cancers as well. However, sigmoidoscopy had no effect on mortality from cancer of the proximal colon (adjusted odds ratio = 0.96; 95% CI, 0.61 to 1.50), suggesting that confounding was not the reason for the apparent benefit.

---

***Clinical Trials.***    The most rigorous design for assessing the benefit of a diagnostic test is a clinical trial, in which subjects are randomly assigned to receive or not to receive the test. Then a variety of outcomes can be measured and compared in the two groups. Randomized trials minimize or eliminate confounding and selection bias and allow measurement of all relevant outcomes such as mortality, morbidity, cost, and satisfaction. Standardizing the testing and intervention process enables others to reproduce the results.

Unfortunately, randomized trials of diagnostic tests are often not practical, especially for diagnostic tests already in use in the care of sick patients. Randomized trials are generally more feasible and important for tests that might be used in large numbers of apparently healthy people, such as new screening tests for cancer.

Randomized trials, however, may bring up ethical issues about withholding potentially valuable tests. Rather than randomly assigning subjects to undergo a test or not, one approach to minimizing this ethical concern is to randomly assign some subjects to receive an intervention that increases the use of the test, such as frequent postcard reminders and assistance in scheduling. The primary analysis must still follow the "intention-to-treat" rule—that is, the entire group that was randomized to receive the intervention must be compared with the entire comparison group. However, this rule will tend to create a conservative bias; the observed efficacy of the intervention will underestimate the actual efficacy of the test, because some subjects in the control group will get the test and some subjects in the intervention group will not. This problem can be addressed in secondary analyses that assume all the difference between the two groups is due to different rates of testing. The actual benefits of testing in the subjects as a result of the intervention can then be estimated algebraically (18).

## Analysis

Analysis of studies of the effect of testing on outcome are those appropriate to the specific design used—odds ratios for case-control studies, risk ratios or hazard ratios for cohort studies or experiments. A convenient way to express the results is to project the results of the testing procedure to a large cohort (e.g., 100,000), listing the number of initial tests, follow-up tests, people treated, side effects of treatment, costs, and lives saved.

# ■ PITFALLS IN THE DESIGN OR ANALYSIS OF DIAGNOSTIC TEST STUDIES

As with other types of clinical research, errors in the design or analyses of studies of diagnostic tests are common. Some of the most common and serious of these, along with steps to avoid them, are outlined below.

### Inadequate Sample Size

A basic principle is that if there are plenty of instances of what the investigator is trying to measure, the sample size is likely to be adequate. However, if the disease or outcome being tested for is rare, this may require testing a very large number of people. Many laboratory tests, for example, are not expensive, and a yield of 1% or less might justify doing them, especially if they can diagnose a serious treatable illness. On the other hand, to conclude that a test is not useful, the upper CI for the yield should be low enough to conclude that the test will not be worthwhile.

For example, Sheline and Kehr (19) retrospectively reviewed routine admission laboratory tests, including the Venereal Disease Research Laboratory (VDRL) test, for 252 psychiatric patients and found that the laboratory tests identified one patient with previously unsuspected syphilis. If this patient's psychiatric symptoms were indeed due to syphilis, it would be hard to argue that it was not worth the $3,186 spent on VDRLs to make this diagnosis. But if the true rate of unsuspected syphilis were close to the 0.4% seen in this study, a study of this sample size could easily have found no cases. In that case, the upper limit of the 95% CI would have been 1.2%—high enough to temper an inappropriate conclusion that the VDRL test was not warranted.

### Inappropriate Exclusion

Excluding patients from the numerator without excluding similar patients from the denominator is a common error. The basic rule is that if any patients who test positive are excluded from the numerator, similar patients must also be excluded from the denominator. In a study of routine laboratory studies of emergency department patients with new seizures (20), for example, 11 of 136 patients (8%) had a correctable laboratory abnormality (hypoglycemia, hypocalcemia, etc.) as a sole or contributory cause for their seizure. In nine of the 11 patients, however, the abnormality was suspected on the basis of the history or physical examination. The authors thus reported that only two of 136 patients (1.5%) had abnormalities not suspected on the basis of the history or physical examination. But if all patients with suspected abnormalities are excluded from the numerator, then similar patients must be excluded from the denominator as well. The correct denominator for this proportion is thus not all 136 patients tested, but only those who were not suspected of having any laboratory abnormalities on the basis of their medical history or physical examination.

## Institution-Specific Results

Generalizability is especially important when a study suggests that a test is not helpful in clinical practice. For example, just because pathologists in a study cannot agree on what constitutes an abnormal Pap smear does not mean that pathologists elsewhere would have the same problem. In some cases, investigators are motivated to study questions that seem particularly problematic in their own institution. The results obtained may be internally valid but of little interest elsewhere.

Nongeneralizable findings can also occur in institutions that do exceptionally well. For example, it is possible that the value of abdominal ultrasonography in children with belly pain reported by Carrico et al. (11) is greater than would be found elsewhere, because of the particular skill of their ultrasonographers.

## Dropping Borderline or Uninterpretable Results

Sometimes a test may fail to give any answer at all, such as if the assay failed, the test specimen deteriorated, or the test result fell into a gray zone of being neither positive nor negative. It is not usually legitimate to ignore these problems, but how to handle them depends on the specific research question and study design. In studies dealing with the expense or inconvenience of tests, failed attempts to do the test are clearly important results. On the other hand, for most other studies of diagnostic tests instances of failure of the test to provide a result should be divided into those that likely are and are not related to characteristics of the patient. Thus patients whose specimens were lost or in whom the assays failed for reasons unrelated to the patient can be excluded.

Patients with "nondiagnostic" imaging studies or a borderline result on a test need to be counted as having had that specific result on the test. In effect, this may change a dichotomous test to an ordinal one—positive, negative, and indeterminate. ROC curves can then be drawn and likelihood ratios can be calculated for the "indeterminate" as well as positive and negative results.

## ■ SUMMARY

1. The usefulness of **medical tests** can be assessed using designs that address a series of increasingly stringent questions (Table 12.1). For the most part, standard observational designs provide descriptive statistics with confidence intervals.
2. The subjects for a study of a diagnostic test should be chosen from patients who have a **spectrum** of disease and nondisease that reflects the anticipated use of the test in clinical practice.
3. If possible, the investigator should **blind** those interpreting the test results from other information about the patients being tested.
4. Measuring the **reproducibility** of a test, including the **inter-** and **intraobserver variability,** is often a good first step in evaluating a test.
5. Studies of the **accuracy of tests** require the choice of a **gold standard** for determining if a patient has, or does not have, the disease or outcome being studied.
6. The results of studies of the accuracy of diagnostic tests can be summarized using **sensitivity** and **specificity, ROC curves,** and **likelihood ratios.** Studies of the accuracy of prognostic tests can be summarized with **risk ratios** or **hazard ratios.**

7. Studies of the effects of tests on **clinical decisions** and the **feasibility, costs, and risks** of tests are often most useful when they suggest a test should not be done.

8. The most rigorous way to study a diagnostic test is to do a **clinical trial,** in which subjects are randomly assigned to receive or not to receive the test, and outcomes, such as mortality, morbidity, cost, and satisfaction, are compared. However, there may be practical and ethical impediments to such trials, and with appropriate attention to possible biases and confounding, **observational studies** of these questions can be helpful.

# EXERCISES

1. You are interested in studying the erythrocyte sedimentation rate (ESR) as a test for pelvic inflammatory disease (PID) in women with abdominal pain.
   a. To do this you'll need to assemble groups of women who do and do not have PID. What would be the best way to sample these women?
   b. How might the results be biased if you used final diagnosis of PID as the gold standard and those assigning that diagnosis were aware of the ESR?
   c. You find that the sensitivity of an ESR greater than 20 is 90%, but the specificity is only 50%. On the other hand, the sensitivity of an ESR greater than 50 is only 75%, but the specificity is 85%. Which cutoff should you use?

2. You are interested in studying the yield of computed tomography (CT) head scans in children presenting to the emergency department with head injuries. You use a database in the radiology department to find reports of all CT scans done on patients less than 18 years old and ordered from the emergency department (ED) for head trauma. You then review the ED records of all that had an abnormal CT scan to determine whether the abnormality could have been predicted from the physical examination.
   a. Out of 200 scans, 10 show intracranial injuries. However, you determine that in eight of the 10, there had been either a focal neurologic examination or altered mental status. Since only two patients had abnormal scans that could not have been predicted from the physical examination, you conclude that the yield of ''unexpected'' intracranial injuries is only two in 200 (1%) in this setting. What is wrong with that conclusion?
   b. What's wrong with using intracranial injuries as the outcome variable for this diagnostic yield study?
   c. What would be some advantages of studying the effects of the test on medical decision making, rather than just the diagnostic yield?

# References

1. Watson JE, Evans RW, Germanowski J, et al. Quality of lipid and lipoprotein measurements in community laboratories. *Arch Pathol Lab Med* 1997;121:105–9.

1a. Bland JM, Altman DG. Statistical methods for assessing agreement between two methods of clinical measurement. *Lancet* 1986;1:307–10.

2. Falahati A, Sharkey SW, Christensen D, et al. Implementation of serum cardiac troponin I as marker for detection of acute myocardial infarction. *Am Heart J* 1999;137:332–7.

3. Sawaya GF, Washington AE. Cervical cancer screening: which techniques should be used and why? *Clin Obstet Gynecol* 1999;42:922–38.

4. Kerlikowske K, Grady D, Barclay J, et al. Positive predictive value of screening mammography by age and family history of breast cancer. *JAMA* 1993;270:2444–50.

5. Sackett D, Haynes R, Guyatt G, et al. *Clinical epidemiology: a basic science for clinical medicine.* Boston: Little, Brown, 1991.

6. Fletcher RH, Wagner EH. *Clinical epidemiology: the essentials,* 3rd ed. Baltimore: Williams & Wilkins, 1996.

7. Friedland DJ. *Evidence-based medicine: a framework for clinical practice.* Stamford, CT: Appleton & Lange, 1998.

8. Pantell RH, Newman TB, Takayam JI, et al. The PROS febrile infant study. In preparation.

9. Kleinbaum DG. *Survival analysis: a self-learning text.* New York: Springer, 1996.

10. Siegel DL, Edelstein PH, Nachamkin I. Inappropriate testing for diarrheal diseases in the hospital. *JAMA* 1990;263:979–82.

11. Carrico CW, Fenton LZ, Taylor GA, et al. Impact of sonography on the diagnosis and treatment of acute lower abdominal pain in children and young adults. *Am J Roentgenol* 1999;172:513–6.

12. Laupacis A, Sackett DL, Roberts RS. An assessment of clinically useful measures of the consequences of treatment. *N Engl J Med* 1988;318:1728–33.

13. Bodegard G, Fyro K, Larsson A. Psychological reactions in 102 families with a newborn who has a falsely positive screening test for congenital hypothyroidism. *Acta Paediatr Scand Suppl* 1983;304:1–21.

14. Rubin SM, Cummings SR. Results of bone densitometry affect women's decisions about taking measures to prevent fractures. *Ann Intern Med* 1992;116:990–5.

15. Waye JD, Lewis BS, Yessayan S. Colonoscopy: a prospective report of complications. *J Clin Gastroenterol* 1992;15:347–51.

16. Psaty BM, Koepsell TD, Lin D, et al. Assessment and control for confounding by indication in observational studies. *J Am Geriatr Soc* 1999;47:749–54.

17. Selby JV, Friedman GD, Quesenberry CJ, et al. A case-control study of screening sigmoidoscopy and mortality from colorectal cancer. *N Engl J Med* 1992;326:653–7.

18. Sheiner LB, Rubin DB. Intention-to-treat analysis and the goals of clinical trials. *Clin Pharmacol Ther* 1995;57:6–15.

19. Sheline Y, Kehr C. Cost and utility of routine admission laboratory testing for psychiatric inpatients. *Gen Hosp Psychiatry* 1990;12:329–34.

20. Turnbull TL, Vanden Hoek TL, Howes DS, et al. Utility of laboratory studies in the emergency department patient with a new-onset seizure. *Ann Emerg Med* 1990;19: 373–7.

# ■ APPENDIX 12.1. CALCULATION OF KAPPA TO MEASURE INTEROBSERVER AGREEMENT

When there are two observers or when the same observer repeats a measurement on two occasions, the agreement can be summarized in a "*c* by *c*" table, where *c* is the number of categories that the measurement can have. For example, consider two observers listening for an S4 gallop on cardiac exam (Table 12.A). They record it as either present or absent. The simplest measure of interobserver agreement is the concordance rate—that is, the proportion of observations on which the two observers agree. The concordance rate can be obtained by summing the numbers along the diagonal from the upper left to the lower right and dividing it by the total number of observations. In this example, out of 100 patients there were 10 patients in whom both observers heard a gallop, and 75 in whom neither did, for a concordance rate of $(10 + 75)/100 = 85\%$.

When the observations are not evenly distributed among the categories (e.g., when the proportion "abnormal" on a dichotomous test is substantially different from 50%), the concordance rate can be misleading. For example, if the two observers each hear a gallop on five patients but do not agree on which patients have the gallop, their observed agreement will still be 90% (Table 12.B). In fact, if two observers both know an abnormality is uncommon, they can have nearly perfect agreement just by never or rarely saying that it is present.

To get around this problem, another measure of interobserver agreement, called

## ■ TABLE 12.A
Interobserver Agreement on Presence of an S4 Gallop

|  | Gallop Heard by Observer 1 | No Gallop Heard by Observer 1 | Total, Observer 2 |
|---|---|---|---|
| **Gallop heard by observer 2** | 10 | 5 | 15 |
| **No gallop heard by observer 2** | 10 | 75 | 85 |
| **Total, observer 1** | 20 | 80 | 100 |

Note: The *concordance rate* is the percentage of the time two observers agree with one another. In this example, both observers either heard or did not hear the gallop in $(10 + 75)/100 = 85\%$ of cases.

## ■ TABLE 12.B
High Agreement When Both Observers Know Gallops are Uncommon

|  | Gallop Heard by Observer 1 | No Gallop Heard by Observer 1 | Total, Observer 2 |
|---|---|---|---|
| **Gallop heard by observer 2** | 0 | 5 | 5 |
| **No gallop heard by observer 2** | 5 | 90 | 95 |
| **Total, observer 1** | 5 | 95 | 100 |

Note: When both observers know that an abnormality is uncommon, they will have a high concordance rate, even if they do not agree on which subjects are abnormal. In this case the observers agree 90% of the time, even though they do not agree at all on who has a gallop.

*kappa* ($\kappa$), is sometimes used. Kappa measures the extent of agreement beyond what would be expected from knowing the *"marginal values"* (i.e., the row and column totals). Kappa ranges from $-1$ (perfect disagreement) to 1 (perfect agreement). A kappa of 0 indicates that the amount of agreement was exactly that expected by chance. $\kappa$ is estimated as:

$$\frac{\text{Observed agreement (\%)} - \text{Expected agreement (\%)}}{100\% - \text{Expected agreement (\%)}}$$

The "expected" proportion in each cell is simply the proportion in that cell's row (i.e., the row total divided by the sample size) times the proportion in that cell's column (i.e., the column total divided by the sample size). The expected agreement is obtained by adding the expected proportions in the cells along the diagonal of the table, in which the observers agreed.

For example, in Table 12.1, the observers appear to have done quite well: They have agreed 85% of the time. But how well did they do compared with agreement by chance? By chance alone they will agree about 71% of the time: (20% × 15%) + (80% × 85%) = 71%. Since the observed agreement was 85%, kappa is (85% − 71%)/(100% − 71%) = 0.48—respectable, if somewhat less impressive than 85% agreement. But now consider Table 12.B. Although the observed agreement was 90%, the expected agreement is (5% × 5%) + (95% × 95%) = 90.5%. Thus kappa is (90% − 90.5%)/(100% − 90.5%) = −0.05%—a tiny bit worse than chance alone.

When there are more than two categories of variable, it is important to distinguish between ordinal variables, which are intrinsically ordered, and nominal variables, which are not. For ordinal variables, kappa fails to capture all the information in the data, because it does not give partial credit for coming close. For example, if a radiograph can be classified as "normal," "questionable," and "abnormal," having one observer call it normal and the other call it questionable is better agreement than if one says it is normal and the other says it is abnormal. To give credit for partial agreement, a weighted kappa* should be used.

---

*The formula for weighted kappa is the same as that for regular kappa except that observed and expected agreement are summed not just along the diagonal, but for the whole table, with each cell first multiplied by a weight for that cell. Any weighting system can be used, but the most common are $w_{ij} = 1 - |i - j|/(c - 1)$ and $w_{ij} = 1 - [(i - j)/(c - 1)]^2$ where $w_{ij}$ is the weight for the number in $i^{th}$ row and the $j^{th}$ column and $c$ is the number of categories.

# 13 Research Using Existing Data: Secondary Data Analysis, Ancillary Studies, and Systematic Reviews

Norman Hearst, Deborah Grady,
Hal V. Barron, and
Karla Kerlikowske

**M**any research questions can be answered quickly and efficiently using data that have already been collected. There are three general approaches to using existing data. **Secondary data analysis** is the use of existing data to investigate research questions other than the main ones for which the data were originally gathered. **Ancillary studies** add measurements of a small number of variables to a study, often in a subset of the participants, to answer a separate research question. **Systematic reviews** combine the results of multiple previous studies that have addressed a given research question to calculate a summary estimate of effect. Making creative use of existing data is an especially effective way for new investigators with limited time and resources to begin to answer important research questions.

## ■ ADVANTAGES AND DISADVANTAGES

The main advantages of using existing data are speed and economy. A research question that might otherwise require much time and money to investigate can sometimes be answered rapidly and inexpensively. For example, in the Multiple Risk Factor Intervention Trial (MRFIT), a large heart disease prevention trial, information about the smoking habits of the wives of the study subjects was recorded to examine whether this influenced the men's ability to quit smoking. After the study was over, one of the investigators realized that the data provided an opportunity to investigate the health effects of passive smoking (a more important research question!). A twofold excess in the incidence of heart disease was found in nonsmoking men married to smoking wives when compared with similar nonsmoking men married to nonsmoking wives (1).

Existing data sets also have limitations. The selection of which data to collect, the quality of data gathered, and how data were recorded are all predetermined. The investigator may have to settle for a variable that is not what he would prefer to have measured (e.g., history of hypertension, a dichotomous historical variable, in place of actual blood pressure). The quality of the data may be poor, with frequent missing or incorrect values. Important confounders and outcomes may not have been measured or recorded. All these factors contribute to the main disadvantage of using existing data: the investigator has little or no control over the data.

# ■ SECONDARY DATA ANALYSIS

## Individual Data Sets

Secondary data sets are of two types: individual and aggregate. Individual data, in which separate information is available for each subject, may come from previous research studies, medical records, health care billing files, death certificates, and many other sources. In such a data set, associations between characteristics can be measured among individual members of the study sample, much as an investigator would do if gathering his own data.

One major category of individual data that may be useful to the clinical researcher is data collected in a **previous research study,** often at the investigator's institution. Many studies collect more data than the investigators can analyze and contain interesting findings that have gone unnoticed. Access to such data is controlled by the study's principal investigator; the new researcher should therefore seek out information about the work of senior investigators at his institution. One of the most important ways a good mentor can be helpful to a new investigator is by providing access to interesting data.

The second category includes large regional and national data sets that are publicly available and do not have a principal investigator. Computerized databases of this sort are a rapidly growing phenomenon and as varied as the reasons people have for collecting information. We will give two examples that deserve special mention, and readers can locate others in their own settings and areas of interest.

Tumor registries are government-supported agencies that collect complete statistics on cancer incidence, treatment, and outcome in defined geographic areas. These registries currently include about 15% of the U.S. population, and the area of coverage is expected to increase during the coming years. One of the purposes of these registries is to provide data to outside investigators. Combined data for all the registries are available from the Surveillance, Epidemiology, and End Results (SEER) Program (see the SEER Web site).

Death certificate registries can be used to follow the mortality of any cohort. The **National Death Index** includes all deaths in the United States since 1978. This can be used to ascertain the vital status of subjects of an earlier study or of those who are part of another data set that includes important predictor variables. An example is the follow-up of men with coronary disease who were treated with high-dose nicotinic acid (or placebo) to lower serum cholesterol in the Coronary Drug Project: Although there was no difference in death rates at the end of the 5 years of randomized treatment, a mortality follow-up 9 years later using the National Death Index revealed a significant difference (2). Whether an individual is alive or dead is public information, so follow-up was complete even for men who had dropped out of the study. This was the first demonstration that cholesterol intervention can reduce total mortality.

The National Death Index can be used when any two of three basic individual identifiers (name, birth date, and Social Security number) are known. Ascertainment of the fact of death is 99% complete with this system, and additional information from the death certificates (notably cause of death) can then be obtained from state records. On the state and local level, many jurisdictions now have computerized vital statistics systems, in which individual data (such as information from birth or death certificates) are entered as they are received.

## Aggregate Data Sets

When individual data are not available, aggregate data sets can sometimes be useful. The term **aggregate data** means that information is available only for groups of subjects (e.g., death rates from cervical cancer in each of the 50 states). With such data, associations can only be measured among these groups by comparing group information on a risk factor (such as tobacco sales) with the rate of an outcome. Studies using aggregate data are called **ecologic studies.**

The advantage of aggregate data is its availability. Its major drawback is the fact that associations are especially susceptible to confounding: Groups tend to differ from each other in many ways, not all of which are causally related. Furthermore, associations observed in the aggregate do not necessarily hold for the individual. For example, sales of cigarettes may be greater in states with high suicide rates, but the individuals who commit suicide may not be the ones doing most of the smoking. This situation is referred to as the **ecologic fallacy.** Aggregate data are most appropriately used to test the plausibility of a new hypothesis or to generate new hypotheses. Interesting results can then be pursued in another study that uses individual data.

## Getting Started

Secondary data analysis can begin in two ways. An investigator may start with a research question of interest to him and try to find a data set that can answer the question. This is the usual approach to clinical research (Chapter 2). The other approach, unique to secondary data analysis, is to begin with a data set and consider questions in the investigator's area of interest and expertise that it can answer. The challenge here is to discover meaningful findings among piles of information.

With either approach, the help of a senior colleague experienced in clinical research is invaluable. An experienced researcher has defined areas of interest in which he stays current and is aware of the important questions that need research. In secondary data analysis, this person can help not only in choosing a research question and designing a protocol, but also in identifying and gaining access to the appropriate database.

## Finding Research Questions to Fit the Data

The process of finding research questions to fit the data, which can be particularly useful to a new investigator who has not yet settled on an area of interest, is summarized in Table 13.1. The investigator first identifies an available data set and familiarizes himself with the information that has been gathered. It may be useful to make a written list or flowchart of all the data collected, including the timing of variables that were measured more than once. The next step is to look

> ■ **TABLE 13.1**
> Steps in Finding Research Questions to Fit an Existing Database
>
> 1. Choose a database.
> 2. Become thoroughly familiar with the database. Make a flow sheet of all vari-
>    ables and how they were measured.
> 3. Identify pairs or groups of variables whose association may be of interest.
> 4. Review the literature and consult experts to determine if these research ques-
>    tions would be novel and important.
> 5. Formulate specific hypotheses and settle on the statistical methods.
> 6. Analyze the data.

for pairs or groups of variables whose relation might be of interest. A brainstorming session involving others familiar with the data may help.

Especially in large cohort studies and clinical trials, relationships among many
variables may never be assessed as part of the original study, simply because the
investigators do not find time to analyze all combinations. For example, in the
CARDIA cohort study of the antecedents of coronary risk factors, an investigator
noticed that blood pressure was measured both sitting and standing. This led to
the questions, "Was there any relation between a postural change in blood pressure
at baseline and the subsequent incidence of hypertension?" and "Was there any
difference between African Americans and whites in this regard?" The answer
to both questions was yes. An orthostatic increase in systolic blood pressure
predicted the 8-year incidence of diastolic hyptertension, especially among African
Americans (3).

Large national data sets provide a similar opportunity. The National Health and
Nutrition Examination Survey (NHANES) includes medical histories, nutritional
questionnaires, and physical examinations performed on a probability sample of
the U.S. population (4). The National Center for Health Statistics, which collects
the NHANES data, encourages outside investigators to perform analyses, such
as examining potential risk factors for diseases. Any scientist can arrange to
purchase, at nominal cost, a computer file that includes any specified set of variables.

## Finding Data Sets to Fit a Research Question

Many investigators prefer the approach of seeking a data set that can answer
questions that emerge in a topic area of interest to them (Table 13.2). This approach

> ■ **TABLE 13.2**
> Steps in Finding Databases to Fit a Specified Research Question
>
> 1. Choose a research question and review the literature thoroughly.
> 2. List combinations of predictor and outcome variables whose relationship
>    might help answer the research question.
> 3. Identify databases that might include the variables of interest.
> 4. Become familiar with each of these databases and consult with individuals
>    who know them well.
> 5. Choose the best database(s) and gain access to the data.
> 6. Formulate specific hypotheses and settle on the statistical methods.
> 7. Analyze the data.

is less constrained, leaving the investigator free to choose among an array of research questions and data sets. After choosing a research topic and becoming familiar with the literature in that area (including a thorough literature search and advice from a senior mentor), the next step is to investigate whether candidate research questions can be addressed with an existing database. It is important to do this carefully, spending days or weeks in an effort to find the best prospect, rather than rushing into something that will take months or years before ultimately being unsuccessful.

The best solution may be close at hand, a database (often attached to a candidate mentor) at the home institution. For example, a University of California, San Francisco (UCSF) fellow noticed in a review article about Lp(a), a little-known coronary disease risk factor, that one of the few interventions known to lower the level of this lipoprotein was estrogen. Knowing that HERS, a major clinical trial of hormone treatment to prevent coronary disease, was being managed at UCSF, the fellow approached the investigators with this interest. Since no one else had specifically planned to examine the relationship between hormone treatment, Lp(a), and coronary heart disease events, the fellow mastered the literature and designed an analysis plan (Appendix 13.1). After receiving permission from the HERS study leadership, he worked with coordinating center statisticians, epidemiologists, and programmers to carry out an analysis that he then wrote up and published (5).

Sometimes it is necessary to venture further afield. Working from a list of predictor and outcome variables whose relation might help to answer the research question, the next step is to locate databases that include these variables. Two great allies in this effort are the telephone and the Internet. Phone calls or e-mail messages to the authors of previous studies or to government officials might result in access to files containing useful data. It is essential to conquer any anxiety that the investigator may feel about contacting strangers to ask for help. Most people are surprisingly cooperative, either by providing data themselves or by suggesting other places to try.

It is sometimes possible to link two databases, one supplying information on the predictor variable and one on the outcome variable. This is relatively straightforward for ecologic studies, as long as both data sets use the same boundaries for the groups being compared (e.g., zip codes, states). Sources of individual data are more difficult to link unless both data sets include the same unique individual identifiers, such as Social Security number.

Once the data for answering the research question have been located, the next challenge is to obtain permission to use them. It is a good practice to use official letterhead on correspondence and to adopt any institutional titles that are appropriate (e.g., instead of "I'm an epidemiology student at . . .," say, "I'm calling from the Department of Epidemiology at . . ."). If someone suggested the contact, it is usually helpful to mention that person's name.

The investigator should be very specific about what information is sought and should confirm the request in writing. It is a good idea to keep the size of the request to a minimum and to offer to pay any cost of preparing the data. If the data set is controlled by another group of researchers, the investigator can suggest a collaborative relationship. In addition to providing an incentive to share the data, this can engage a coinvestigator who is familiar with the database. It is wise to clearly define such a relationship early on, including who will be first author of the planned publications. Serious arrangements of this sort will benefit from a face-to-face meeting.

Here is an example of the use of secondary data in a **natural experiment** that included randomization. In a natural experiment, people have received an intervention in the past for reasons unrelated to research, and a database is available with which to assess an outcome that might have been affected by this assignment. We studied the effect of the 1970 to 1972 draft lottery (involving 5.2 million 20-year-old men assigned randomly by date of birth) on delayed mortality (assessed by state death certificate registries) (6). The predictor variable in this study (date of birth) was a proxy for military service during the Vietnam era. Men who had been randomly assigned to be eligible for the draft had significantly greater mortality from suicide and motor vehicle accidents in the 10 years after they would have returned from the military. The study was done for less than $2,000 (not including the investigators' time), yet it was a more unbiased approach to examining the delayed effect of military service on specific causes of death than other studies of this topic with much larger budgets.

## Use of Large Community-Based Data Sets

Secondary data can be especially useful for studies to evaluate patterns of utilization and clinical outcomes of medical treatment. This approach can complement the information available from randomized trials and examine questions that trials cannot answer. The types of existing data include (a) **administrative and clinical databases** such as those developed by Medicare, the Veterans Administration, Kaiser Permanente Medical Group, and the Duke Cardiovascular Disease Databank, and (b) **registries** such as the San Francisco mammography registry and the National Registry of Myocardial Infarction (NRMI). Information from any of these sources (many of which can be found on the Web) can be very useful for studying rare outcomes and for assessing real-world utilization and effectiveness of an intervention that has been shown to work in a clinical trial setting (Example 13.1).

---

**Example 13.1. The National Registry of Myocardial Infarction (NRMI)**

Large data sets are especially useful for studying rare events. For example, the NRMI was used to examine the risk factors for intracranial hemorrhage after recombinant tissue-type plasminogen activator (tPA) was given for acute myocardial infarction in patients receiving usual care (7). The registry included 71,073 patients who received tPA; among these, 673 had intracranial hemorrhage confirmed by computed tomography or magnetic resonance imaging. A multivariate analysis showed that a tPA dose exceeding 1.5 mg/kg was significantly associated with developing an intracranial hemorrhage. Given that the overall risk of developing an intracranial hemorrhage was less than 1%, a clinical trial collecting primary data to examine this outcome would have been prohibitively large and expensive.

---

Another valuable contribution from this type of secondary data analysis is a better understanding of the difference between efficacy and effectiveness. The randomized clinical trial is the gold standard for determining the **efficacy** of a therapy under highly controlled circumstances in selected clinical settings. In the "real world," however, patients and treatments are often different. The choice of drugs and dosage by the treating physician and the adherence to medications by the patient are much more variable. These factors often act to make the new therapy less effective than demonstrated in trials. Assessing the **effectiveness** of treatments in actual practice can sometimes be accomplished through studies using secondary data. For example, primary angioplasty has been demonstrated to be superior to thrombolytic therapy in clinical trials of treating patients with acute myocardial infarction (8). But this may only be true when success rates for angioplasty are as good as those achieved in the clinical trial setting. Secondary analysis of a community data set has shown no benefit of primary angioplasty over thrombolytic therapy (9,10).

Secondary data analysis is often the best approach for studying the utilization of accepted therapies. Although clinical trials can demonstrate efficacy of a new therapy, this benefit can only occur if the therapy is adopted by practicing physicians. Understanding **utilization rates,** addressing regional variation and use in specific populations (such as the elderly, ethnic minorities, the economically disadvantaged, and women), can have major public health implications. For example, despite convincing data that angiotensin-converting enzyme inhibitors decrease mortality in patients with MI, a secondary analysis of community data has shown that many patients with clear indications for such therapy do not receive it (11,12).

As with other types of research, secondary data analyses are more convincing when an association found in one data set can be duplicated in another collected using a different approach or a different patient population. This reduces the chance that the association observed in the first database was a result of chance or bias. For example, Vaccarino et al. performed a retrospective cohort study using existing data from 15 Connecticut hospitals and found a higher mortality after MI in women compared with men in younger age groups but not in those who were older (13). Subsequently, a similar analysis in a larger and more diverse database found a similar interaction (14).

# ■ ANCILLARY STUDIES

Research with secondary data requires that the data needed to answer a research question are already available. In an **ancillary study,** the investigator adds a small number of measurements to an existing study to answer a different research question. For example, in the HERS trial of the effect of hormone therapy on risk for coronary events in 2,763 elderly women, an investigator added measurement of the frequency and severity of urinary incontinence. Adding a one-page questionnaire created a large trial of the effect of hormone therapy on urinary incontinence, with essentially no additional time or expense (15).

Ancillary studies have many of the **advantages** of secondary data analysis with fewer constraints. They are both inexpensive and efficient, and the investigator can design a few key ancillary measurements specifically to answer the research question. Ancillary studies can be added to any type of study, including cross-sectional and case-control studies, but large prospective cohort studies and randomized trials are particularly well suited to such studies.

Ancillary studies in randomized trials have the problem that the measurements may be most informative when added before the trial begins, and it may be difficult for an outsider to identify trials in the planning phase. Even when a variable was not measured at baseline, however, a single measurement during or at the end of the trial can produce useful information. By adding cognitive function measures at the end of the HERS trial, the investigators were able to compare the cognitive function of elderly women treated with hormone therapy for 4 years with the cognitive function of those treated with placebo (16). In the absence of a baseline measurement, *change* in cognitive function between the two groups (usually a more powerful outcome) could not be compared; however, the comparison at the end of the study preserved the value of randomization and produced an important null finding (16).

A good opportunity for ancillary studies is provided by the **banks of stored serum, DNA, images,** and so on, that are found in most large clinical trials and cohort studies. The opportunity to propose new measurements using these specimens can be an extremely cost-effective approach to answering a novel research question, especially if it is possible to make these measurements on a subset of specimens using a nested case-control design. In HERS, for example, it was possible to examine whether the excess number of thromboembolic events in the hormone-treated group was due to an interaction with Leiden factor V deficiency by genetic analyses of fewer than 100 cases and controls.

In most large prospective cohort studies, the investigators periodically add new measurements, providing an excellent opportunity for ancillary studies. For example, an ongoing prospective cohort study of risk factors for osteoporotic fractures among 9,700 elderly women (Study of Osteoporotic Fractures) included multiple measures of health and functional ability. By adding a measure of nursing home placement, an investigator was able to evaluate risk factors for institutionalization among elderly women.

## Getting Started

Opportunities for ancillary studies should be actively pursued, especially by new investigators with limited time and resources. A good place to start is to identify studies with research questions that include either the predictor or the outcome variable of interest. For example, investigators interested in the effect of weight loss on pain associated with osteoarthritis might start by identifying trials of interventions (such as diet, exercise, behavior change, or drugs) for weight loss. Such studies can be identified by searching lists of studies funded by the federal government, by contacting pharmaceutical companies that manufacture drugs for weight loss, and by talking with experts in weight loss who are familiar with ongoing studies. To create an ancillary study, the investigator would simply add a measure of arthritis symptoms among subjects enrolled in these studies. Alternatively, he might identify studies that have joint pain as an outcome, and add change in weight as an ancillary measure.

After identifying a study that provides a good opportunity for ancillary measures, the next step is to obtain the cooperation of the study investigators. Most researchers are happy to add ancillary measures to an established study if they address an important question and do not substantially interfere with the conduct of the main study. For example, most researchers would be enthusiastic about adding a brief questionnaire or a measurement that participants find unintrusive and interesting. Investigators will be more reluctant to add measures that require a lot of the participant's time (cognitive function testing) or are dangerous or unpleasant (colonoscopy).

Generally, formal permission from the principal investigator or the appropriate study committee is required to add an ancillary study. Most large, multicenter studies have established procedures requiring a written application. The proposed ancillary study is generally reviewed by a committee that can approve, reject, or revise the ancillary study. Many ancillary measures require funding, and the ancillary study investigator must find a way to pay these costs. Of course, the cost of an ancillary study is much less than the cost of conducting the same study independently. Some large studies may have their own mechanisms for funding ancillary studies, especially if the research question is important and considered relevant by the funding agency.

The **disadvantages** of ancillary studies are few. In some cases there may be practical problems in obtaining official permission to perform the study, training those who will make the measurements, and obtaining separate informed consent from participants. Because the ancillary study investigator may not have designed or conducted the main study, it may also be difficult to obtain access to the full database for analysis. These issues, including a clear understanding of authorship of scientific papers that result from the ancillary study and the rules governing their preparation and submission, need to be clarified before starting the study.

# ■ SYSTEMATIC REVIEWS

**Systematic reviews** identify completed studies that address a research question, and evaluate the results of these studies to arrive at conclusions about a body of research. In contrast to other approaches to reviewing the literature, systematic reviews use a well-defined and uniform approach to identify all relevant studies, display the results of eligible studies, and, when appropriate, calculate a summary estimate of the overall results. The statistical aspects of a systematic review (calculating summary effect estimates and variance, statistical tests of heterogencity, and statistical estimates of publication bias) are called **meta-analysis.**

A systematic review can be a good opportunity for a new investigator. Although it takes a surprising amount of time and effort, a systematic review generally does not require substantial financial or other resources. Completing a good systematic review requires that the investigator become intimately familiar with the literature regarding the research question. For new investigators, this detailed knowledge of published studies is invaluable. Publication of a good systematic review can also establish a new investigator as an "expert" on the research question. Moreover, the findings, with power enhanced by the larger sample size available in the combined studies and peculiarities of individual study findings revealed by comparison with the others, often represent an important scientific contribution. Systematic review findings can be particularly useful for developing practice guidelines.

The elements of a good systematic review are listed in Table 13.3. Just as for

---

**■ TABLE 13.3**
Elements of a Good Systematic Review

1. Clear research question
2. Comprehensive and unbiased identification of completed studies
3. Definition of inclusion and exclusion criteria
4. Uniform and unbiased abstraction of the characteristics and findings of each study
5. Clear and uniform presentation of data from individual studies
6. Calculation of a summary estimate of effect and confidence interval based on the findings of all eligible studies when appropriate
7. Assessment of the heterogeneity of the findings of the individual studies
8. Assessment of potential publication bias
9. Subgroup and sensitivity analyses

other studies, the methods for completing each of these steps should be described in a written protocol before the systematic review begins.

## The Research Question

As with any research, a good systematic review has a well-formulated, clear research question that meets the usual FINER criteria (feasible, interesting, novel, ethical, and relevant; see Chapter 2). Feasibility depends largely on the prior existence of a set of studies of the question. The research question should describe the disease or condition of interest, the population and setting, the intervention and comparison treatment (for trials), and the outcomes of interest. For example, *"Among persons admitted to an intensive care unit unstable angina, does treatment with aspirin plus intravenous heparin reduce the risk of myocardial infarction and death during the hospitalization more than treatment with aspirin alone (17)?"*

## Identifying Completed Studies

Systematic reviews are based on a comprehensive and unbiased search for completed studies. The search should follow a well-defined strategy established before the results of the individual studies are known. The process of identifying studies for potential inclusion in the review and the sources for finding such articles should be explicitly documented before the study. Searches should not be limited to MEDLINE, which includes only about half of all published English-language clinical research studies and often does not list non-English-language references. Depending on the research question, other electronic databases such as AIDSLINE, CANCERLIT, and EMBASE can be included, as well as manual review of the bibliography of relevant published studies, previous reviews, evaluation of the Cochran Collaboration database, and consultation with experts.

## Criteria for Including and Excluding Studies

The protocol for a systematic review should provide a good rationale for including and excluding studies, and these criteria should be established a priori. Criteria for including or excluding studies from meta-analyses typically designate the period during which studies were published, the population that is acceptable for study, the disease or condition of interest, the intervention to be studied, whether blinding is required (for trials), acceptable control groups, required outcomes, maximal acceptable loss to follow-up, and minimal acceptable length of follow-up. Once these criteria are established, each potentially eligible study should be reviewed for eligibility independently by two or more investigators, with disagreements resolved by another reviewer or by consensus. When determining eligibility, it may be best to blind reviewers to the date, journal, authors, and results of trials.

Published systematic reviews should list studies that were considered for inclusion and the specific reason for excluding a study. For example, if 30 potentially eligible trials are identified, these 30 trials should be fully referenced and reasons should be given for each exclusion.

## Collecting Data from Eligible Studies

Data should be abstracted from each study in a uniform and unbiased fashion. Generally, this is done independently by two or more abstractors using predesigned forms that include variables that define eligibility criteria, design features, the population included in the study, the number of individuals in each group, the intervention (for trials), the main outcome, secondary outcomes, and outcomes in subgroups. The data abstraction forms should include any data that will subsequently appear in tables describing the studies included in the systematic review or in tables or figures presenting the outcomes. When the two abstractors disagree, a third abstractor may settle the difference, or a consensus process may be used. The process for abstracting data from studies for the systematic review should be clearly described in the manuscript.

The published reports of some studies that might be eligible for inclusion in a systematic review may not include important information, such as design features, risk estimates, and standard deviations. Often it is difficult to tell if design features such as blinding were not implemented or were just not described in the publication. The reviewer can sometimes calculate relative risks and confidence intervals from crude data presented from randomized trials, but it is generally unacceptable to calculate risk estimates and confidence intervals based on crude data from observational studies unless there is sufficient information to adjust for potential confounders. Every effort should be made to contact the authors to retrieve important information that is not included in the published description of a study. If this information cannot be calculated or obtained, the study findings are generally excluded.

## Presenting the Findings Clearly

Systematic reviews generally include three types of information. First, important characteristics of each study included in the summary review are presented in tables. These often include the study sample size, number of outcomes, length of follow-up, characteristics of the population studied, and methods used in the study. Second, the review displays the results of the individual studies (risk estimates and confidence intervals) in a figure. Finally, in the absence of significant heterogeneity (see below), the review presents summary estimates and confidence intervals based on the findings of all the included studies as well as sensitivity and subgroup analyses.

The summary effect estimates represent the main outcomes of the systematic review but should be presented in the context of all the information abstracted from the individual studies. The characteristics and findings of individual studies included in the systematic review should be displayed clearly in tables and figures so that the reader can form opinions that do not depend solely on the statistical summary estimates.

## Meta-Analysis: Statistics for Systematic Reviews

***Summary Effect Estimate and Confidence Interval.***    Once all completed studies have been identified, those that meet the inclusion and exclusion criteria have been chosen, and data have been abstracted from each study, a summary estimate (summary relative risk, summary odds ratio, etc.) and confidence interval may be calculated. The summary effect is essentially an average effect weighted by the size of each study. Methods for calculating the summary effect and confidence interval are discussed in Appendix 13.1.

***Heterogeneity.***    Combining the results of several studies is not appropriate if the studies differ in clinically important ways, such as the intervention, outcome, controls, blinding, and so on. It is also inappropriate to combine the findings if the results of the individual studies differ widely. Even if the methods used in the studies appear to be similar, the fact that the results vary markedly suggests that something important was different in the individual studies. This variability in the findings of the individual studies is called **heterogeneity** (and the study findings are said to be **heterogeneous**); if there is little variability, the study findings are said to be **homogeneous.**

How can the investigator decide if the studies used the same methods and had similar findings? First, he can review the individual studies to determine if there are substantial differences in study design, study populations, intervention, or outcome. Then he can examine the results of the individual studies. If some trials report a substantial beneficial effect of an intervention and others report considerable harm, heterogeneity is clearly present.

Sometimes, however, it is more difficult to decide if heterogeneity is present. For example, if one trial reports a 50% risk reduction for a specific intervention but another reports only a 30% risk reduction, is heterogeneity present? Statistical approaches (tests of homogeneity) have been developed to help answer this question (Appendix 13.1).

## Assessment of Publication Bias

Publication bias occurs when published studies are not representative of all studies that have been done, usually because positive results tend to be submitted and published more often than negative results. There are two main ways to deal with publication bias. **Unpublished studies can be identified** and the results included in the summary estimate. Unpublished results may be identified by querying investigators and reviewing abstracts, meeting presentations, and doctoral theses. The results of unpublished studies can be included with those of the published trials in the overall summary estimate, or sensitivity analyses can determine if adding these unpublished results substantially changes the summary estimate determined from published results. However, including unpublished results in a systematic review is problematic for several reasons. It is often difficult to identify unpublished studies and even more difficult to abstract the required data. Frequently, inadequate information is available to determine if the study meets inclusion criteria for the systematic review or to evaluate the quality of the methods. For these reasons, unpublished data are not often included in meta-analyses.

Alternatively, the extent of potential **publication bias can be estimated** and this information used to temper the conclusions of the systematic review. Publication bias exists when unpublished studies have different findings from published studies. Unpublished studies are more likely to be small (large studies usually get published, regardless of the findings) and to have found no association between the risk factor or intervention and the outcome (markedly positive studies usually get published, even if small). If there is no publication bias, there should be no association between a study's size and findings. A strong correlation between study outcome and sample size suggests publication bias. In the absence of publication bias, a plot of study sample size (or study weight) versus outcome (e.g., log relative risk) should have a bell or funnel shape with the apex near the summary effect estimate.

The funnel plot in Fig. 13.1A suggests that there is little publication bias because small studies with both negative and positive findings were published. The plot in Fig. 13.1B, on the other hand, suggests publication bias because the distribution appears truncated in the corner that should contain small, negative studies.

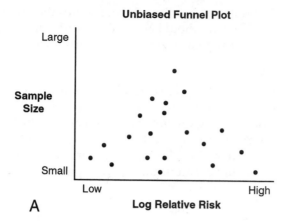

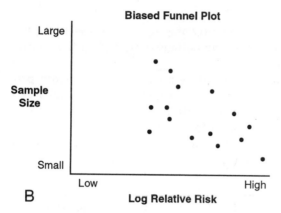

■ **FIGURE 13.1**

**A:** Funnel plot suggestive of minimal publication bias since there are studies with a range of large and small sample sizes, and low relative risks are reported by some smaller studies. **B:** Funnel plot suggestive of publication bias since the smaller studies primarily report high relative risks.

When substantial publication bias is likely, summary estimates should not be calculated or should be interpreted cautiously. Every reported systematic review should include some discussion of potential publication bias and its effect on the summary estimates.

## Subgroup and Sensitivity Analyses

**Subgroup analyses** may be possible using data from all or some subset of the studies included in the systematic review. For example, in a systematic review of the effect of postmenopausal estrogen therapy on endometrial cancer risk, some of the studies presented the results by duration of estrogen use. Subgroup analyses of the results of studies that provided such information demonstrated that longer duration of use was associated with higher risk for cancer (18).

**Sensitivity analyses** indicate how "sensitive" the findings of the meta-analysis are to certain decisions about the design of the systematic review or inclusion of certain studies. For example, if the authors decided to include studies with a slightly different design or methods in the systematic review, the findings are strengthened if the summary results are similar whether or not the questionable studies are included. Systematic reviews should generally include sensitivity analyses if any of the design decisions appear questionable or arbitrary.

### Garbage In, Garbage Out

The biggest drawback to a systematic review is that it can produce a very reliable-appearing summary estimate based on the results of individual studies that are of poor quality. The process of assessing quality is complex and problematic. We favor relying on relatively strict criteria for good study design when setting the inclusion criteria. If the individual studies that are summarized in a systematic review are of poor quality, no amount of careful analysis can prevent the summary estimate from being unreliable.

## ■ SUMMARY

### Secondary Data Analysis

1. Secondary data analysis has the **advantage** of greatly reducing the time and cost of doing research and the **disadvantage** of providing the investigator with little or no control over the data.
2. One good source of data for secondary analysis is an **existing project** at the investigator's institution; another is the large number of **databases** now available from many sources. Although **individual data are preferable,** aggregate data can also sometimes be useful for ecologic analysis.
3. Investigators may begin either by looking for research questions to fit an existing database or by looking for a database that can answer a particular research question.
4. Large community-based data sets are useful for studying the **effectiveness** and **utilization** of an intervention in the community, and for discovering **rare adverse events**.

### Ancillary Studies

1. A clever ancillary study can answer a new research question with **little cost and effort.** As with secondary data analyses, the investigator **cannot control the design,** including the population and many of the variables measured, but he is able to **specify a few key additional measurements.**
2. Good opportunities for ancillary studies may be found in **cohort studies** or **clinical trials** that include either the predictor or outcome variable for the research question of interest. **Stored banks of serum, DNA, images,** and so on, provide the opportunity for cost-effective nested case-control designs.
3. Most large studies have written procedures that allow investigators (including outside scientists) to propose and carry out ancillary studies.

### Systematic Reviews

1. A good systematic review, like any other study, requires a complete **written protocol** before the study begins. The protocol should include the **research question,** methods for **identifying all eligible studies,** methods for **abstracting data** from the studies, and **statistical methods.**
2. The statistical aspects of a systematic review, termed **meta-analysis,** include the **summary effect estimate and confidence interval,** tests for evaluating **heterogeneity** and **potential publication bias,** and planned **subgroup** and **sensitivity analyses.**

3. The **characteristics** and **findings** of individual studies should be displayed clearly in tables and figures so that the reader can form opinions that do not depend solely on the statistical summary estimates.

4. The biggest drawback to a systematic review is that the results can be no more reliable than the **quality** of the underlying studies upon which it is based.

# EXERCISES

**1.** The research question is, "Do Latinos in the United States have higher rates of gallbladder disease than whites, African Americans, or Asian Americans?" What existing databases might enable you to determine race-, age- and sex-specific rates of gallbladder disease at low cost in time and money?

**2.** A research fellow became interested in the controversial question of whether high serum triglyceride levels increase risk for coronary heart disease. Because of the expense and difficulty of conducting a study to generate primary data, he wanted an existing database that contained the variables he needed to answer his research question but was generated for other reasons (so that it was unlikely that someone else had already studied the research question with that data set). He found an investigator at his institution who had access to the database of a large multicenter randomized controlled trial of the effects of interventions on several risk factors for coronary heart disease (the Multiple Risk Factor Intervention Trial).

Fortunately, the MRFIT investigators agreed to allow him access to the data. The necessary predictors and outcome measures were present in the database. The fellow and his advisor then requested the analyses that they wanted from the MRFIT Coordinating Center.

**a.** What are the advantages of this approach to study this question?

**b.** What are the disadvantages of this approach?

# References

1. Svendsen KH, Kuller LH, Martin MJ, et al. Effects of passive smoking in the Multiple Risk Factor Intervention Trial (MRFIT). *Am J Epidemiol* 1987;126:783–95.

2. Canner PL. Mortality in CDP patients during a nine-year post-treatment period. *J Am Coll Cardiol* 1986;8:1245–55.

3. Thomas R, Hulley S. Personal communication.

4. See National Health and Nutrition Examination Survey (NHANES) website.

5. Shlipak M, Simon J, Vittinghoff E, et al. Estrogen and progestin, lipoprotein (a), and the risk of recurrent coronary heart disease events after menopause. *JAMA* 2000;283:1845.

6. Hearst N, Newman TB, Hulley SB. Delayed effects of the military draft on mortality: a randomized natural experiment. *N Engl J Med* 1986;314:620–4.

7. Gurwitz JH, Gore JM, Goldberg RJ, et al. Risk for intracranial hemorrhage after tissue plasminogen activator treatment for acute myocardial infarction. Participants in the National Registry of Myocardial Infarction 2. *Ann Intern Med* 1998;129:597–604.

8. Weaver WD, Simes RJ, Betriu A, et al. Comparison of primary coronary angioplasty and intravenous thrombolytic therapy for acute myocardial infarction: a quantitative review. *JAMA* 1997;278:2093–8 [published erratum appears in *JAMA* 1998;279:1876].

9. Every NR, Parsons LS, Hlatky M, et al. A comparison of thrombolytic therapy with

primary coronary angioplasty for acute myocardial infarction. Myocardial Infarction Triage and Intervention Investigators. *N Engl J Med* 1996;335:1253–60.

10. Tiefenbrunn AJ, Chandra NC, French WJ, et al. Clinical experience with primary percutaneous transluminal coronary angioplasty compared with alteplase (recombinant tissue-type plasminogen activator) in patients with acute myocardial infarction: a report from the Second National Registry of Myocardial Infarction (NRMI- 2). *J Am Coll Cardiol* 1998;31:1240–5.

11. Barron HV, Bowlby LJ, Breen T, et al. Use of reperfusion therapy for acute myocardial infarction in the United States: data from the National Registry of Myocardial Infarction 2. *Circulation* 1998;97:1150–6.

12. Barron HV, Michaels AD, Maynard C, et al. Use of angiotensin-converting enzyme inhibitors at discharge in patients with acute myocardial infarction in the United States: data from the National Registry of Myocardial Infarction 2. *J Am Coll Cardiol* 1998;32:360–7.

13. Vaccarino V, Horwitz RI, Meehan TP, et al. Sex differences in mortality after myocardial infarction: evidence for a sex-age interaction. *Arch Intern Med* 1998;158:2054–62.

14. Vaccarino V, Parsons L, Every NR, et al. Sex-based differences in early mortality after myocardial infarction. National Registry of Myocardial Infarction 2 Participants. *N Engl J Med* 1999;341:217–25.

15. Grady D, Brown J, Vittinghoff E, et al. Postmenopausal hormone therapy for urinary incontinence, in press.

16. Grady D, Yaffe K, Kristof M, et al. Effect of postmenopausal hormone therapy on cognitive function: the Heart and Estrogen/Progestin Replacement Study, in press.

17. Oler A, Whooley M, Oler J, et al. Heparin plus aspirin reduces the risk of myocardial infarction or death in patients with unstable angina. *JAMA* 1996;276:811–15.

18. Grady D, Gebretsadik T, Kerlikowske K, et al. Hormone replacement therapy and endometrial cancer risk: a meta-analysis. *Obstet Gynecol* 1995;85:304–13.

# ■ APPENDIX 13.1. STATISTICAL METHODS FOR META-ANALYSIS

## Summary Effects and Confidence Intervals

The primary goal of meta-analysis is to calculate a summary effect size and confidence interval. An intuitive way to do this is to multiply each trial relative risk (an effect estimate) by the sample size (a weight that reflects the accuracy of the relative risk), add these products, and divide by the sum of the weights. In actual practice, the inverse of the variance of the effect estimate from each individual study ($1/\text{variance}_i$) is used as the weight for each study. The inverse of the variance is a better estimate of the accuracy of the effect estimate than the sample size because it takes into account the number of outcomes and their distribution. The weighted mean effect estimate is calculated by multiplying each study weight ($1/\text{variance}_i$) by the log of the relative risk (or any other risk estimate, such as the odds ratio, risk difference, etc.), adding these products, and dividing by the sum of the weights. Small studies generally result in a large variance (and a wide confidence interval around the risk estimate) and large studies result in a small variance (and a narrow confidence interval around the risk estimate). Thus, in a meta-analysis, large studies get a lot of weight (1/small variance) and small studies get little weight (1/big variance).

To determine if the summary effect estimate is statistically significant, the variability of the estimate of the summary effect is calculated. There are various formulas for calculating the variance of summary risk estimates (1,2). Most use something that approximates the inverse of the sum of the weights of the individual studies (1/sum weights). The variance of the summary estimate is used to calculate the 95% confidence interval around the summary estimate ($\pm 1.96 \times \text{variance}^{1/2}$).

## Random- versus Fixed-Effect Models

There are multiple statistical approaches available for calculating a summary estimate (2). The choice of statistical approach is usually dependent on the type of outcome (relative risk, risk reduction, difference score, etc.) and does not usually make much difference. However, one statistical issue that can affect the outcome of a meta-analysis of clinical trials is whether a fixed-effect or random-effect model is chosen. The fixed-effect model simply calculates the variance of a summary estimate based on the inverse of the sum of the weights of each individual study. The random-effect model adds variance to the summary effect in proportion to the variability of the results of the individual studies. Summary effect estimates are generally similar using either the fixed- or random-effect model, but the variance of the summary effect is greater in the random-effect model to the degree that there is heterogeneity among studies, and the confidence interval around the summary effect is correspondingly larger and more likely not to be statistically significant. Many journals now require authors to use a random-effect model because it is considered "conservative" (i.e., investigators are less likely to find a statistically significant result than when using the fixed-effect model). Meta-analyses should state clearly whether they used a fixed- or random-effect model.

## Statistical Tests of Homogeneity

Tests of homogeneity assume that the findings of the individual trials are the same (the null hypothesis) and use a statistical test (test of homogeneity) to determine if the data (the individual study findings) refute this hypothesis. A chi square test is commonly used (1). If the data do support the hypothesis ($P >$ 0.10), the investigator accepts that the studies are homogeneous. If the data do not support the hypothesis ($P < 0.10$), he rejects the null hypothesis and assumes that the study findings are heterogeneous (apples and oranges). In other words, there are meaningful differences in the populations studied or in the nature of the predictor or outcome variables.

All meta-analyses should report a test of homogeneity with a $P$-value. These tests are not very powerful and it is hard to reject the null hypothesis and prove heterogeneity when the sample size—the number of individual studies—is small. For this reason, a $P$-value somewhat higher than the typical value of 0.05 is typically used as a cutoff. If substantial heterogeneity is present, it is inappropriate to combine the results of trials into a single summary estimate.

## References

1. Petitti D. *Meta-analysis, decision analysis and cost effectiveness analysis.* New York: Oxford University Press, 1994.
2. Cooper H, Hedges LV. *The handbook of research synthesis.* New York: Russell Sage Foundation, 1994.

# SECTION III

# Implementation

# 14 Addressing Ethical Issues

## Bernard Lo

**R**esearch with human participants raises ethical concerns because people accept risks and inconvenience primarily to advance scientific knowledge and to benefit others. Public willingness to participate in clinical research and to support it with federal funding depends on a trust that such research is conducted according to strict ethical standards. In this chapter, we begin by reviewing ethical principles and the federal regulations about informed consent and institutional review boards in the United States. We then turn to a number of ethical considerations including scientific misconduct, conflict of interest, authorship, and confidentiality.

## ■ ETHICAL PRINCIPLES

Three ethical principles guide research with human participants (1). The principle of **respect for persons** requires investigators to obtain informed consent from research participants, to protect participants with impaired decision-making capacity, and to maintain confidentiality. Research participants are not passive sources of data, but individuals whose rights and welfare must be respected.

The principle of **beneficence** requires that the research design be scientifically sound and that the risks of the research be acceptable in relation to the likely benefits. Risks to participants include not only physical harm from tests or treatments but also psychosocial harm, such as breaches of confidentiality, stigma, and discrimination. The risks of participating in the study can be reduced, for example, by screening potential participants to exclude those likely to suffer adverse effects, using data from procedures that are carried out in the course of clinical care, and monitoring participants for adverse effects.

The principle of **justice** requires that the benefits and burdens of research be distributed fairly. Vulnerable populations, such as people with poor access to health care, those with impaired decision-making capacity, and residents of nursing homes, may lack the capacity to make informed or free choices about participating in research. Such populations may seem attractive if access and follow-up are especially convenient, but vulnerable populations should not be targeted for research if other populations would also be suitable.

Justice also requires equitable access to the benefits of research. Traditionally, clinical research has been regarded as risky and potential subjects have been thought of as guinea pigs who needed protection from dangerous interventions that would confer little or no benefit. Increasingly, however, clinical research is regarded as providing access to potentially life-saving new therapies for human immunodeficiency virus (HIV) infection, cancer, and organ transplantation. Patients who seek promising new drugs for fatal conditions want increased access to clinical research, not greater protection (2). Children, women, and members of ethnic minorities have been historically underrepresented in clinical research. As a result, the evidence base for clinical care for such patients is weak. Clinical researchers, particularly researchers funded by the National Institutes of Health, must have adequate representation of children, women, and members of ethnic minorities in studies or else justify why they are underrepresented.

# ■ FEDERAL REGULATIONS FOR RESEARCH ON HUMAN SUBJECTS

**Federal regulations** are intended to ensure that clinical research is conducted in an ethically acceptable manner (3). They apply to all federally funded research in the United States and to research that will be submitted to the Food and Drug Administration in support of a new drug or device application. In addition, many universities require that all research on human subjects conducted by affiliated faculty and staff comply with these guidelines, including research funded privately or conducted off-site.

These federal regulations define research as "systematic investigation designed to develop or contribute to generalizable knowledge" (3). Research is therefore distinguished from unproven clinical care that is directed toward benefiting the individual patient and not toward publication. It is also distinguished from program evaluations that will not be applied in other settings.

Researchers who have questions about these federal regulations should consult their institutional review board (IRB) and read the full text of federal regulations, which are available on the Web site of the Office of Health Research Protection (OHRP) of the Department of Health and Human Services. The federal regulations provide two main protections for human subjects, IRB approval and informed consent.

## Institutional Review Board Approval

Federal regulations require that research on human subjects be approved by an IRB. The **IRB mission** is to ensure that the research is ethically acceptable and that the welfare and rights of research participants are protected. Although most IRB members are researchers, IRBs must also include community members and people knowledgeable about legal and ethical issues concerning research.

When approving a research study, the IRB must determine that

- Risks to participants are minimized.
- Risks are reasonable in relation to anticipated benefits and the importance of the knowledge that may be expected to result.
- Selection of participants is equitable.
- Informed consent will be sought from participants or their legally authorized representatives.
- Confidentiality is adequately maintained (3).

The IRB system is decentralized. Each local IRB implements federal regulations using its own forms and guidelines, and there is no appeal to a higher body. As a result, the protocol for a multicenter study may be approved by the IRB of one institution and not by the IRB of another institution. Usually this situation can be resolved through discussions that clarify perceived problems or through modifications to the protocol.

---

■ **TABLE 14.1**

What Research Is Exempt from IRB Review?

Surveys, interviews, or observations of public behavior unless
    Subjects can be identified, either directly or through identifiers
    Disclosure of subjects' responses could place them at risk for legal liability or
        damage their reputation, financial standing, or employability.
Studies of existing records, data, or specimens, provided that
    Samples exist and are publicly available (e.g., data tapes released by state
        and federal agencies)
    Information is recorded by the investigator in such a manner that subjects can-
        not be identified, either directly or through identifiers. Coded data is consid-
        ered identifiable if the codes could be broken with the cooperation of
        others.
Research on normal educational practices

---

IRBs have been criticized for several reasons (4, 5). They may place undue emphasis on consent forms and fail to scrutinize the research design. Review of the scientific merit of the research (which must be adequate for the research to be ethical) is usually beyond the expertise of the IRB and is left to the funding agency. Although IRBs need to review any protocol revisions and monitor adverse events, they do not check whether research was actually carried out in accordance with the approved protocols. Many IRBs lack the resources and expertise to adequately fulfill their mission of protecting research participants. For these reasons federal regulations and IRB approval should be regarded only as a minimal ethical standard for research. Ultimately, the **judgment and character of the investigator** are the most essential elements for ensuring that research is ethically acceptable.

***Exceptions to IRB Review.*** IRBs may **exempt** from review certain types of research (Table 14.1). The ethical justification for such exemptions is that almost all people would consent to such research and that obtaining consent from each subject would make such studies prohibitively expensive or difficult. Most surveys, interviews, and observations of public behavior are exempt; however, surveys dealing with topics that could place respondents at risk for legal liability or could damage their reputation, financial standing, or employability. For example, surveys are not exempt if they deal with risk factors for human immunodeficiency virus, alcohol use, or mental illness would not be exempt. Research with existing data, records, or specimens may not be exempted from IRB review if information is coded in ways that could be broken with the cooperation of others.

An IRB may allow certain research to undergo **expedited review** by a single reviewer rather than the full committee (Table 14.2). The Department of Health and Human Services publishes a list of types of research that are eligible for expedited review (6), which can be obtained at the OHRP website. These are listed in Table 14.2.

The concept of minimal risk to participants plays a key role in federal regulations. **Minimal risk** is defined as that "ordinarily encountered in daily life or during the performance of routine physical or psychological tests." Both the magnitude and probability of risk must be considered. Because this concept is not more precisely defined, the IRB must make a judgment whether any given project may be considered minimal risk.

■ **TABLE 14.2**
What Research May Undergo Expedited IRB Review?

Research that involves no more than minimal risk and is one of the categories of
    research listed by the OHRP as eligible for expedited review
    Collection of specimens through venipuncture
    Collection of specimens through noninvasive procedures routinely employed in
    clinical practice, such as electrocardiograms and magnetic resonance im-
    aging. However, procedures using x-rays must be reviewed by the full IRB
    Research involving data, records, or specimens that have been collected or
    will be collected for clinical purposes and research using surveys or interviews
    if they are not already exempt from IRB review
Minor changes in previously approved research

## Informed Consent

As part of the informed consent process, investigators must disclose information
that will be relevant to the potential participant's decision about whether or not
to participate in the research. Crucial questions are the following: Why is the
research being done? What will participants do in the course of the research?
What are the risks and benefits of participating? Specifically, investigators must
discuss the following with potential participants (Appendix 14.1):

1. **The nature of the research project.** The prospective subject should be told
   explicitly that research is being conducted, what the purpose of the research
   is, and how participants are being recruited. The actual study hypothesis need
   not be stated.
2. **The procedures of the study.** Participants need to know what they will be
   asked to do in the research project. On a practical level, they should be told how
   much time will be required and how often. Procedures that are not standard care
   should be identified as such. Alternative procedures or treatments that may
   be available outside the study should be discussed. If the study involves blinding or randomization, these concepts should be explained in terms the participant can understand.
3. **The risks and potential benefits of the study and the alternatives to participating in the study.** Medical, psychosocial, and economic harms and benefits
   should be described in lay terms. Also, potential participants need to be told
   the alternatives to participation, especially if effective care is available outside
   the study. Concerns have been voiced that often the information provided to
   participants does not realistically portray the likelihood and nature of risks
   and benefits (7). For example, research on new drugs is sometimes described
   as offering clinical benefits to participants. However, most promising new
   interventions, despite encouraging preliminary results, show no significant
   advantages over standard therapy. Often participants have a "therapeutic misconception" that the research intervention is effective treatment (8). Investigators should make it clear that it is not known whether the study drug is
   more effective than standard therapy and that promising drugs may cause
   serious harm.
4. **Procedures to maintain confidentiality.** Strategies for protecting confidentiality
   include coding research data, storing it in locked cabinets, and limiting personnel who can access data. However, investigators should not make unqualified
   promises of confidentiality. Confidentiality may be breached if data are inadvertently disclosed, if research records are subpoenaed, or if conditions are identi-

fied that legally must be reported. Researchers have a moral and legal obligation to break confidentiality to prevent harm in such situations as child abuse, certain infectious diseases (e.g., AIDS and tuberculosis), and serious threats of violence by psychiatric patients. In projects where information about such situations can be foreseen, the protocol should specify how field staff should respond, and participants should be informed of these plans.

Research records may be subpoenaed. Investigators can forestall this possibility by obtaining confidentiality certificates from the Public Health Service if the research project involves sensitive information, such as sexual attitudes or practices, use of alcohol or drugs, illegal conduct, mental health, or any information that could reasonably lead to stigma or discrimination (9). These certificates allow the investigator to withhold names or identifying characteristics of the participants from people not connected with the project, even if faced with a subpoena or court order. The research need not be federally funded. There are exceptions to the protections of the certificates, such as authorized audits by funding agencies or the Food and Drug Administration.

5. **Assurances that participation in the research is voluntary.** Participants must be told that declining to participate in the study will not compromise their medical care and that they may withdraw from the project at any time.

6. **Consent forms.** Written consent forms are generally required to document that the process of informed consent—discussions between an investigator and the subject—has occurred. (For an example see Appendix 14.2.) Both the discussions and the consent forms should avoid technical jargon and complicated sentences that may not be understood. IRBs have been criticized for excessive focus on consent forms rather than on whether potential participants have understood pertinent information. Providing information over several visits and using audiotapes or videotapes may enhance participants' understanding. In research that involves substantial risk, investigators should consider assessing whether participants have appreciated the disclosed information.

   Informed consent or written consent forms can be waived in some situations (Table 14.3). Under these provisions, individual informed consent is often waived for health services research and epidemiologic research that carry out secondary analyses of existing data.

7. **Subjects who lack decision-making capacity.** When participants are not capable of giving informed consent, permission to participate in the study should be obtained from the subject's legally authorized representative. More important, the protocol should be subjected to additional scrutiny, to ensure that the research question could not be studied in a population that is capable of giving consent.

***Research Participants Who Require Additional Consideration.*** Federal regulations impose additional requirements in some situations where informed consent is impossible or suspect (3). Under these circumstances, the protocol

---

■ **TABLE 14.3**
When May Informed Consent Be Waived or Altered?

The research presents no more than minimal risk to participants
The waiver or alteration would not adversely affect the rights and welfare of participants
The research is otherwise not practical

should be subjected to additional scrutiny, to ensure that the research question could not be studied in a population that is capable of giving consent. These additional requirements are to ensure that vulnerable people, such as those outlined in the following paragraphs, are not taken advantage of in research.

1. **Children.** Investigators must obtain both the permission of the parents and the assent of the child when developmentally appropriate. In addition, research on children involving more than minimal risk is circumscribed, unless it presents the prospect of direct benefit to the child. If the research offers no such prospect, it may still be permitted, provided that there is only a minor increase over minimal risk and that the research is likely to yield generalizable knowledge about the child's disorder or condition.
2. **Prisoners.** Prisoners may not feel free to refuse to participate in research and may be unduly influenced by cash payments or parole considerations. Federal regulations limit the types of research that are permitted and require stricter IRB review and Department of Health and Human Services approval.
3. **Pregnant women, fetuses, and embryos.** Extra protections and restrictions are required when research is carried out on fetuses and embryos or pregnant women.
4. **People with impaired decision-making capacity.** Individuals with impaired decision-making capacity or mental illnesses such as Alzheimer's disease or schizophrenia may not be competent to consent to research. They may also be vulnerable if they are institutionalized. Recently, some research projects have been severely criticized for withdrawing effective medications from with people with mental illness or administering drugs to provoke psychiatric symptoms, without adequate consent procedures or follow-up. The National Bioethics Advisory Commission has recommended additional federal safeguards for research on people with mental disorders that may impair decision-making capacity, including more explicit determinations of decision-making capacity and greater restrictions on research of greater than minimal risk that offers no prospect of direct benefit to participants (10).

## ■ RESPONSIBILITIES OF INVESTIGATORS

### Scientific Misconduct

In several highly publicized cases, researchers enrolled ineligible patients in clinical trials, made up research data, and altered research data to produce favorable results (11–14). Such conduct is unethical, may yield incorrect answers to the research question, undermines public confidence in research, and threatens public support of federally funded research (15).

The federal government has proposed to define **research misconduct** narrowly as fabrication, falsification, and plagiarism (16). **Fabrication** is making up results and recording or reporting them. **Falsification** is manipulating research materials, equipment, or procedures or changing or omitting data or results so that the research record misrepresents the actual findings. **Plagiarism** is appropriating another person's ideas, results, or words without giving appropriate credit.

The federal definition of misconduct requires perpetrators to act intentionally in the sense that they have some awareness that their conduct is wrong. This definition of research misconduct excludes honest error or legitimate scientific differences of opinion, which are a normal part of the research process. The federal definition also excludes other wrong actions, such as double publication, failure to share research materials, and sexual harassment (17). Such inappropriate behavior should be dealt with by the research leader and institution.

When research misconduct is alleged, both the funding agency and the investigator's institution have the responsibility to carry out a fair and timely inquiry or investigation. During an investigation both whistleblowers and accused scientists have rights that must be respected. Whistleblowers need to be protected from retaliation, and accused scientists need to be told the charges and given an opportunity to respond. Punishment for proven research misconduct may include suspension of a grant, debarment from future grants, and other administrative, criminal, or civil procedures.

## Conflicts of Interest

Researchers may have conflicting interests that might impair their objectivity and undermine public trust in research (18). Even the perception of a conflict of interest may be deleterious (19).

*Types of Conflict of Interest.*   The following are some types of conflict of interest:

1. **Dual roles for clinician-investigators.** An investigator may be the personal physician of an eligible research subject. Such patients may fear that their future care will be jeopardized if they decline to participate in the research, or they may not distinguish between research and treatment. Furthermore, what is best for a particular patient may not be what is best for the research project. In some cases, it may be better for the patient not to enroll in the study or to drop out of the study and receive individualized care that differs from the research protocol. An investigator, however, may attempt to persuade his patient to enroll or continue in the study in order to serve the research objectives. In this situation, the welfare of the patient should be paramount, and the physician must do what is best for the patient.
2. **Financial conflicts of interest.** Studies of new drugs are commonly funded by pharmaceutical companies and biotechnology firms (20). The companies have an obvious interest in proving that the drugs are effective and safe. The ethical concern is that financial ties may lead to bias in the design and conduct of the study, the overinterpretation of positive or failure to publish negative results (18). If investigators or family members hold stock or stock options in the company making the drug or device under study, they may reap huge financial rewards if the treatment is shown to be effective, in addition to their compensation for conducting the study. Furthermore, investigators may lose well-paying consulting arrangements if the drug proves ineffective.

*Responding to Conflicting Interests.*   Researchers can respond to some conflicts of interest by substantially eliminating the potential for bias. Other situations, however, have such great potential for conflict of interest that they should be avoided. The following are some ways of responding to the problem of conflict of interest:

1. **Minimize conflicting interests.** In well-designed clinical trials, several standard precautions help keep competing interests in check. Investigators can be blinded to the intervention a subject is receiving, to prevent bias in assessing outcomes. An independent data and safety monitoring board, whose members have no

conflict of interest, can review interim data and terminate the study if the data provide convincing evidence of benefit or harm. The **peer review** process for grants, abstracts, and manuscripts also helps eliminate biased or falsified research.

Physicians should separate the roles of investigator in a research project and clinician caring for a patient whenever possible. Another member of the research team should handle consent discussions and follow-up visits that are part of the study.

If research is funded by a pharmaceutical company, investigators need to ensure that the contract gives them **unrestricted access to the primary data and statistical analysis,** and the **freedom to publish findings** whether or not the drug is found to be effective (21,22). The investigator has an ethical obligation to take responsibility for all aspects of the research, ensuring that the work is done rigorously. The sponsor should be able to review the manuscripts, make suggestions, and ensure that patent applications have been filed before the article is submitted to a journal. However, the sponsor must not have power to veto or censor publication (22).

2. **Disclose competing and conflicting interests.** Conflicts of interest need to be disclosed to potential participants in research. In a landmark court case, the California Supreme Court declared that physicians need to "disclose personal interests unrelated to the patient's health, whether research or economic, that may affect the physician's professional judgment" (23). Medical journals commonly require authors to disclose such conflicts of interest when manuscripts are submitted or published (24,25). Although disclosure itself is a small step, it may deter investigators from practices that are difficult to justify.

3. **Ban certain situations that lead to conflicts of interest.** Researchers in clinical trials and members of data safety monitoring boards, as well as their families, should not hold stock or stock options in the manufacturer of the therapies they are studying in a clinical trial (26,27). Many universities and multicenter trials require investigators to agree to these restrictions.

## Authorship

Authorship of scientific papers results in prestige, promotions, and grants for researchers. Thus investigators are eager to receive credit for publications. However, researchers are less eager to take responsibility for problems with published articles (28). In several cases of scientific misconduct, coauthors of manuscripts containing fabricated, falsified, or plagiarized data denied knowledge of the misconduct. The rise in multiple-authored papers has made it more difficult to assign accountability for published articles.

Problems with authorship include honorary authorship and ghost authorship. **Honorary authorship** refers to authors who have made only trivial contributions to the paper. **Ghost authorship** refers to authors who made substantial contributions to the paper but are not listed as authors; ghost authors are often employees of pharmaceutical companies or public relations officers. These abuses of authorship are common. In one study, 26% of authors did not make substantial contributions to the project (29). Such honorary authors were more common in papers with greater numbers of authors. Most often guest authors provided access to the study site and such resources as patients, reagents, laboratory assistance, or funding (29). In another study, 21% of articles had honorary authors and 13% had ghost authors (30).

Medical journals have set **criteria for authorship** (31). Authors must make substantial contributions to (a) the conception and design of the project, or the data analysis and interpretation, and (b) the drafting or revising of the article; they must also give final approval of the manuscript. Mere acquisition of funding, data collection, or supervision of a research group does not justify authorship, although it warrants a gracious acknowledgment. Because there is no agreement on criteria for first, middle, or last author, it has been suggested that the contributions of each author to the project be described in the published article (32).

Disagreements commonly arise over who should be an author or over the order of authors. These issues are best discussed explicitly and decided at the beginning of a project. If collaborators do not carry out the tasks that justify their role as authors, changes in authorship should be negotiated when decisions are made to shift responsibilities for the work. Detailed suggestions have been made for how to carry out such negotiations diplomatically (33).

# ■ OTHER ETHICAL ISSUES

## Randomized Clinical Trials

Although randomized blinded trials are the most rigorous design for evaluating interventions, they present special ethical concerns because treatment is determined by chance. The ethical basis for assigning treatment by randomization is the judgment that both arms of the protocol are in **equipoise.** That is, current evidence does not prove that either arm is superior (34). Furthermore, individual subjects, often with advice from their physicians, must find randomization acceptable. If physicians believe strongly that one arm of the trial is superior and can provide the same treatment offered in that arm outside the study, they cannot recommend that their patients enter the trial.

The appropriate interventions for control groups also raise ethical concerns. According to the **principle of nonmaleficence,** it is problematic to withhold from the control group therapies that are known to be effective. However, placebo controls may still be justified in short-term studies that do not offer serious risks to subjects, such as studies of mild hypertension and mild pain. Potential subjects need to be informed of effective interventions that are available outside the research study. Dilemmas about the control group are particularly difficult when the research participants have such poor access to care that the research project is the only practical way for them to receive adequate health care. For such vulnerable people, care available in a research study may represent an undue inducement. Ethically, it is preferable to avoid including such vulnerable people as research participants, unless the study concerns problems particularly prevalent in that population.

It may be unethical to continue a clinical trial after it has been demonstrated that one therapy is safer or more effective. Furthermore, it would be wrong to continue a trial that will not answer the research question in an acceptable time frame, because of low enrollment, low incidence of outcome events, or high dropout rates. The periodic analysis of interim data in a clinical trial by an independent **data and safety monitoring board** can determine whether a trial should be terminated prematurely. The researchers themselves should not carry out such interim analyses, because they may have a conflict of interest. Procedures for examining interim data and statistical stopping rules should be specified in the protocol (Chapter 11).

Clinical trials in developing countries present additional ethical dilemmas (Chapter 18).

## Research on Previously Collected Specimens and Data

Research on previously collected specimens and data offers the potential for significant discoveries. For example, DNA testing on stored biologic specimens may identify genes that increase the likelihood of developing a disease or responding to a particular treatment. There are many reasons to allow such research without informed consent from participants. Research on previously collected specimens and data offers no physical risks to participants. Moreover, requiring consent from participants can make the research impossible to carry out or prohibitively expensive.

However, such research also raises ethical concerns. When samples were collected in the context of clinical care, such as tumor specimens removed at surgery, patients who signed a general consent form allowing these specimens to be used in research may have had little idea of what kind of research might be carried out later. Breaches of confidentiality may occur and may lead to stigma and discrimination. Even if individual participants are not harmed, groups may be harmed. Historically, genetics research in the United States led to eugenics abuses, such as forced sterilization of people with mental retardation or psychiatric illness (35). Furthermore, participants may object to the use of data and samples in certain ways (36). For instance, for religious reasons some individuals may not want their biologic materials to be used in contraception research. Similarly, some people may not want their specimens used in research to identify a gene that predisposes to criminal behavior.

The National Bioethics Advisory Commission recommended that research using coded samples be eligible for waiver of informed consent if the study adequately protects the confidentiality of personally identifiable information (36). When biologic specimens are collected in the future, consent forms should allow participants to agree to certain broad categories of future research on the specimens. For example, participants might agree to allow their specimens to be used in future research on related conditions or for any kind of future study.

## Genetic Research

The growing use of DNA analysis in clinical research poses particular ethical concerns regarding confidentiality. Researchers need to determine whether they will disclose the results of investigational genetics tests to subjects. If the test results are sufficiently valid and accurate to be disclosed, subjects should be offered the option of receiving or not receiving their results; and they should receive genetic counseling before any disclosure. In addition, researchers need to decide whether to recommend that relatives seek testing or clinical follow-up. In some cases, subjects may be estranged from relatives and may not wish to inform them. In such situations, the privacy of the subject needs to be respected. Breaching confidentiality is justified only when the breach allows third parties to take actions that are highly likely to reduce a significant risk of serious harm (37). In research projects, these criteria will seldom be met.

Clinical trials of gene "therapy" highlight concerns regarding conflicts of interest and informed consent, as dramatized in a case in which an asymptomatic participant died in a Phase I trial (38). The principal investigator headed a biotechnology company that developed the gene therapy technique under study. Critics charged that conflicts of interest led investigators to discount evidence about the adverse effects of the intervention, to downplay risk during the informed consent process, and to disregard laboratory abnormalities in the subject who died. In addition, volunteers may not appreciate that a Phase I study is not intended to provide direct therapeutic benefit to them as participants.

## Payment to Research Participants

Participants in clinical research deserve compensation for their time and effort and for out-of-pocket expenses such as transportation and child care. Practically speaking, compensation may be needed to enroll and retain participants. The widespread practice is to offer higher payment for studies that are very inconvenient or risky. However, payment also raises ethical concerns about undue inducement to participate in research. If participants are paid more to participate in riskier research, poor people may be induced to undertake risks that they would consider unacceptable in their better judgment. To avoid undue influence, it has been suggested that compensation be based on actual expenses and the time of participants, at an hourly rate for unskilled labor (39).

## ■ SUMMARY

1. Investigators must ensure that their projects observe the ethical principles of **respect for people, beneficence,** and **justice.**
2. Investigators must ensure that research meets applicable **federal regulations. Informed consent** from participants and **IRB review** are the key features of these regulations.
3. During the informed consent process, investigators must explain to potential participants the **nature** of the project and its **procedures;** the potential **risks, benefits,** and **alternatives;** ways **confidentiality** will be addressed; and the voluntary nature of the research.
4. **Vulnerable** populations, especially **children, prisoners, pregnant women,** and people with **impaired mental capacity,** require special attention in research design and in informed consent.
5. Investigators must have **ethical integrity.** They must not commit **scientific misconduct,** including fabrication, falsification, or plagiarism. They should deal appropriately with authorship and with **conflicts of interest** caused by conflicting goals of safeguarding human subjects, advancing scientific knowledge, and accruing personal gain.
6. In randomized clinical trials, the intervention arms must be in **equipoise,** control groups must receive **appropriate interventions,** and there must be mechanisms for **stopping the trial** if one intervention has been found safer or more effective.
7. **Genetic research** and research that is carried out on **previously collected** specimens and data have special ethical issues.
8. **Payments** to research participants should not exceed a level that compensates them for expenses.

## EXERCISES

> **1.** You are evaluating a new urinary catheter for safety and effectiveness. You hope that this new catheter, which is more flexible than those currently available, will be associated with less discomfort and fewer bladder infec-

tions. You propose that the new catheter be evaluated in patients in a nursing home. Your protocol requires that a randomly selected sample of patients with chronic urinary catheters be switched to the new device the next time their catheters need changing. Your outcomes are nurses' evaluation of patient discomfort and a urine culture after 2 weeks.

   **a.** What are the advantages and disadvantages of conducting the study in a nursing home?

   **b.** The participants using the new catheter need a catheter, and the measurement of outcomes is only minimally invasive. Is approval from an IRB needed? Is consent from research participants needed?

   **c.** If consent is needed, what procedures would you use?

2. You are conducting a randomized clinical trial to evaluate a new chemotherapy regimen for treatment of inoperable non–small-cell lung cancer. Patients with inoperable lung cancer will be randomized to the new regimen or no active care. It is hoped that the new regimen will improve disease-free survival and overall survival.

   **a.** What evidence will the committee on human subjects require before approving your protocol?

   **b.** What material should be included in the informed consent form?

   **c.** What training would you provide to the people obtaining informed consent?

3. You are running a clinical trial to evaluate a new arthritis medication. Subjects are enrolled by physicians in practice, who obtain baseline and follow-up data. These physicians are paid for each participant they enroll. In reviewing the data, you note that one physician has enrolled ten participants during the past month, a far greater number than any other physician and greater than expected.

   **a.** What are some possible reasons for this finding?

   **b.** What action would be appropriate for you to take?

# References

1. National Commission for the Protection of Human Subjects of Biomedical and Behavioral Research. *The Belmont Report: ethical principles and guidelines for the protection of human subjects of biomedical and behavioral research.* Washington, DC: U.S. Government Printing Office, 1979.

2. Levine C, Dubler NN, Levine RJ. Building a new consensus: ethical principles and policies for clinical research on HIV/AIDS. *IRB* 1991;13:1–17.

3. Protection of human subjects. 45 CFR 46 (1998).

4. U.S. General Accounting Office. *Continued vigilance critical to protecting human subjects.* Washington, DC: Government Accounting Office, 1996.

5. Office of the Inspector General. *Institutional review boards: their role in reviewing approved research.* Washington, DC: Department of Health and Human Services, 1998.

6. Protection of human subjects: categories of research that may be reviewed by the Institutional Review Board (IRB) through an expedited review procedure. 63 Fed Reg 60, 364 (1998).

7. Advisory Committee on Human Radiation Experiments. *Final report.* New York: Oxford University Press, 1998.

8. Appelbaum PS. False hopes and best data: consent to research and the therapeutic misconception. *Hastings Center Rep* 1987;17:20–4.

9. Wolf L, Lo B. Using the law to protect the confidentiality of sensitive research data. *IRB* 1999;21:4–7.

10. National Bioethics Advisory Commission. *Research involving persons with mental disorders*

*that may affect decision-making capacity.* Rockville, MD: National Bioethics Advisory Commission, 1998.

11. Culliton B. Coping with fraud: the Darsee case. *Science* 1983;220:31–5.
12. Relman AS. Lessons from the Darsee affair. *N Engl J Med* 1983;308:1415–7.
13. Engler RL, Covell JW, Friedman PJ. Misrepresentation and responsibility in medical research. *N Engl J Med* 1987;317: 1383–9.
14. Angell M, Kassirer J. Setting the record straight in the breast-cancer trials. *N Engl J Med* 1994;330:1448–50.
15. Dingell JD. Shattuck lecture—misconduct in medical research. *N Engl J Med* 1993;328:1610–5.
16. Proposed federal policy on research misconduct to protect the integrity of the research record. 64 Fed Reg 55, 722 (1999).
17. Friedman PJ. Advice to individuals involved in misconduct accusations. *Acad Med* 1996;71:716–23.
18. Relman AS. Economic incentives in clinical investigation. *N Engl J Med* 1989;320:933–4.
19. Thompson DF. Understanding financial conflicts of interest. *N Engl J Med* 1993;329:573–6.
20. American Federation for Clinical Research guidelines for avoiding conflict of interest. *Clin Res* 1990;38:239–40.
21. Hillman AL, Eisenberg JM, Pauly MV, et al. Avoiding bias in the conduct and reporting of cost-effectiveness research sponsored by pharmaceutical companies. *N Engl J Med* 1991;324:1362–5.
22. Rennie D, Flanagin A. Thyroid storm. *JAMA* 1997;277:1238–43.
23. *Moore* v. *Regents of University of California,* 51 Cal.3d 120; Cal. Rptr. 146, 793 P.2d 479 (1990).
24. Rennie D, Flanagin A. Conflicts of interest in the publication of science. *JAMA* 1991;266:266–7.
25. Angell M, Kassirer JP. Editorials and conflicts of interest. *N Engl J Med* 1996;335:1055–6.
26. Healy B, Campeau L, Gray R, et al. Conflict-of-interest guidelines for a multicenter clinical trial of treatment after coronary-artery bypass-graft surgery. *N Engl J Med* 1989;320:949–51.
27. Topol EJ, Armstrong P, Van de Werf F, et al. Confronting the issues of patient safety and investigator conflict of interest in an international trial of myocardial reperfusion. *J Am Coll Cardiol* 1992;19:1123–8.
28. Rennie D, Flanagin A. Authorship! Authorship! Guests, ghosts, grafters, and the two-sided coin. *JAMA* 1994;271:469–71.
29. Shapiro DW, Wenger NS, Shapiro MS. The contributions of authors to multiauthored biomedical research papers. *JAMA* 1994;271:438–42.
30. Flanagin A, Carey LA, Fontranarosa PB, et al. Prevalence of articles with honorary authors and ghost authors in peer-reviewed medical journals. *JAMA* 1998;280:222–4.
31. Lundberg GD, Glass RM. What does authorship mean in a peer-reviewed medical journal? *JAMA* 1996;276:75.
32. Rennie D, Yank V, Emanuel L. When authorship fails: a proposal to make contributors accountable. *JAMA* 1997;278:579–85.
33. Browner WS. *Publishing and presenting clinical research.* Baltimore: Lippincott Williams & Wilkins, 1999:125–32.
34. Freedman B. Equipoise and the ethics of clinical research. *N Engl J Med* 1987;317:141–5.
35. Kevles DJ. *In the name of eugenics.* Berkeley: University of California Press, 1985:96–112.
36. National Bioethics Advisory Commission. *Research on human stored biologic materials.* Rockville, MD: National Bioethics Advisory Commission, 1999.
37. Lo B. *Resolving ethical dilemmas: a guide for clinicians,* 2nd ed. Philadelphia: Lippincott Williams & Wilkins, 2000:42–51.
38. Marshall E. Gene therapy on trial. *Science* 2000;288:951–57.
39. Dickert N, Grady C. What's the price of a research subject? Approaches to payment for research participation. *N Engl J Med* 1999;341:198–203.

# ■ APPENDIX 14.1. CHECKLIST FOR INFORMED CONSENT

### ■ The nature of the research project

Explicit statement that the project involves research
Identification of investigators
Purposes of the research
Procedure for selection of subjects

### ■ Procedures of the study

Time required
Assignment of treatments
Explanation of randomization and blinding
Procedures that are experimental rather than standard care

### ■ Benefits and harms of procedures

Probability and magnitude of benefits and harms
Procedures to maximize benefits and minimize harms
Alternative procedures or treatments available outside the study
Potential costs
Information about results that will or will not be disclosed to subjects

### ■ Procedures to maintain confidentiality

### ■ Assurances and contact information

Assurances that participation in research is voluntary
Assurance that subject may decline to participate or withdraw at any time without penalty
Explicit offer to answer questions or provide further information
Directions on whom to contact with questions about the study and the rights of research subjects, or about injuries resulting from the research

# ■ APPENDIX 14.2. EXAMPLE OF A CONSENT FORM
## Consent to Participate in a Research Study

***Title of Research Study.***   Hypertension Arrhythmia Reduction Trial (HART)

***Investigator.***   Dr. Maya Aaron, Department of Medicine, University of California, San Francisco, phone (415) 476-XXXX.

***Purpose and Background.***   This is a study of the side effects of different medicines for high blood pressure (hypertension), particularly the risk of irregularities of the heartbeat (arrhythmias). The purpose of this research is to learn which of two commonly prescribed treatments for high blood pressure causes the fewest irregularities of the heartbeat.

***Procedures.***   If I agree to participate, the following things will happen:

1. I will answer some questions about my medical history. This will take about 15 minutes.
2. I will have an ordinary physical examination to confirm that I have mild hypertension. This will take about 20 minutes.
3. I will have blood drawn with a needle from my arm for potassium and other tests. The needle often causes discomfort lasting less than a minute; occasionally a bruise or minor infection may occur, but these are very unlikely.
4. I will have an electrocardiogram (ECG) and an echocardiogram. These are not painful, do not involve needles, and are not dangerous. The electrocardiogram, which traces my heart rhythm, takes about 2 or 3 minutes. The echocardiogram, which measures heart dimensions, takes about 10 or 15 minutes.
5. I will have continuous recording of my heart rhythm for 24 hours. For this, I will wear a portable recorder about the size of a book on a strap over my shoulder for 24 hours. This test is not painful, does not involve needles, and is not dangerous.
6. I will then be given some pills to take twice a day. The pills will be either hydrochlorothiazide (a commonly prescribed medicine for high blood pressure), or hydrochlorothiazide with potassium (a commonly prescribed combination), or a placebo (an inactive sugar pill). The choice of medicine will be determined by chance, not by the research doctor. Neither I nor the research doctor will know which drug I am taking, although in case of an emergency it can be revealed. I will take this medicine for 2 months.
7. While I am taking the medicine I will have my blood pressure checked each month. At the end of the 2 months I will have a second 24-hour recording of my heart rhythm. I will also have blood drawn again and answer some questions about side effects.

***Benefits.***   There may be no direct benefit to me from participating in the study. However, I may find out the safest way to treat my high blood pressure. I will receive several heart tests free.

***Risks.***   My blood pressure may rise during the 2 months I am taking a drug or placebo. The risk of developing medical complications, such as a heart attack or stroke, are very small. Steps have been taken to reduce any risk. My blood pressure will be checked periodically, and if it rises above a certain level, it will be measured a second time the next day. If my blood pressure remains above this level, I will be treated with known medicine.

The medicine that I am given may cause side effects that are bothersome but rarely serious. I may experience dizziness, tiredness, weakness, or impotence.

**Reimbursement.** I will be paid $25 for the first time and $50 for the second time I complete the 24-hour continuous recording of my heart rhythm. If I am injured as a result of being in this study, treatment will be available. The costs of such treatment may be paid by the University of California, depending on a number of factors. The University does not normally provide any other form of compensation for injury. For further information about this, I may call the Committee on Human Research at (415) 476-XXXX.

**Alternatives.** The medicines used in this study are standard treatments for high blood pressure that can be obtained without participating in the study.

**Confidentiality.** The results of all the study tests will be discussed with me and sent to my personal physician (unless I wish otherwise). Except for this disclosure, all information obtained in this study will be considered confidential and used only for research purposes. My identity will be kept confidential insofar as the law allows.

**Questions.** _____, the research assistant, has discussed this information with me and offered to answer my questions. If I have further questions, I can contact him at 476-XXXX or Dr. Aaron, the director of the study, at 476-XXXX.

**Right to Refuse or Withdraw.** My participation in the study is entirely voluntary, and I am free to refuse to take part or withdraw at any time without affecting or jeopardizing my future medical care.

**Consent.** I agree to participate in this study. I have been given a copy of this form and had a chance to read it.

Signature:

_____

Date:

_____

Signature of clinician:

_____

# Designing Questionnaires and Data Collection Instruments

## Steven R. Cummings, Anita L. Stewart, and Stephen B. Hulley

**M**uch of the data in clinical research is gathered using questionnaires or interviews. For many studies, the validity of the results depends on the quality of these instruments. In this chapter we will describe the components of good questionnaires and interviews and outline procedures for developing them.

## ■ DESIGNING GOOD QUESTIONS AND INSTRUMENTS

### Open-Ended and Closed-Ended Questions

There are two basic types of questions, open-ended and closed-ended, which serve somewhat different purposes.

**Open-ended questions** are particularly useful when it is important to hear what respondents have to say in their own words. An example of an open-ended question is the following:

1. What habits do you believe increase a person's chance of having a heart attack?

_____

_____

Open-ended questions leave the respondent free to answer with fewer limits imposed by the researcher. They are often used in exploratory phases of question design because they facilitate understanding a concept as respondents express it. Phrases and words used by respondents can form the basis for more structured items in a later phase. The chief disadvantage of open-ended questions is that they usually require qualitative methods to code and analyze the responses, which take more time and subjective judgment than coding closed-ended questions.

**Closed-ended questions** are more common and form the basis for most standardized measures. These questions ask respondents to choose from one or more preselected answers, such as the following:

2. Which one of the following do you think increases a person's chance of having a heart attack the most? (Check one.)
   ☐ Smoking
   ☐ Being overweight
   ☐ Stress

Since closed-ended questions provide a list of possible alternatives from which the respondent may choose, they are quicker and easier to answer and the answers are easier to tabulate and analyze. In addition, the list of possible answers often helps clarify the meaning of the question. Finally, closed-ended questions are well suited for use in multi-item scales designed to produce a single score (see later).

Closed-ended questions have several disadvantages. They lead respondents in certain directions and do not allow them to express their own, potentially unique, answers. Moreover, the potential responses listed by the researcher may not include an answer that is most appropriate for a particular respondent. This last problem can be minimized by conducting a pretest using an open-ended version of the questions to collect potential responses and using these responses to expand the list of potential answers to the question. Whenever there is a chance that the set of answers is not **exhaustive** (i.e., does not include all possible options), it is important to include an option such as "Other (please specify)" or "None of the above." When a single response is desired, the set of possible responses should also be **mutually exclusive** (i.e., the categories should not overlap) to ensure clarity and parsimony.

When the question allows more than one answer, instructing the respondent to mark "all that apply" is not ideal. This does not force the respondent to consider each possible response, and a missing item may represent either an answer that does not apply or an overlooked item. It is better, therefore, to ask respondents to mark each possible response as either "yes" or "no":

3. Which of the following increases the chance of having a heart attack?

|  | Yes | No | Don't know |
|---|---|---|---|
| Smoking | ☐ | ☐ | ☐ |
| Being overweight | ☐ | ☐ | ☐ |
| Stress | ☐ | ☐ | ☐ |

**The visual analog scale (VAS)** is another option for recording answers to closed-ended questions using lines or other drawings. The participant is asked to mark a line at a spot, along the continuum from one extreme to the other, that best represents his characteristic. It is important that the words that anchor each end describe the most extreme values for the item of interest. For convenience of measurement, the lines are often 10 cm long and the score is the distance, in centimeters, from the lowest extreme. Example 15.1 is an example of a visual analog scale for pain with a participant's rating.

Visual analog scales are attractive because they rate characteristics on a continuous scale; they may be more sensitive to change than ratings based on categorical lists of adjectives. An alternative approach is to provide numbers to circle instead of a line. This may be easier to score, but some participants may find it difficult to understand, so it is important to explain and give examples of how to answer the question.

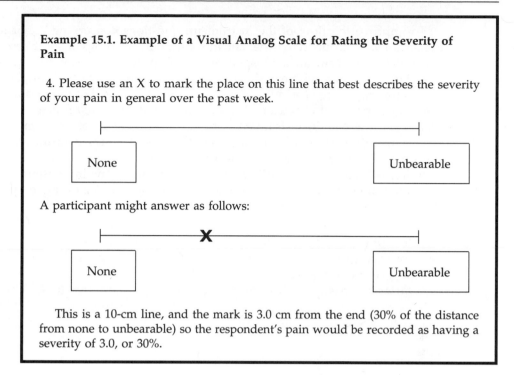

**Example 15.1. Example of a Visual Analog Scale for Rating the Severity of Pain**

4. Please use an X to mark the place on this line that best describes the severity of your pain in general over the past week.

None                                     Unbearable

A participant might answer as follows:

**X**

None                                     Unbearable

This is a 10-cm line, and the mark is 3.0 cm from the end (30% of the distance from none to unbearable) so the respondent's pain would be recorded as having a severity of 3.0, or 30%.

## Formatting

On questionnaires, it is customary to describe the purpose of the study and how the data will be used in a brief statement on the cover. Similar information is usually presented at the beginning of an interview as part of obtaining consent. To ensure accurate and standardized responses, all instruments must have instructions specifying how they should be filled out. This is true not only in self-administered questionnaires, but also for the forms that interviewers use to record responses.

Sometimes it is helpful to provide an example of how to complete a question, using a simple question that is easily answered (see box).

**Example 15.2. Instructions on How to Fill Out a Questionnaire that Assesses Dietary Intake (from the Study of Osteoporotic Fractures).**

These questions are about your usual eating habits during the past 12 months. Please mark your usual serving size and write down how often you eat each food in the boxes next to the type of food.

For example, if you drink a medium (6 oz.) glass of apple juice about three times a week, you would answer:

Apple Juice    ☐ Small (3 oz)        ☒ time(s) per        ☐ Day
               ☒ Medium (6 oz)                            ☒ Week
               ☐ Large (9 oz)                             ☐ Month
                                                          ☐ Year

To improve the flow of the instrument, questions concerning major subject areas should be grouped together and introduced by headings or short descriptive statements. To warm up the respondent to the process of answering questions, it is helpful to begin with emotionally neutral questions such as self-rated health or functioning. More sensitive questions can then be placed in the middle. Questions about personal characteristics such as income or sexual function are often placed at the end of the instrument. For each question or set of questions, particularly if the format differs from that of other questions on the instrument, instructions must indicate clearly how to respond.

If the instructions include different time frames, it is sometimes useful to repeat the time frame at the top of each new set of questions. For example, questions such as

5. How often have you visited a doctor during the past year?
6. How many times have you been treated as a patient in an emergency department during the past year?
7. During the past year, how many times were you admitted to the hospital?

can be shortened as follows:

8. During the past year, how many times have you
   a. Visited a doctor?
   b. Been a patient in an emergency department?
   c. Been admitted to a hospital?

The visual design of the instruments should make it as easy as possible for respondents to complete all questions in the correct sequence. If the format is too complex, respondents or interviewers may skip questions, provide the wrong data, and even refuse to complete the instruments.

On questionnaires a neat format with plenty of space is more attractive and easier to use than one that is crowded or cluttered. Although investigators often assume that a questionnaire will appear shorter by having fewer pages, the task is more difficult when more questions are crowded onto a page. Response scales should be spaced widely enough so that it is easy to circle or check the correct number without the mark accidentally including the answer above or below. When an open-ended question is included, the space for responding should be big enough to allow respondents with large handwriting to write comfortably in the space. People with visual problems, including many elderly subjects, will appreciate large type (e.g., font size 14) and high contrast (black on white).

Possible answers to closed-ended questions should be lined up vertically and preceded by boxes or brackets to check, or by numbers to circle, rather than open blanks:

9. How many different medicines do you take every day? (Check one)

☐ None
☐ 1–2
☐ 3–4
☐ 5–6
☐ 7 or more

Sometimes the investigator may wish to follow up certain answers with more detailed questions. This is best accomplished by a branching question. Respondents' answers to the initial question, often referred to as a "screener," determine whether they are directed to answer additional questions or skip ahead to later questions. For example:

10. Have you ever been told that you have high blood pressure?

    ☐ Yes
    ☐ No

If yes, how old were you when you were first told that you had high blood pressure?
_____years old
If no, go to question 11.

**Branching questions** save time and allow respondents to avoid irrelevant or redundant questions. Directing the respondent to the next appropriate question is done by using arrows to point from response to follow-up questions and including directions such as "Go to question 11" (see Appendix 15.1).

## Wording

Every word in a question can influence the validity and reproducibility of the responses. The objective should be to construct questions that are simple, are free of ambiguity, and encourage accurate and honest responses without embarrassing or offending the respondent.

*Clarity.* Questions must be as clear and specific as possible. In general, concrete words are preferred over abstract words. For example, to measure the amount of exercise respondents get, asking, "How much exercise do you usually get?" is less clear than "During a typical week, how many hours do you spend exercising (e.g., vigorous walking or sports)?"

*Simplicity.* Questions should use simple, common words that convey the idea and avoid technical terms and jargon. For most people, for example, it is clearer to ask about "drugs you can buy without a doctor's prescription" than to ask about "over-the-counter medications": Sentences should also be simple, using the fewest words and simplest grammatical structure that convey the meaning.

*Neutrality.* Avoid "loaded" words and stereotypes that suggest that there is a most desirable answer. Asking, "During the last month, how often did you drink too much alcohol?" will discourage respondents from admitting that they drink a lot of alcohol. "During the last month, how often did you drink more than five drinks in one day?" is a more factual, less judgmental (and less ambiguous) question.

Sometimes it is useful to set a tone that permits the respondent to admit to behaviors and attitudes that may be considered undesirable. For example, when asking about a patient's compliance with prescribed medications, an interviewer or a questionnaire may use an introduction: "People sometimes forget to take medications their doctor prescribes. Do you ever forget to take your medication?"

Wording of these introductions can be tricky. It is important to give respondents permission to admit certain behaviors without encouraging them to exaggerate.

Collecting information about potentially sensitive areas like sexual behavior or income is especially difficult. Some people feel more comfortable answering these types of questions in self-administered questionnaires than in interviews, but a very skillful interviewer can sometimes reveal open and honest answers. In personal interviews, it may be useful to put potentially embarrassing responses on a card so that the respondent can answer by simply pointing to a response.

## Setting the Time Frame

Many questions are designed to measure the frequency of certain habitual or recurrent behaviors, like drinking alcohol or taking medications. To measure the frequency of the behavior it is essential to have the respondent describe it in terms of some unit of time, such as the number of cans of beer drunk during a day. If the behavior is usually the same day after day, such as taking one tablet of a diuretic every morning, the question can be very simple: "How many tablets do you take a day?"

Many behaviors change from day to day, season to season, or year to year. To measure these, the investigator must first decide what aspect of the behavior is most important to the study: the average or the extremes. For example, a study of the effect of chronic alcohol intake on the risk of cardiovascular disease may need a measurement of average consumption during a period of time. On the other hand, a study of the role of alcohol in the occurrence of falls may need to know how frequently the respondent drank enough alcohol to become intoxicated.

Questions about average behavior can be asked in two ways: asking about "usual" or "typical" behavior or counting actual behaviors during a period of time. For example, an investigator may determine average intake of beer by asking respondents to estimate their usual intake:

12. About how many beers do you have during a typical week (one beer is equal to one 12-oz. can or bottle, or one large glass)?
   _____ beers per week

This format is simple and brief. It assumes, however, that respondents can accurately average their behavior into a single estimate. Since drinking patterns often change markedly over even brief intervals, the respondent may have a difficult time deciding what is a typical week. Faced with questions that ask about usual or typical behavior, people often report the things they do most commonly and ignore the extremes. Asking about drinking on typical days, for example, will underestimate alcohol consumption if the respondent drinks unusually large amounts on weekends.

An alternative approach is to quantify exposure during a certain period of time.

13. During the last 7 days, how many beers did you have (one beer is equal to one 12-oz. can or bottle, or one large glass)?
   _____ beers in the last 7 days

The goal is to ask about the shortest recent segment of time that accurately represents the characteristic over the whole period of interest for the research question. The best length of time depends on the characteristic. For example, patterns of sleep can vary considerably from day to day, but questions about sleep habits during the past week may adequately represent patterns of sleep during an entire year. On the other hand, the frequency of unprotected sex varies greatly from week to week so that questions about unprotected sex should cover much longer intervals.

Choosing the time period involves trade-offs. Focusing on a recent and brief period of time, such as the past week, may improve the respondent's recall and ability to average. On the other hand, the period of time defined in the question may not be typical of the rest of the year. If the period included holidays or special occasions, for example, this may overestimate the respondent's usual use of alcohol. When asking about actual behavior, the longer the time period, the more difficult it is for respondents to remember and the more they tend to bias their answer toward recent modes of behavior.

Using diaries or calendars may be a more accurate approach if the behavior is irregular. This approach allows the investigator to calculate an average daily score of the object or behavior being assessed. The use of diaries assumes, however, that the time period assessed was typical.

## Avoid Pitfalls

***Double-Barreled Questions.***   Each question should contain only one concept. Questions that use the words *or* or *and* sometimes lead to unsatisfactory responses. Consider this question that was designed to assess caffeine intake: "How many cups of coffee or tea do you drink during a day?" Coffee contains much more caffeine than tea and differs in other ways, so a response that combines the two beverages is not as precise as it could be. When a question attempts to assess two things at one time, it is better to break it into two separate questions. "(1) How many cups of coffee do you drink during a typical day?" and "(2) How many cups of tea do you drink during a typical day?"

***Hidden Assumptions.***   Sometimes questions make assumptions that may not apply to all people who participate in the study. For example, a standard depression item asks how often respondents have felt this way in the past week: "I felt that I could not shake off the blues even with help from my family." This assumes that respondents have families and ask for emotional support; for those who do not have a family or who do not seek help from their family, it is difficult to answer the question.

***The Question and Answer Options Don't Match.***   It is important that the question match the options for the answer, a task that seems simple but is often done incorrectly. For example, the question, "Have you had pain in the last week?" is sometimes matched with response options of "never," "seldom," "often," "very often," which is grammatically incorrect and can be confusing to respondents. (The question should be changed to "How often have you had pain in the last week?" or the answer should be changed to "yes" or "no.") Another common problem occurs when questions about intensity are given agree/disagree options. For example, a respondent may be given the statement "I am sometimes depressed" and then asked to respond with "agree" or "disagree." For those who are often depressed, it is unclear how to respond; disagreeing with this statement could mean that the person is often depressed or never depressed. In such a case, it is usually clearer to use a simple question about how often the person feels depressed matched with options about frequency (never, sometimes, often).

## Scales and Scores to Measure Abstract Variables

It is difficult to quantitatively assess abstract concepts, such as quality of life, from single questions. Thus abstract characteristics are commonly measured by generating scores from a series of questions that are organized into a scale.

Using multiple items to assess a concept may have other advantages over single questions or several questions asked in different ways that cannot be combined. Compared with the alternative approaches, multi-item scales can increase the range of possible responses (e.g., a multi-item quality-of-life scale might generate scores that range from 1 to 100 while a single question rating quality of life might produce four or five responses from "poor" to "excellent"). A disadvantage of multi-item scales is that they produce results (e.g., quality of life = 46.2) that are difficult to understand intuitively.

Likert scales are commonly used to quantify attitudes, behaviors, and domains of health-related quality of life. These scales provide respondents with a list of statements or questions and asks them to select a response that best represents the rank or degree of their answer. Each response is assigned a number of points.

14. For each item, circle the one number that best represents your opinion:

|  | Strongly Agree | Agree | Neutral | Disagree | Strongly Disagree |
|---|---|---|---|---|---|
| a. Smoking in public places should be illegal. | 1 | 2 | 3 | 4 | 5 |
| b. Advertisements for cigarettes should be banned. | 1 | 2 | 3 | 4 | 5 |
| c. Public funds should be spent for antismoking campaigns | 1 | 2 | 3 | 4 | 5 |

An investigator can compute an overall score for a respondent's answers by simply summing the score for each item, or averaging the points for all nonmissing items. For example, a person who answered that he or she strongly agreed that smoking in public places should be illegal (one point) and advertisements for cigarettes be banned (one point) but disagreed that public funds should be spent for antismoking advertising (four points) would have a total score of 6. Simply adding up or averaging item scores assumes that all the items have the same weight and that each item is measuring the same general characteristic.

The **internal consistency** of a scale can be tested statistically using measures such as Cronbach's alpha (1) that assess the overall consistency of a scale. Cronbach's alpha is calculated from the correlations between scores on individual items. Values of this measure above 0.70 are usually acceptable, and 0.80 or more is excellent. Lower values for internal consistency indicate that some of the individual items may be measuring different characteristics.

## Creating New Questionnaires and Scales

Sometimes an investigator needs to measure a characteristic for which there is no standard questionnaire or interview approach. When no adequate measure can be found of a concept that is important to the research, it is necessary to create new questions or develop a new scale. The task can range from the creation of a single new question about a minor variable in one study (e.g., "How frequently do you cut your toenails?") to developing and testing a new multi-item scale for measuring the primary outcome (such as sexual quality of life) for a major study or line of investigation. At the simplest end of this spectrum, the investigator may use good judgment and basic principles of writing good questions to develop an item that should then be pretested to make sure it is clear and produces appropriate answers. At the other extreme, developing a new instrument to measure an important concept (such as sexual function in women) may need a systematic approach that can take years from initial draft to final product.

The latter process often begins by generating potential items for the instrument from interviews with individuals and "**focus groups**" (small groups of people who are relevant to the research question and who are invited to spend 1 or 2 hours discussing specific topics pertaining to the study with a group leader). Once the instrument has been drafted, the next step is to invite critical review by peers, mentors, and experts. The investigator then proceeds with the iterative sequence of pretesting, revising, shortening, and validating that is described in the next section. The development of the National Eye Institute Visual Function Questionnaire illustrates this process (Example 15.3).

Because the creation and validation of new multi-item instruments is time-consuming, it should generally only be undertaken for variables that are central to a study, and when existing measures are inadequate or inappropriate for the people who will be included in the study.

---

**Example 15.3. Development of a New Multi-Item Instrument**

The National Eye Institute Visual Function Questionnaire exemplifies the painstaking development and testing of a multi-item instrument. Mangione and colleagues devoted several years to creating and testing the scale because it was intended to serve as a primary measurement of outcome of many studies of eye disease (2–4). They began by interviewing patients with eye diseases about the ways that the conditions affected their lives. Then they interviewed focus groups of patients with the diseases and analyzed transcripts of these sessions to choose relevant questions and response options. They produced and pretested a long questionnaire that was then administered to hundreds of participants in several studies. They used data from these studies to identify items that made the largest contribution to variation in scores from person to person and to shorten the questionnaire from 51 to 25 items.

---

# ■ STEPS IN ASSEMBLING THE INSTRUMENTS FOR THE STUDY

There are several steps in developing a set of instruments for a particular study. These include listing variables that may be appropriate to the study; collecting existing instruments and developing new ones; formatting the instrument to be clear, attractive, and easy to follow; and pretesting it to estimate the time needed for administration and to examine the distribution and validity of the responses.

## Make a List of Variables

Before designing an interview or questionnaire instrument, the researcher should write a detailed list of the information to be collected and concepts to be measured in the study. It can be helpful to list the role of each item (e.g., predictors, outcomes, and potential confounders) in answering the main research questions.

## Collect Existing Measures

Assemble a file of questions or instruments that are available for measuring each variable. One practical approach is to create a folder for each variable to be measured and then to find and file copies of candidate questions or instruments for each item. It is important to use the best possible instruments to measure the main predictors and outcomes of a study, so most of the effort of collecting alternative instruments should focus on these major variables.

There are several sources for instruments. A good place to start is to collect instruments from other investigators who have conducted studies that included measurements of interest. Many standard instruments have been compiled and reviewed in books, review articles, and electronic sources such as CD-ROMs or Web sites. There are collections of instruments on the Web that can be found by searching for key terms such as "health outcomes questionnaires." Instruments can also be found by examining published studies of similar topics and by calling or writing the authors.

Borrowing instruments from other studies has the advantage of saving development time and allowing results to be compared with those of other studies. On the other hand, existing instruments may not be entirely appropriate for the question or the population, or they may be too long. It is ideal to use existing instruments without modification. However, if some of the items are inappropriate (as may occur when a questionnaire developed for one cultural group is applied to a different setting), it may be necessary to delete, change, or add a few items.

If a good established instrument is too long, the investigator can contact those who developed the instrument to see if they have shorter versions. Deleting items from established scales risks changing the meaning of scores so that results cannot be compared with results from studies that used the intact scale. Shortening a scale can also diminish its reproducibility or its sensitivity to detect changes. However, it may be possible to delete sections or "subscales" that are not essential to the study while leaving other parts intact.

## Compose a Draft

The first draft of the instrument should include more questions about the topic than will eventually be included in the instrument. The first draft should be formatted just as a final questionnaire would be.

## Revise

The investigator should read the first draft carefully, attempting to answer each question as if he were a respondent and trying to imagine all possible ways to misinterpret questions. The goal is to identify words or phrases that might be confusing or misunderstood by even a few respondents and to find abstract words or jargon that could be translated into simpler, more concrete terms. It should also identify questions that are complex (e.g., contain the terms *and* or *or*) that can be split into two or more questions. It is useful to have colleagues and experts in questionnaire design review the instrument. In addition to considering the content of the items, they should also address the issue of clarity.

## Shorten the Set of Instruments for the Study

Studies usually collect more data than will be analyzed. Long interviews, questionnaires, and examinations may tire respondents and thereby decrease the accuracy and reproducibility of their responses. When the instrument is sent by mail, people are less likely to respond to long questionnaires than to short questionnaires. It is important to resist the temptation to include additional questions or measures "just in case" they might produce interesting data. Questions that are not essential to answering the main research question increase the amount of effort involved in entering, cleaning, and analyzing data. Time devoted to unnecessary or marginally valuable data can detract from other efforts and decrease the overall quality and productivity of the study.

To decide if a concept is essential, it is useful to think ahead to analyzing and reporting the results of the study. Sketching out the final tables will help to ensure that all needed variables are included and to identify those that are less important. If there is any doubt about whether an item or measure will be used in later analyses, it is usually best to leave it out.

### Pretest

Pretests should be done to clarify, refine, and time the instrument. For key measurements, large pretests may be valuable to find out whether each question produces an adequate range of responses and to test the validity and reproducibility of the instrument (Chapter 17).

### Validate

Questionnaires and interviews can be assessed for validity (roughly equivalent to accuracy) and for reproducibility (precision) in the same fashion as any other type of measurement (Chapter 4). The process starts with choosing questions that have **face validity,** a subjective but important judgment that the items are assessing the characteristics that the investigator wants to assess. The accuracy of new instruments can then be compared with "**gold standard**" measurements of the condition of interest. An alternative, when no gold standard is available, is to compare the responses of two groups of patients who are believed to have very different levels of the condition of interest; the questions are often the most valid ones that yield the largest differences between those groups. Ultimately, the **predictive validity** of an instrument can be assessed by correlating measurements with future outcomes.

If an instrument is intended to measure change, then its responsiveness can be tested by applying it to patients before and after receiving effective treatments or to participants in randomized trials of interventions considered effective by other measures of outcome. For example, a new instrument designed to measure quality of life in people with impaired visual acuity might include questions that have face validity (e.g., "Are you able to read a newspaper without glasses or contact lenses?"). Answers could be compared with the responses to an existing validated instrument (Example 15.3) among patients with severe cataracts and among those with normal eye examinations. The responsiveness of the instrument to change could be tested by comparing responses of patients with cataracts before and after curative surgery. The process of validating new instruments is time-consuming and expensive, and worthwhile only if existing instruments are inadequate for the research question or population to be studied.

## ■ ADMINISTERING THE INSTRUMENTS

### Questionnaires versus Interviews

There are two basic approaches to collecting data about attitudes, behaviors, knowledge, health, and personal history. Questionnaires are instruments that respondents administer to themselves, and interviews are those that are administered verbally by an interviewer. Each approach has advantages and disadvantages.

**Questionnaires** are generally a more efficient and uniform way to administer simple questions, such as those about age or habits of tobacco use. Questionnaires are less expensive than interviews and do not require as much time from research staff. **Interviews** are usually the better approach for collecting answers to complicated questions that require explanation or guidance, and interviewers can make sure that instruments are answered completely. Interviews may be necessary when participants will have variable abilities to read and understand questions. However, interviews are more costly and time-consuming, and they have the disadvantage that the responses may be influenced by the relationship between the interviewer and the respondent. Both types of instruments can be standardized, but interviews are inevitably administered at least a little differently each time. Both methods of collecting information are susceptible to errors caused by imperfect memory; both are also affected by the respondent's tendency to give socially acceptable answers, although not necessarily to the same degree.

The choice of which method to use is often dictated by practical considerations; interviews may be prohibitively expensive or logistically impossible. When both methods are feasible, the choice generally involves trade-offs between cost effectiveness and the complexity of the questions to be answered.

## Interviewing

The skill of the interviewer can have a substantial impact on the quality of the responses. **Standardizing** the interview procedure from one interview to the next is the key to maximizing reproducibility. The interview must be conducted with uniform wording of questions and uniform nonverbal signals during the interview. Interviewers must be careful to avoid introducing their own biases into the responses by changing the words or the tone of their voice. This requires practice and training.

For the interviewer to comfortably read or recite the questions verbatim, the interview should be written in language that resembles common speech. Questions that sound unnatural or stilted when they are said aloud will encourage interviewers to improvise their own, more natural but less standardized way of asking the question.

Sometimes it is necessary to follow up on a respondent's answers to encourage him to give an appropriate answer or to clarify the meaning of a response. This "**probing**" can also be standardized by writing standard phrases in the margins or beneath the text of each question. For example, a question about how many cups of coffee respondents drink on a typical day may cause some respondents to say "I'm not sure; it's different from day to day." The instrument may include a standard follow-up "probe," such as, "Do the best you can; tell me approximately how many you drink on a typical day."

Interviews can be conducted in person or over the telephone. **Computer-assisted telephone interviewing** (CATI) can reduce some of the costs associated with interviews while retaining most of their advantages. The interviewer reads the questions to the respondent as they appear on the computer screen, and answers are entered directly into a database as they are keyed in. This enables immediate checking of out-of-range values. In-person interviews, however, may be necessary if the study requires direct observation of participants or physical examinations, or if potential participants do not have telephones (e.g., the homeless). Some elderly and ill persons are best reached through in-person interviews where they are living.

## Methods of Administering Questionnaires

There are several methods of administering questionnaires. They can be given to subjects in person or administered through the mail, by e-mail, or via a Web site. Distributing questionnaires in person allows the researcher to explain the instructions before the subject starts answering the questions. When the research requires the participant to visit the research site for examinations, questionnaires can also be sent in advance of an appointment and answers checked for completeness by staff before the participant leaves.

**Diaries** or calendars are special forms of self-administration and can be used to keep track of events, behaviors, or symptoms that happen episodically (such as falls) or that vary from day to day (such as pain following surgery). This may be valuable when the timing or duration of an event is important or the occurrence is easily forgotten. For example, diaries have been used to measure the number of days of vaginal bleeding and the duration of limited activity after fractures. However, this approach can be time-consuming for participants and can lead to more missing data than the more common retrospective questions.

**Electronic questionnaires** have several advantages. Questionnaires sent by e-mail allow respondents to respond immediately, and the electronic data are easy to compile and enter directly into databases. Questionnaires posted on Web sites can produce very clean data because answers can be automatically checked for missing and out-of-range values, the errors pointed out to the respondent, and the responses accepted only after the errors are corrected. Mailed questionnaires may reach a broader population but are less likely to be returned. All questionnaires are less likely to be completed by those with limited literacy or lower education.

## ■ SUMMARY

1. For many clinical studies, the quality of the results depends on the quality and appropriateness of the **questionnaires** and **interviews.** Investigators should take the time and care to make sure the **instruments** are as **valid** and **reproducible** as possible before the study begins.
2. **Open-ended questions** are useful for exploring new areas, and **closed-ended questions** are easier to answer and analyze. The response options to a closed-ended question should be **exhaustive and mutually exclusive.**
3. Questions should be **clear, simple, neutral,** and **appropriate** for the population that will be studied. Investigators should examine potential questions from the viewpoint of potential participants, looking for **ambiguous terms** and common pitfalls such as **double-barreled questions, hidden assumptions,** and **answer options that do not match the question.**
4. The instrument should be **easy to read,** and interview questions should be comfortable to read out loud. Questions should be preceded by clear instructions and examples if needed. The **format** should be spacious and uncluttered, with instructions and arrows that direct the respondent or interviewer.
5. To measure abstract variables, such as attitudes or health status, questions can be combined into **multi-item scales** to produce a total score. Such scores assume that the questions measure a single characteristic and that the responses are **internally consistent.**

6. An investigator should search out and use **existing instruments** that are known to produce valid and reliable results. When it is necessary to modify existing measures or devise a new one, the investigator should start by collecting existing measures to be used as potential models and sources of ideas.

7. The whole set of measurements to be used in a study should be **pretested** and timed before the study begins. For new measures, small initial pretests can improve the clarity of questions and instructions; later, larger tests can test and refine the new instrument's range, reproducibility, validity (by comparison to gold standard measurements), and responsiveness to change.

8. **Self-administered questionnaires** are more economical than **interviews,** they are more readily standardized, and the added privacy can enhance the validity of the responses. Interviews, on the other hand, can ensure more complete responses and enhance validity through improved understanding. Administration of instruments by **computer-assisted telephone interviewing, e-mail,** and **Internet** can enhance the efficiency of a study.

# EXERCISES

1. As part of a study of alcohol and muscle strength, an investigator plans to use the following item for a self-response questionnaire to determine current use of alcohol:

   "How many drinks of beer, wine, or liquor do you drink each day?"

   _____ 0
   _____ 1–2
   _____ 3–4
   _____ 5–6
   _____ 7–8

   Briefly describe at least two problems with the item.

2. Write a short series of questions for a self-response questionnaire that will better assess current alcohol use.

3. Comment on the advantages and disadvantages of a self-response questionnaire versus a structured interview to assess risky sexual behavior.

# References

1. Bland JM, Altman DG. Cronbach's alpha. *BMJ* 1997;314:572.
2. Mangione CM, Berry S, Spritzer K, et al. Identifying the content area for the 51-item National Eye Institute Visual Function Questionnaire: results from focus groups with visually impaired persons. *Arch Ophthalmol* 1998;116:227–33.
3. Mangione CM, Lee PP, Pitts J, et al. Psychometric properties of the National Eye Institute Visual Function Questionnaire (NEI-VFQ). NEI-VFQ Field Test Investigators. *Arch Ophthalmol* 1998;116:1496–504.

## ■ APPENDIX 15.1. AN EXAMPLE OF A QUESTIONNAIRE ABOUT SMOKING

The following items are taken from a self-administered questionnaire used in our Study of Osteoporotic Fractures. Note that the branching questions are followed by arrows that direct the subject to the next appropriate question, that the form is precoded with the data entry instructions (the small numbers in the boxes), and that the format is uncluttered with the responses consistently lined up on the left of each next area.

1. Have you smoked at least 100 cigarettes in your entire life?

☐ Yes ⟶ 
2. About how old were you when you smoked your first cigarette?

☐☐ years old

☐ No

3. On the average over the entire time since you started smoking, about how many cigarettes did you smoke per day?

☐☐ cigarettes per day

4. Have you smoked any cigarettes in the past week?

☐ Yes ⟶ 5. About how many cigarettes per day did you smoke in the past week?

☐☐ cigarettes per day

☐ No

Please skip to next page, question #7

6. How old were you when you stopped smoking?

☐☐ years old

Please go to question #7

7. Have you ever lived for at least a year in the same household with someone who smoked cigarettes regularly?

☐ Yes ⟶ 8. For about how many years, in total, have you lived with someone who smoked cigarettes regularly at the time?

☐☐ years

☐ No

9. On the average over the entire time you lived with people who smoked, about how many cigarettes a day were smoked while you were at home?

☐☐ cigarettes per day

10. Do you now live in the same household with someone who smokes cigarettes regularly?

☐ Yes

☐ No

11 etc.

# Data Management

## Deborah Grady, Thomas B. Newman, and Eric Vittinghoff

In the last chapter we discussed how to develop questionnaires, measurement instruments, and data collection forms. The next step is to convert the completed data collection forms into an accurate, complete data set in a format that can be analyzed statistically. In this chapter we will consider the practical issues of how to do this.

The steps in data management are described in Table 16.1. The first step is to define or **code each variable**—assign a name and define the variable format and the range of permitted responses. Investigators should **set up the database** before the study begins. This includes determining the hardware and software that will be used to manage the data, the format of the database, and how data will be entered and edited. After a thorough test of data management procedures, data entry and editing for the study begins. A record is kept of any changes in the database, and regular backups are made with storage in remote locations. At the end of the study, analyses are carried out, and the original data (either on paper or, preferably, electronically) are archived and stored.

## ■ DEFINING THE VARIABLES

### Names

Using the data collection forms, each variable should be identified and given a name. This variable name will subsequently be used to identify variables in the database and for analysis. Table 16.2 illustrates names that might be set up for the questionnaire on smoking (see Appendix 15.1). Each variable has an abbreviated name that is self-explanatory; for example, "eversmo" is more informative than "question 1" and makes it easier to read analysis output. Variable names should be short but understandable and consistent. For example, a variable that collects data on the age at which a participant began to smoke cigarettes might be coded as "aastsmo." Similarly, another variable that collects data on whether a participant reports smoking cigarettes at the current time might be coded "cursmo." If information on current smoking is collected at baseline and visits 1 to 4, the variables might be coded as "cursmo0," "cursmo1," "cursmo2," and so on. If this convention is used, then each measurement that is repeated at

247

■ **TABLE 16.1**
Steps in Data Management

Define each variable
Set up the study database and data dictionary
Test data management procedures before the study begins
Enter the data; identify and correct errors
Document changes in the original data
Back up the dataset regularly
Create a dataset for analysis
Archive and store the original data, the final database, and the study analyses

more than one visit is labeled similarly. For example, height at baseline and height at visit 1 would be named "height0" and "height1." In many software packages, this convention also allows the data programmer to efficiently request the values of multiple height measurements as "height0-height4," rather than typing in five names. In addition, some packages make it possible to attach longer "labels" to variables, further increasing the interpretability of analysis output. For example, if the variable "aastsmo" is labeled "Age at which subject started smoking," a table of the distribution of age at which subjects started smoking would carry both the variable name and the label.

Abbreviations should also be used consistently. For example, if "aastsmo" is the name for a variable measuring age at starting to smoke, then age at menopause should be labeled "aamenop." It is a good idea to name all variables using lower case, which is easier to type and eliminates mistakes that can occur if software programs are case sensitive. Some software programs allow only eight characters for variable names—check before naming!

■ **TABLE 16.2**
Naming and Formatting the Variables for the Questionnaire in Appendix 15.1 in a Data Dictionary, and Setting Up the Guidelines for Editing

| Question No. | Variable Name | Type | Format | Permitted Values | Logic Checks |
|---|---|---|---|---|---|
| 1 | eversmo | integer | No<br>Yes<br>Missing | = 0<br>= 1<br>= .a | |
| 2 | aastsmo | integer | 7 to 59<br>Missing<br>Don't know<br>Does not apply | = 7–59<br>= .a<br>= .b<br>= .c | .c if and only if response to #1 is 0. |
| 3 | avgcigs | integer | 0 to 100<br>Missing<br>Don't know<br>Does not apply | = 0–100<br>= .a<br>= .b<br>= .c | .c if and only if response to #1 is 0. |
| 4 | cursmo | integer | No<br>Yes<br>Missing<br>Does not apply | = 0<br>= 1<br>= .a<br>= .c | .c if and only if response to #1 is 0. |
| 5 | aastopsmo | integer | 7 to 59<br>Missing<br>Don't know<br>Does not apply | = 7–59<br>= .a<br>= .b<br>= .c | .c if and only if response to #4 is 0; must be ≥ response to #2. |

Some measurements are not collected on data forms, such as biochemical measurements that are produced by a laboratory. In this case, the data may be transferred electronically by the laboratory and merged with the main database. Such variables must also be defined and described in a data dictionary.

## Format and Range of Permissible Values

For each variable, the **data dictionary** should include the type, format, and the permissible values that can be entered in the database. Variable types include continuous, integer, and free text. Free text data must be coded for analysis, a procedure that is time-consuming and prone to errors. For example, medications used during a study are often collected as text data. If the researcher knows in advance that he will be interested in whether the patient is taking a diuretic, it is best to have a yes/no item for diuretic use on the data collection form. If the data on medications are free text, the researcher will need to parse the text for strings of characters, such as "furos" or "Lasix," to identify subjects who took furosemide. A frequency tabulation of all text strings indicating medications should then be scanned to make sure no other strings likely indicating furosemide have been missed. Sometimes it is helpful to include free text that will not be analyzed to provide salient information about the participant or the visit that can then be visually scanned by the staff investigating records. For example, a "notes" field might include the text "subject grossly obese; wt is 440 pounds" to clarify the extreme value for a subject whose weight is entered as 200 kilograms.

**Consistent rules** should be used to code variables. In Table 16.2, for example, if "eversmo" is answered on the data form as yes or no, the data code might be 0 or 1, where 0 represents *no* and 1 represents *yes*. It is good practice to be consistent when coding dichotomous variables. In particular, 0 should always represent *no* or *absent*, and 1 should always represent *yes* or *present*. With this coding, the average value of the variable is interpretable as the proportion with the attribute.

Once each variable has been named and the type and format defined, a range of permitted values can be assigned. For dichotomous variables only two discrete values (plus missing) are allowable. For continuous variables, deciding on the allowable range may be more difficult. The purpose of defining variable ranges is to guide data editing. Values outside the defined range must be checked for accuracy. If the range set for continuous variables is too wide, inaccurate values may not be identified. In contrast, if the range is set too narrow, many accurate values will need to be checked and verified.

**Missing data** should be assigned a value that is not a possible numeric value because analysis programs treat the code as data. For example, if missing data are coded "99", a subject who has a missing value for age will actually be analyzed as if age is 99 years. Missing data are often coded ".". It is best to code "don't know" differently from missing data because the implications for editing and analyzing the data are different. In addition, some variables are supposed to be missing because the data are not applicable. For example, if a subject reports never smoking, the variables for age at starting to smoke and number of cigarettes per day should be missing. Some software programs allow several codes for missing, such as ".a" for missing, ".b" for don't know, and ".c" for values that are not applicable. In the analysis, all these values are treated as missing, but the reason the data are missing is retained.

| ■ **TABLE 16.3** Functions Required for Data Entry, Management, and Analysis | |
| --- | --- |
| **Function** | **Options** |
| Data entry | Keyboard    Directly into database    Via interface into database Machine read Voice recognition |
| Data editing | Manual Automatic Interactive |
| Establish relational tables | Manual Relational database software |
| Generate reports | Manual Spreadsheet, graphic and statistical software |
| Perform statistical analysis | Spreadsheet and statistical analysis software |

# ■ CREATING THE STUDY DATABASE AND DATA DICTIONARY

The functions required for entering, editing, managing, and analyzing data are shown in Table 16.3. For small studies, these functions can be accomplished simply using spreadsheet software. Large, complex databases may require multiple types of integrated software custom-programmed to meet the goals of the specific study.

## Simple Databases

Perhaps the most common and easily accessible approach to creating a simple database is to use a **spreadsheet** program and then transfer the data to statistical software for analysis (Table 16.4). Spreadsheets arrange data in a matrix of rows (for the study subjects) and columns (for the variables) called a **table or flat file**. The easiest way to enter data in a spreadsheet program is using a keyboard to enter values directly into the appropriate cell (row and column) of the table. Data editing in a spreadsheet is generally a simple matter of comparing the values in the database with the values written on the data collection forms. Spreadsheets generally do not provide good tools for creating a data entry interface or for performing automatic or interactive data editing.

| ■ **TABLE 16.4** Some Software Programs Used in Database Design, Data Management, and Analysis | |
| --- | --- |
| **Spreadsheet** Excel **Relational database** Oracle Microsoft SQL Server **Enterprise manager** Oracle Microsoft SQL Server | **Statistical analysis** Statistical Analysis System (SAS) Statistical Package for the Social Sciences (SPSS) Stata **Machine readable forms** Teleform **Interface builder** Microsoft Access Power Builder Visual Basic |

Note: This table provides examples of software packages but makes no attempt to be comprehensive or to recommend specific software.

Spreadsheet programs can produce simple reports and calculate basic statistics. However, it is typically easier and more efficient to transfer the database after entry and editing into a statistical program for data analysis. Data transfer is generally quick and easy, as most statistical analysis programs can read data directly from spreadsheets.

## Complex Databases

Most large and more complex studies use **relational databases** for data entry, editing, and management. Some of these packages also provide powerful interface builders for data entry. **Interfaces** allow the data entry screen to be formatted to resemble the data form, facilitating data entry. Data can then be entered uncoded and automatically translated by the program into the correct data format in the database. Interface builder software can also be used with other software to perform this function.

Relational database programs typically allow the investigator to easily perform **double data entry** in which the data are entered twice and discrepant values are identified for correction. **Automatic range** and **logic edits** can also be established, and editing can be done interactively, so that the data entry operator is prompted to correct missing, out-of-range or illogical values at the time of data entry. These software packages can also be programmed so that data entry can be done via machine-readable forms or voice recognition.

A relational database includes multiple related tables. For example, in a study of the effect of smoking on lung cancer risk, separate tables (related by subject ID) might contain demographic variables, variables related to smoking history, occupational exposures, and incidence of lung cancer. Additional subtables might contain data on severity of the cancer (size, stage, grade, and histologic type), information on genetic markers found in the cancers, and surgical outcome for those subjects who underwent surgery. The same information could be stored in one large table, but many of the cells would be inapplicable, since only a minority of the subjects will develop lung cancer. This type of relational database allows efficient data editing and management, since only the tables involved in specific editing procedures are used. In contrast to spreadsheet programs, relational database software provides powerful tools to ensure that related tables are complete and accurate across complex databases. For example, relational database programs can prompt to make sure that a subject with lung cancer has complete data in related tables for severity, genetic features, and treatment. Furthermore, reclassification of a lung cancer as another condition could prompt correction or deletion of entries in the related cancer tables.

Relational database software provides powerful and flexible programming tools, the ability to handle multiple related data tables and to produce flexible and complex reports. However creating and customizing the program may require substantial time and expertise, and the complexity of the editing and checking parameters makes modifications difficult if there are changes in the data collection forms. The statistical analysis capability of relational databases is limited, and data are usually transferred to another software package for data analysis.

## Statistical Analysis Software and Enterprise Managers

The strength of **statistical analysis software,** of course, is to perform statistical analyses. Some of these packages also provide basic data entry and editing modules, but it is generally easier to enter and perform basic data editing using either spreadsheet or relational database software and subsequently transfer the data for analysis. Statistical analysis software also provides very powerful graphic and report generation functions.

**Enterprise management software** is used by most pharmaceutical companies and professional research organizations. This software allows the user to perform uniform procedures on multiple study databases simultaneously.

## Data Dictionary

The **data dictionary** is a document that includes a description of study variables and data management procedures. For each variable, it includes the variable location (form or questionnaire name and question number), name, label, type, format, permissible range of values, and additional edits to be performed, such as logic and consistency checks. The data dictionary should be created before any data are collected, but additions to the dictionary will occur throughout the study. Definitions for redefined and derived variables used for analysis should also be included.

## Test the Data Management System Before the Study Begins

The entire database system (forms, coding, data entry, data editing, query management, and data transfer) should be tested using dummy data. Test forms can be completed and the data entered, edited, and transferred for analysis using the methods planned for the study. Dummy data forms can include variable values that are missing, out of range, and illogical to make sure that the data editing system is correctly identifying errors. When malfunctions are identified, they should be corrected and the system retested until it works correctly.

## ■ ENTERING THE DATA AND CORRECTING ERRORS

Data should be recorded directly on forms that have been specifically designed for data collection. Such forms can be created on paper or as computer screens that resemble forms. It is important to record the data directly on the forms at the time the measurements are made (rather than keeping notes on scraps of paper as an intermediary step) to minimize the possibility of losses or transcription errors. The completed forms are then edited by a staff member while the study subject is still present, looking for omissions, illegible entries, and gross errors that can be corrected on the spot. Changes to paper data forms should be documented by crossing out the erroneous data (not erasing it) and writing in the correct data, the date of change, and the identification number of the staff person who made the change.

## Enter the Data

The goals of data entry are to enter the data efficiently and accurately into the database. Data entry should be done within several days of data collection. Entering the data promptly prevents backlogs from accumulating, allows early identification of data collection problems, minimizes the possibility of losses, and permits the investigator to examine periodic reports that keep track of his study. It also generates queries regarding missing, out-of-range, or illogical values at a time when it may still be possible to return to the source of the data and correct any errors.

***Keyboard Data Entry.***   A simple method is to enter data manually on a keyboard directly into the database. Using a spreadsheet, this process requires the data entry operator to translate answers on data forms (such as "yes") to codes in the database ("1"). For example, suppose a participant answers the question, "Have you ever smoked more than five cigarettes in your life?" by checking a box corresponding to "no." The data entry operator is required to find the proper cell in the spreadsheet (identified by the participant's identification number and the variable name "eversmo") and enter "0," the coded value for "no." Preprinting the variable codes on the paper form can facilitate coding, but the process of translating the data to coded values is tedious and prone to error. Direct keyboard data entry is most commonly performed by study staff, but this service is also available from commercial businesses.

Keyboard data entry can also be accomplished using various interfaces on the computer screen. An interface can be constructed to resemble or be identical to paper forms. Using this approach, data can be entered uncoded. For example, when entering the response for "eversmo," the data entry operator might see a replica of the form on the screen. At the question, "Have you ever smoked more than five cigarettes in your life?" the data entry operator notes that the participant checked the box for "no" on the paper form and then clicks on the same box displayed on the computer screen. This entry is then automatically converted by the program to the correct code.

Some data entry systems allow study subjects to enter their own response directly to the database using hand-held, laptop, or desktop computers. These systems are efficient because there are no intermediary steps between the subject's response and data entry, and no paper forms are required. This approach may be particularly useful for gathering sensitive information that study participants may be reluctant to discuss with interviewers. However, data entry by the subjects produces no source documents, so that checking for data entry errors is impossible. Also, subjects must be taught to use the data entry system and may not understand it well enough to be accurate. A major advantage of this system is its suitability for subjects to enter data directly to the study database from their homes, using a variety of Web-based access devices.

***Machine-Readable Forms.***   Machine-readable forms can be created using special software. When scanned or faxed, the handwritten information on these forms is read into the database. The obvious advantage is that manual data entry is not required. However, these systems are more difficult and costly to design and maintain. Because the software currently does not read text very accurately, machine-readable forms must be completed carefully, typically requiring that "bubbles" be filled in for categorical variables and that text be written clearly in block letters inside specific spaces. For this reason, machine-readable forms are often completed by trained study staff, rather than by study participants. Machine reading is improving quickly, however, and it may soon be possible for study participants to complete these forms.

***Distributed Data Entry.***   Data from studies that take place at multiple sites need to be entered into a central database. The simplest way to do this is to mail the data forms to a central location and manually enter the data. This approach is relatively slow and cumbersome. Alternatively, data can be entered at each site (either via keyboard or using machine-readable forms) and transferred to a central database via fax, e-mail, or the Internet. This **distributed data entry** facilitates the

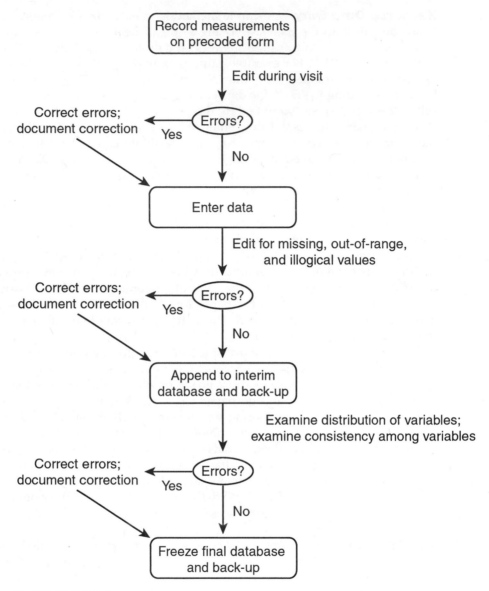

**■ FIGURE 16.1**
Schematic diagram of a system for data management.

timely entry of data and permits interactive editing by the staff who will correct the errors. However, the programs may be complex to design and maintain, and require that study staff at multiple sites be trained to perform data entry. The same system can also be used to send data-editing queries (see later) to the sites, and for study-wide communication.

## Identify and Correct Errors in the Data

Errors in the database should be identified and corrected during each step of creating and analyzing the database (Fig. 16.1). At the **data entry stage**, errors can be minimized by training data entry personnel and emphasizing the importance of accurate data. **Double data entry** is a traditional approach to minimize data entry errors. The data are entered twice; the database program compares the two values for each variable and presents a list of values that do not match. Discrepant entries are then checked on the original data forms and corrected. Double data entry identifies data entry errors at the cost of doubling the time required for data entry. An alternative is to recheck or reenter a random proportion of the data. If the error rate is acceptably low, additional data editing is unlikely to be worth the effort and cost.

Most software programs that are used to enter data from machine-readable forms provide a verification step. After the data forms are scanned or faxed, an image of the completed form and the data as they will appear in the database are presented on a computer screen. The person who is verifying the data must approve each coded value before it becomes part of the database. Systems for collecting data from machine-readable forms generally handle some types of data so well (bubbles, check boxes) that verification is not required, but accuracy should be tested before the study begins and retested during data collection. Machine-readable systems may be less accurate for other types of data, such as text, and verification may be necessary.

After ensuring accurate entry, data are edited or cleaned. **Data editing** includes checking to make sure that the variables are not missing, are within the permitted range, and are logically consistent with other variables. The data dictionary establishes the basis for editing the data. In Table 16.2 the column labeled "permitted values" specifies the values that will be used for range checks. For example, "aastsmo" can only have values between 7, the earliest age the investigator believes plausible for the onset of smoking, and 59, the upper age limit specified by the inclusion criteria for subjects in his study of middle-aged women. The column in Table 16.2 labeled "logic checks" specifies the rules for a different kind of editing. Here the internal consistency of responses in several fields can be checked. For example, the answer to question 2 ("aastsmo") should not be missing if the subject has indicated in question 1 that she smokes.

Detection of potential errors in the data should generate a written or electronic **query,** including the name of the variable and the reason that it may be incorrect. Queries are sent to study staff, who can respond to them by checking original source documents or data forms, interviewing the participant, or repeating the measurement. Resolution of queries should include the outcome of the query, the date, and the identification number of the person who responded. The response to a query may be to accept the variable value (a participant is really 7 feet, 2 inches tall), correct it (the participant is actually 6 feet, 2 inches tall), or confirm that it is missing.

A final step in editing data is to examine extreme values, using software programs to display the lowest and highest values for each variable. Rechecking the accuracy of these outliers is a common data edit. If data are being collected by several investigators from different clinics or locations, means and medians should also be compared across sites. Substantial differences by investigator or site can indicate systematic differences in measurement or data collection.

Data editing and cleaning should give higher priority to more important variables. For example, in a randomized trial, the most important variable is the outcome, and no errors should be tolerated. In contrast, errors in other variables, such as the date of a visit, will not substantially impact the results of analyses. Data editing is an iterative process (Fig. 16.1). After errors are identified and corrected, editing procedures should be repeated until very few important errors are identified. At this point, the edited database is declared final or "**frozen**," so that no further changes are permitted even if errors are discovered.

## Document Changes in the Original Data

A system should be developed for keeping track of identified data errors, queries, and the resulting changes in the database. A person who is unfamiliar with the study should be able to re-create the final database using the original data and detailed **documentation** of how the database was changed in response to data editing.

# ■ CREATING A DATASET FOR ANALYSIS

Several steps are required to prepare a dataset for analysis. Generally, a copy of the data-base is transferred to statistical analysis software. Variables are often redefined and new variables created. For example, continuous variables may be dichotomized (blood pressure above a cutpoint defined as hypertension), new categories created (specific drugs grouped as antibiotics), and derived variables defined (years of smoking × number of packs of cigarettes per day = pack years). It is desirable to decide how missing data will be handled. "Don't know" is often recoded as a special category, combined with "no," or excluded as missing. Many responses that are "not applicable" (such as the number of live births for women who report never being pregnant) are recoded as the appropriate response ("0" live births) for analysis.

When multiple manuscripts are written based on the same database, it is desirable to use the same definitions of variables and handle missing data in the same way for each analysis. For example, it may be puzzling for readers if the number of diabetic participants in the study varies. This could easily happen if diabetes is defined as self-reported diabetes in one analysis and reported use of hypoglycemic medications in another.

The database should be completely edited and frozen before any final analyses for publication begin. All procedures used to create an analysis-ready dataset should be clearly defined in the data dictionary and in a well-documented data management program.

# ■ BACKING UP AND ARCHIVING THE DATASET

As the database begins to accumulate, it is important to make a copy at regular intervals. **Backing up** the dataset guards against catastrophic losses. Storing the backup in a different building (e.g., in the investigator's home) or even in a different city guards against loss from natural disasters.

At the end of the study the original data, data dictionary, final database, and the study analyses should be **archived** for several years. Such archives allow the investigator to respond to questions about the integrity of the data or analyses and to perform further analyses to address new research questions.

# ■ SUMMARY

1. It is important to develop and test the data management system before the study begins.
2. Variables should be named using **systematic abbreviations,** and the format and range of permissible values assigned.

3. The study **data dictionary** includes variable names, format, permissible values, logic checks, derived variables, and any other data management rules.
4. Data should be entered into the database as soon as possible after collection. The accuracy of data entry can be improved by using **double data entry** and data entry interfaces that include **automatic** and **interactive editing features.**
5. **Data editing** should occur as soon as possible after data entry and includes checks for missing, out-of-range, and illogical values, and examination of extreme values.
6. It is important to document the reason for changes in the original data.
7. Datasets should be **backed up regularly** and stored in more than one location.
8. The original data, the final study database, and the study analyses should be archived and stored for several years after the end of the study.

# Implementing the Study: Pretesting, Quality Control, and Protocol Revisions

## Stephen B. Hulley and Steven R. Cummings

**M**ost of this book has dealt with the left-hand side of the clinical research model (Fig. 17.1), addressing matters of design. In this chapter we turn to the right-hand, implementation side.

First, there is the issue of **pretesting.** Even the best of plans thoughtfully assembled in the armchair may work out differently in practice. The response rates for acquiring or following subjects may be far lower than anticipated, and the measurements may turn out to be impractical. It is best to discover these problems in pilot studies that guide appropriate changes in the protocol before the study begins.

Second, there is the issue of **quality control.** Many investigators give insufficient attention to the task of implementing the study because it is tedious and less intellectually stimulating than the design and analysis phases. As a result, the conclusions of a well-designed study can be marred by carelessness and other errors in implementation. The solution is to develop systems for maximizing the completeness and quality of the data once the study is in progress.

These two aspects of implementation also lead to a difficult topic: whether to **change the study protocol** after the study has begun. No matter how good the pretests, the investigator will inevitably discover, once the study is under way, a better way to apply the intervention or measure the outcome. This chapter addresses the painful issue of when to tinker with the study protocol and when to leave it alone.

## ■ PRETESTING

The nature and timing of pilot studies that pretest the study methods depend on the needs of the study. The purpose is to guide the development of a study protocol that will produce better answers to the research questions at a lower cost in time and money. In general, small pilot studies that take only a few days or weeks serve very well, and a series of small pilot studies is generally more useful than one very large one.

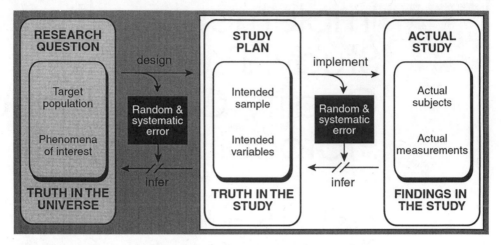

■ **FIGURE 17.1**
Implementing a research project.

## Finalizing the Study Protocol

The main reason for pretesting is to guide decisions about how to design the recruitment, measurement, and intervention approaches. **Pilot studies** of the methods for recruiting the study subjects can provide estimates of the number of subjects who are available and willing to enroll, and test the efficiency of different recruitment approaches. They can also give the investigator an idea of the nature of the populations he will be sampling—the distributions of age, sex, race, and other characteristics that may be important to the study.

Pilot studies are also important in developing the approaches to measuring variables. **Small exploratory pretests** are used to examine alternatives at an early stage. The investigator can spend a few hours looking through clinic charts to see if the desired information has been systematically recorded in previous years. He can select a small convenience sample of subjects to test a new questionnaire that includes open-ended responses to form the basis for constructing appropriate categorical responses in the final instrument. He can ask about subjective reactions to each procedure and any discomfort it may have caused, about whether there were questionnaire items that were not understood, and about other ways to improve the study.

Later in the planning process, some studies will benefit from **large pretests** with subjects drawn from the actual population to test the logistics of making the measurements and to refine and validate the instruments. If the study sample will include people of diverse age, sex, race, and cultural background, and if the measurements are sensitive to this diversity, it may be important to include representatives from each major subgroup in the pretest.

Pretests are helpful for studies that involve a new **intervention.** Interventions designed to change behavior, such as a school-based AIDS prevention program, are particularly challenging. Pilot studies also play an important role in testing the systems for **data management.** Entering and editing real data will help the investigator to know whether the data management system works, and tabulating the findings will reveal information on the quality and spread of responses for each questionnaire item.

## Rehearsing the Research Team

Before the study begins, it is a good idea to test all the recruitment and measurement procedures in a full-scale **dress rehearsal.** The purpose is to iron out problems with the final set of instruments and procedures using subjects who will not be counted in the study findings.

Also, if several people will be involved in collecting the data, the principal investigator can take this opportunity to check on the research team and study plan. What appears to be a smooth, problem-free protocol on paper usually reveals logistic and substantive problems in practice, and the dress rehearsal will generate improvements in the approach. The investigator himself can serve as a **mock subject** in order to experience the study and the research team from that viewpoint, or he may put outside experts in this role to solicit professional reactions to the study plan and its implementation.

## ■ QUALITY CONTROL

An unheralded but very important aspect of clinical research is the approach to ensuring the quality and consistency of the data. This topic receives insufficient attention because the data collection phase of a study is usually repetitive and tedious, and because measurements often seem more straightforward than they are. In the absence of appropriate quality control procedures to prevent them, problems with missing or erroneous data are likely to occur.

### Missing Data

Missing data can be disastrous if they affect a large proportion of the measurements, and even a few missing values can sometimes bias the conclusions. A study of the long-term sequellae of an operation that has a delayed mortality rate of 5%, for example, could seriously underestimate this complication if 10% of the patients were lost to follow-up and if death were a common reason for losing them. Erroneous conclusions due to missing data can sometimes be corrected after the fact—in this case by an intense effort to track down the missing patients—but often the measurement cannot be replaced.

There are statistical techniques for inputing a missing value based on other information (from baseline or from other follow-up visits) available for the subject. Although these techniques are useful, particularly for multivariate analysis in which the accumulation of missing data across a number of predictor variables could otherwise lead to large proportions of subjects unavailable for analysis, they do not guarantee conclusions free of nonresponse bias if there are substantial numbers of missing observations. The only good solution is to design and carry out the study in ways that avoid missing data.

### Inaccurate and Imprecise Data

Inaccurate and imprecise data constitute an insidious problem that often remains undiscovered, particularly when more than one person is involved in making the measurements. In the worst case the investigator designs the study and leaves the collection of the data to his research assistants. When he returns to analyze the data, some of the measurements may be seriously biased by the consistent use of an inappropriate technique. After the baseline examinations in a large cardiovascular trial had been completed, for example, a central review of the lung function tests showed that the water levels in the spirometry machines in some clinics had not been kept at an adequate level; the baseline vital capacity results had to be discarded for many subjects (1).

A worse problem arises when errors in the data cannot be detected after the fact. If the interviews are carried out with leading questions or if blood pressure is measured differently in subjects known to be receiving placebo, the database will include serious errors that are undetectable. The investigator will assume that the variables mean what he intended them to mean, and, blissfully ignorant of the problem, may draw conclusions from his study that are wrong.

## Fraudulent Data

Clinical investigators who lead a research team have to keep in mind the possibility of an unscrupulous employee who chooses fabrication of study information as the easiest way to get the job done. Approaches to guarding against such a disastrous event include taking great care in choosing colleagues and staff, developing a strong relationship with them so that the code of ethical behavior is explicitly understood by all, being alert to the possibility of fraud when data are examined, and making an occasional check of the primary source of the data to be sure that they are real.

## Quality Control of Clinical Procedures

The quality control of clinical procedures begins during the planning phase and continues throughout the study (Table 17.1).

***The Operations Manual.***     The operations manual is an expanded version of the methods section of the study protocol. It operationally defines (i.e., specifies exactly) how to recruit study subjects, measure variables, and perform the study. An operations manual is essential for research carried out by several individuals, particularly when there is collaboration among investigators in more than one location. Even when a single investigator does all the work himself, operational

| ■ **TABLE 17.1**  Quality Control of Clinical Procedures | |
| --- | --- |
| Steps that precede the study | Develop a manual of operations      Operational definitions of recruitment and        measurement procedures      Standardized instruments and forms      Approach to managing and analyzing the        data      Quality control systems      Systems for blinding subjects and investi-        gators    Train the research team    Certify the research team |
| Steps during the study | Provide steady and caring leadership    Hold regular staff meetings    Recertify the research team    Periodically review performance    Periodically compare measurements across      technicians |

Note: Clinical procedures include blood pressure measurement, structured interview, chart review.

definitions help to reduce random variation and changes in measurement technique over time.

The contents of an operations manual are illustrated in Appendix 17.1. They include all the instruments and forms used in the study, with instructions on contacting the study subjects; carrying out interviews; filling in, coding, and editing forms; collecting and processing specimens; managing and analyzing the data; and ensuring quality control.

***Training and Certification.*** Studies carried out by a research team benefit from a formal system for training those who will carry out measurements of particular importance and for testing and certifying their competence to do so. In a multicenter clinical trial of antihypertensive treatment, for example, it is important to have accurate and precise measurements of blood pressure (a partially subjective outcome for which there is no feasible gold standard). Members of the team can be trained in a standardized approach to preparing the patient, applying the blood pressure cuff, locating the brachial artery, inflating and deflating the cuff, and recognizing which sounds represent the diastolic blood pressure. They can be required to pass a written test on the relevant section of the operations manual and to obtain satisfactory readings on pretest subjects assessed simultaneously by the instructor using a double stethoscope. This certification procedure can be supplemented during the study by a scheduled program of recertification.

Sometimes **role-playing** is a useful strategy in the process of training interviewers; one member of the research team pretends to be a subject, coming up with challenging responses. Afterward, the investigator leads a discussion of how the interviewer handled the situation and of the alternatives. The training experience should also include real subjects, and it is efficient to use the pretests and dress rehearsal in the training and certification process.

***Leadership and Supervision.*** Quality control in a study that involves more than one person on the research team begins with the integrity and leadership of the principal investigator. He cannot watch every measurement of colleagues and staff, but if he creates a sense that he is aware of all study activities and feels strongly about the accuracy of the data, most people will respond in kind. It is helpful to visit each member of the team from time to time, expressing appreciation. In addition to such intangibles, a good leader is adept in delegating authority appropriately (team members thrive on responsibility and independence) and at the same time setting up a hierarchical system of supervision that ensures sufficient oversight of all aspects of the study.

***Staff Meetings.*** From the outset of the planning phase, the investigator should lead regular meetings with all members of the research team. Meetings should have the agenda distributed in advance, with progress reports from individuals who have been given responsibility for specific areas of the study. These meetings provide an opportunity to discover and solve problems, and to involve everyone in the process of developing the project and its timetable. Regular staff meetings are a great source of morale and interest in the goals of the study.

***Performance Review.*** It is important to set up a system for reviewing the techniques used by each member of the research team. We recommend that supervisors review the way clinical procedures are carried out by periodically sitting in on representative clinic visits or telephone calls. After obtaining the study subject's permission, the supervisor can be quietly present for at least one complete example of every kind of interview or technical procedure each member of his research team performs. This may seem awkward at first (clinicians are used to being alone in a room with a patient and closing the door), but it soon becomes comfortable.

It is helpful to use a standardized checklist (provided in advance) during these observations. Afterward, communication between the supervisor and the research team member can be facilitated by reviewing the checklist; notes can then be filed to record the fact of the visit and the resolution of any quality control issues that were noted. Such discussions are most effective when carried out in a positive and nonpejorative fashion.

Involving **peers** from the research team as reviewers is useful for building morale and teamwork, as well as for ensuring the consistent application of standardized approaches among members of the team who do the same thing. One advantage of using peers as observers in this system is that all members of the research team acquire a sense of ownership of the quality control process. Another advantage is that the observer often learns as much from seeing someone else handle things as the person on the receiving end of the review procedure.

**Periodic Reports.** It is important to tabulate data on the technical quality of the clinical procedures and measurements at regular intervals. This can give clues to the presence of missing, inaccurate, or imprecise measurements. Differences among the members of a blood pressure screening team in the mean levels observed over the past 2 months, for example, can lead to the discovery of differences in their measurement techniques. Similarly, a gradual change over a period of months in the standard deviation of sets of readings can indicate a change in the technique for making the measurement.

Quality control often includes formal efforts to test the validity and reliability of the study measures. Such efforts include collecting particular sets of data twice to examine the concordance between measurements, checking the internal consistency among related responses on a single occasion, and using a gold standard to validate the measure on a sample of the study subjects.

**Special Procedures for Drug Interventions.** Clinical trials that use drugs, particularly those that are blinded, require special attention to the quality control of dispensing the medication. Providing the correct drug and dosage is ensured by carefully planning with the manufacturer and pharmacy the nature of the drug distribution approach, and by overseeing its implementation.

**Quality Control Coordinator.** In large studies it is a good idea to assign one member of the research team to take responsibility for developing appropriate quality control techniques for all aspects of the study and overseeing their use by the team. The goal is to detect possible problems before they occur and prevent them.

## Quality Control of Laboratory Procedures

The quality of laboratory procedures can be controlled using many of the approaches described above for clinical procedures (Table 17.2). In addition, the fact that specimens are being removed from the subjects (creating the possibility of mislabeling) and the technical nature of laboratory tests lead to special strategies.

| ■ **TABLE 17.2** | |
|---|---|
| Quality Control of Laboratory Procedures | |
| Steps that precede the study | Use strategies in Table 17.1 |
| | Establish good labeling procedures |
| Steps during the study | Use strategies in Table 17.1 |
| | Check equipment periodically |
| | Use blinded duplicates or standard pools |

Note: Laboratory procedures include blood tests, x-rays, electrocardiograms, images.

Many of these are beyond the scope of this book (2,3), but several are summarized here.

***Attention to Labeling.*** When a subject's blood specimen or electrocardiogram is mistakenly labeled with another individual's name, it may be impossible to correct or even discover the error later. The only solution is prevention, avoiding transposition errors by carefully checking the subject's name and number when labeling each specimen. A computer can print sets of labels for blood tubes and records; these speed the process of labeling and avoid the digit transpositions that can occur when numbers are handwritten. A good procedure to follow when transferring serum from one tube to another is to label the new tube in advance and hold the two tubes next to each other, reading one out loud while checking the other; this can also be automated with bar codes.

***Blinding.*** The task of blinding the observer is easy when it comes to measurements on specimens that have been taken from the patient, and it is always a good idea to label specimens so that the technician has no knowledge of the study group or the value of other key variables. Even for apparently objective procedures like an automated blood glucose determination, this precaution greatly reduces opportunities for bias and provides a stronger methods section when reporting the results.

***Blinded Duplicates and Standard Pools.*** When specimens or images in a multicenter study are sent to a central laboratory for chemical analysis or interpretation, it may be desirable to send blinded duplicates—a second specimen from a random subset of subjects given a separate and fictitious ID number—through the same system. This strategy gives a measure of the precision of the laboratory techniques and can be designed in a way that tests either the consistency of a single observer or the consistency among observers. Another approach for serum specimens that can be stored frozen is to prepare a pool of serum at the outset and periodically send aliquots through the system that are blindly labeled with a fictitious subject's ID numbers. Measurements carried out on the serum pool at the outset, using the best available technique, establish the concentration of its constituents; the pool is then used as a gold standard during the study, providing estimates of accuracy and precision.

## Quality Control of the Data

The investigator should set up and pretest the data management system before the study begins. This includes designing the forms for recording measurements, choosing computer hardware and software for data editing and management,

■ **TABLE 17.3**
Quality Control of Data Management: Steps That Precede the Study

Be parsimonious: collect only needed variables
Select appropriate computer hardware and software
Plan analyses with dummy tabulations
Design forms that are
   Self-explanatory
   Coherent (e.g., multiple-choice options are exhaustive and mutually exclusive)
   Clearly formatted with boxes for data entry and arrows directing skip patterns
   Printed in lower case using capitals, underlining, and bold font for emphasis
   Esthetic and easy to read
   Pretested and validated
   Labeled on every page with date, name, ID number, and/or bar code
Program computer to flag missing and out-of-range values

and planning dummy tabulations to ensure that the appropriate variables are collected (Table 17.3).

***Designing the Forms.*** The design of the data collection forms will have an important influence on the quality of the data. Designing the data entry system in advance forces the investigator to standardize the responses during the planning stage and reduces error in entering the data. It also reminds him to avoid open-ended responses that will be difficult to enter.

Entries that involve judgment require explicit operational definitions; these should be summarized briefly on the form itself and set out in more detail in the operations manual. The items should be coherent and the sequence of the items should be clearly formatted, with arrows indicating when questions should be skipped. Making the forms readable and esthetic encourages careful attention among those who will use them. Pretesting will ensure clarity of meaning and ease of use. Labeling every page with the date, name, and ID number of the subject safeguards the integrity of the data should pages be separated.

***Collecting and Managing the Data.*** Strategies for enhancing the completeness and accuracy of the data are an important aspect of quality control. For clinical measurements this should be addressed while the subject is still in the clinic, when it is relatively easy to correct errors that are discovered. The strategy is straightforward: a member of the research team edits what is written on the forms, checking the completeness and appropriateness of the entries (Table 17.4). If the editor can be someone fresh, uninvolved in collecting the data, this will increase the likelihood of detecting missing values and other errors.

An important supplement to this hand editing process is the **computerized editing** that is part of the data entry and management systems programmed to flag missing, inconsistent, and out-of-range values (Chapter 16). For small studies in which this is not feasible, an alternative is simply to take a random sample of the original forms and a printout of what is in the database, and compare the two by inspection.

***Periodic Tabulations.*** Inspection of frequency distributions of important variables at regular intervals allows the investigator to assess the completeness and quality of the data at a time when correction of past errors may still be possible (e.g., by calling the participant back in) and when further errors in the remainder

---

**■ TABLE 17.4**

Quality Control of Data Management: Steps During the Study

---

Check for omissions and major errors while subject is still in the clinic
  No errors or transpositions in ID number, name code, date on each page
  All the correct forms for the specified visit have been filled out
  No missing entries or faulty skip patterns (e.g., skip to question _____)
  Entries are legible
  Values of key variables are within permissible range (e.g., resting heart rate
    >50 and <130; values outside these levels would merit rechecking)
  Values of key variables are consistent with each other (e.g., age and birth
    date)
Check accuracy of entries by hand on a random sample
Carry out periodic frequency distributions to discover aberrant values
Create other periodic tabulations to discover errors (see Appendix 17.2)

---

of the study can be prevented. A useful list of topics for quality control reports is provided in Appendix 17.2.

## Collaborative Multicenter Studies

Many research questions require larger numbers of subjects than are available in a single center, and these are often addressed in collaborative studies carried out by research teams that will work in several locations. Sometimes these are all in the same city or state, and a single investigator can oversee all the research teams. Often, however, collaborative studies are carried out by investigators in cities that are thousands of miles apart with separate funding and administrative structures.

Studies of this sort require special steps to ensure that all centers are doing the same study and producing comparable data that can be combined in the analysis of the results. A **coordinating center** establishes a communication network, coordinates the development of the operations manual and other quality control aspects of the trial, trains staff at each center who will make the measurements, and oversees data management, analysis, and publication. Collaborative studies often have distributed data entry systems with computers or scanners connected through the Internet. This puts data entry and editing closer to those who collect it, enhancing their involvement in the quality of the study.

There is also a need for establishing a governance system with a **steering committee** made up of the principal investigators and representatives of the sponsoring institution, and with various subcommittees. One subcommittee needs to be responsible for quality control issues, developing the standardization procedures and the systems for training, certification, and performance review. These tend to be complicated and expensive, providing centralized training for relevant staff from each center and coordinating site visits and data audits by peers from collaborating institutions (Appendix 17.2).

## A Final Thought

A common error in research that bears on quality control is the tendency to collect **too much data.** The fact that the baseline period is the only chance to measure baseline variables leads to a desire to include everything that might conceivably be of interest (e.g., recording routine components of the physical examination that have little relation to the research question and expanding questionnaires to cover peripheral issues in detail). Investigators tend to collect far more data than they will ever analyze or publish.

One problem with this approach is the time consumed by measuring less important things; subjects become tired and annoyed, and the quality of more important measurements deteriorates. Another problem is the added size and complexity of the database, which makes quality control and data analysis more difficult. It is wise to question the need for every variable that will be collected and to eliminate many that are optional. Including a few intentional redundancies can improve the validity of important variables, but parsimony is the general rule.

# ■ PROTOCOL REVISIONS ONCE DATA COLLECTION HAS BEGUN

No matter how extensive the pretesting, further problems in design or measurement techniques inevitably appear once the study has begun. The general rule is to make as few changes as possible after the study has begun. Sometimes, however, protocol modifications can strengthen the study.

## Making Minor Revision

The decision on whether a minor change will improve the integrity of the study is often a trade-off between the benefit that results from the improved methodology and the disadvantages of altering the uniformity of the study and of spending time and money to change the system. Decisions that simply involve making an **operational definition** more specific are relatively easy. For example, in a study that excludes alcoholics, can a recovering alcoholic be included? This decision should simply be made, one way or the other, with adequate communication to ensure that it is applied uniformly at all sites for the remainder of the study.

Other decisions are more difficult. A questionnaire to elicit symptoms of angina pectoris asks if the pain goes away within 10 minutes. Six months into the study the investigator realizes that this does not distinguish the brief sharp pains of a few seconds duration that probably originate in the rib cage from the pain of some minutes duration that could represent an ischemic myocardium. The investigator could change the wording of a question to exclude instances of sharp pain lasting less than 10 seconds. Doing so might produce a variable that is more appropriate for the research question, but it would create a change half way through the study in the nature of what is measured.

This is difficult to deal with in the analysis phase, and it may be best not to make the change. Sometimes it is possible to continue measuring the variable the old way and to add the new approach in addition. The new version of the question should be asked last, so that it will not alter the responses to the original standard set of questions.

Changes in study methods should be noted in writing, making sure that everyone involved in the study is aware of them. These notes should be dated and retained in the operations manual, where they can be retrieved at the end of the study for analysis. It is important to recognize, however, that in the real world of research it is difficult to deal with protocol changes during the analysis phase. The investigator should undertake minor changes without any illusions, realizing that data collected before and after the change will often end up being combined.

## Making Substantive Revisions

Larger changes in the study protocol, such as including different kinds of subjects or changing the intervention, can be a more serious problem. Although there may be good reasons for making these changes, they must be undertaken with a view to analyzing and reporting the data separately if this will lead to a more appropriate interpretation of the findings. The judgments involved are illustrated by the different resolutions of two examples from the Multiple Risk Factor Intervention Trial (MRFIT), a multicenter heart attack prevention study.

The initial inclusion criteria required each participant to have a risk of coronary heart disease in the top 10% of the population, based on the Framingham risk factor data. Experience soon showed that only 6% of the men who were screened met these criteria (because risk factor levels in the population had declined since the Framingham study began and because volunteers tend to be healthier than average). The MRFIT investigators decided one-third of the way through recruitment that changing the entry criterion from the top 10% to the top 15% would enhance the feasibility of recruiting enough subjects and would not compromise the conclusions. This change was noted in reporting the findings (4), but the investigators did not consider it necessary to analyze the data separately for the two phases of the study.

The second example concerns the approach for measuring one of the main end points in the MRFIT, nonfatal myocardial infarction. The approach specified in the protocol was a blinded reading of yearly electrocardiograms. Near the end of the study, the investigators realized that it would also be desirable to use data from hospitalizations for assessing this important outcome. In order not to change the previously established hypothesis, however, the findings for nonfatal heart attack were reported separately for the two ascertainment approaches (5).

These are examples of substantive revisions that enhanced feasibility or the information content of the study without compromising its overall integrity. Tinkering with the protocol is not always so successful. Substantive revisions should only be undertaken after weighing the pros and cons with members of the research team and appropriate advisors. The investigator must then deal with the potential impact of the change when he draws and reports the conclusions.

## ■ SUMMARY

1. The process of designing the study should include a series of **pilot studies** to improve the nature and efficiency of the methods for recruiting subjects, applying the intervention and making measurements. These may begin as **small and informal pretests** and end with **large pilot studies** to refine and validate the methods and with **dress rehearsals** for the research team.

2. Even well-designed studies can yield erroneous conclusions because of missing, inaccurate, or imprecise data. **Quality control** strategies to minimize these problems include the following:

    a. Efforts to enhance the **quality of the clinical procedures**—developing an operations manual, training and certifying the research team in the standard techniques, providing high-quality leadership, meeting regularly with the research team, creating performance review systems, and examining periodic tabulations of the recruitment and measurement data.

    b. Efforts to enhance the **quality of the laboratory procedures**—in addition to the procedures noted above, developing systems for blinding and systematically labeling the specimens taken from the study subjects, and for using standard pools and blinded duplicates.

    c. Efforts to enhance the **quality of the data management**—in addition to the procedures noted above, improving the design of the forms and developing systems to oversee the accuracy of collecting, editing, entering, and analyzing the data.

3. After the study has started, new ideas for improving the study will inevitably tempt the investigator to make changes in the study plan. However, **protocol revisions** after data collection has begun should be undertaken cautiously, and only when they will enhance the study without compromising its overall integrity.

# EXERCISES

**1.** An investigator studied the research question, ``What are the predictors of death following hospitalization for myocardial infarction?'' Research associates collected detailed data from charts and conducted extensive interviews with 120 hospitalized patients followed over the course of 1 year. About 15% of the patients died during the follow-up period. When data collection was complete, one of the research associates entered the data into a computer using a standard database program. When the data entry was complete, the investigator began to run analyses of the data. To his chagrin he discovered that about 10% to 20% of data about some predictor variables was missing, and a large number did not seem to make sense. Only 57% of the sample had been seen at the 1-year follow-up, now more than a year overdue for some subjects. You are called in to consult on the project.

**a.** What can he do now to improve the quality of his data?

**b.** Briefly describe at least three ways that he could reduce missing values and errors in his next study.

## References

1. Townsend MC, Morgan J, Durkin D, et al. Quality control aspects of pulmonary function testing in the MRFIT. *Control Clin Trials* 1986;7:179S–192S.
2. Canner PL, Krol WF, Forman SA. External quality control programs. *Control Clin Trials* 1983;4:441–66.
3. Widdowson BM, Kuehneman M, DuChene AG, et al. Quality control of biochemical data in the MRFIT. *Control Clin Trials* 1986;7:17S–33S.
4. The MRFIT Research Group. MRFIT: risk factor changes and mortality results. *JAMA* 1982;248:1465–77.
5. The MRFIT Research Group. CHD death, nonfatal acute MI and other clinical outcomes in the MRFIT. *Am J Cardiol* 1986;58:1–13.

# ■ APPENDIX 17.1. EXAMPLE OF AN OPERATIONS MANUAL TABLE OF CONTENTS

Chapter 1. Introductory summary
  Specific objectives of the study
  Study design
Chapter 2. Background and rationale
Chapter 3. Organization and policies
  Participating units (clinical centers, laboratories, coordinating center, etc.)
  Administration and governance (committees, funding agency, safety and data monitoring, etc.)
  Policy concerns (publications and presentations, ancillary studies, conflict of interest, etc.)
Chapter 4. Recruitment
  Eligibility and exclusion criteria
  Sampling design
  Recruitment approaches (publicity, referral contacts, screening, etc.)
  Informed consent
Chapter 5. Clinic visits
  Content of baseline visit
  Randomization procedures
  Content and timing of follow-up visits
  Follow-up procedures for non-responders
Chapter 6. Predictor variables
  Measurement procedures
  Intervention and blinding protocol
  Drug handling procedures
  Assessment of compliance
Chapter 7. Outcome variables
  Assessment and adjudication of primary outcomes
  Assessment and management of other outcomes and adverse events
Chapter 8. Quality control
  Overview and responsibilities
  Training in procedures
  Certification in procedures
  Equipment maintenance
  Peer review and site visits
  Periodic reports
Chapter 9. Data management and analysis
  Data collection and recording
  Data entry
  Editing, storage, and backup
  Confidentiality
  Analysis plans
Appendices
  Letters to subjects, primary providers, etc.
  Questionnaires, forms
  Details on procedures, criteria, etc.

N.B. This is a model for a large multicenter study. The manual of operations for a small study can be less elaborate.

# ■ APPENDIX 17.2. QUALITY CONTROL CHECKLISTS

I. Tabulations for monitoring performance characteristics:
  A. Clinic characteristics
    1. Subject recruitment
      a. Number of subjects screened for enrollment; number rejected and tabulation of reasons for rejection
      b. Cumulative graph of number recruited compared with that required to achieve recruitment goal
    2. Patient follow-up
      a. Number of completed follow-up examinations for each expected visit; number seen within specified time frame
      b. Number of dropouts and of patients who cannot be located for follow-up
    3. Data quantity and quality
      a. Number of forms completed, number that generated edit messages, and number of unanswered edit queries
      b. Number of forms missing
    4. Protocol adherence
      a. Number of ineligible subjects enrolled
      b. Summary of data on pill counts and other adherence tests by treatment group
  B. Data center characteristics
    1. Number of forms received and number awaiting data entry
    2. Cumulative list of coding and protocol changes
    3. Timetable indicating completed and unfinished tasks
  C. Central laboratory characteristics
    1. Number of samples received and number analyzed
    2. Number of samples inadequately identified, lost, or destroyed
    3. Number of samples requiring reanalysis and tabulation of reasons
    4. Mean and variance of interaliquot differences over time and secular trend analyses based on repeat determinations of known standards
  D. Reading center characteristics
    1. Number of records received and read
    2. Number of records received that were improperly labeled or had other deficiencies (tabulate deficiencies)
    3. Analyses of repeat readings as a check on reproducibility of readings and as a means of monitoring for time shifts in the reading process
II. Site visit components:
  A. Site visit to clinical center
    1. Private meeting of the site visitors with the clinic director
    2. Meeting of the site visitors with members of the clinic staff
    3. Inspection of examining and record storage facilities
    4. Comparison of data contained on randomly selected data forms with those contained in the computer data file
    5. Review of file of data forms and related records to assess completeness and security against loss or misuse

Tables should contain results for the entire study period, and, when appropriate, for the time period covered since production of the last report. Rates and comparisons among centers should be provided when appropriate.

6. Observation of clinic personnel carrying out specified procedures
7. Check of operations manuals, forms, and other documents on file at the clinic to assess whether they are up-to-date
8. Observation or verbal walkthrough of certain procedures (e.g., the series of examinations needed to determine patient eligibility)
9. Conversations with actual study subjects during or after enrollment as a check on the informed consent process
10. Private conversations with key support personnel to assess their practices and philosophy with regard to data collection
11. Private meeting with the clinic director's chief concerning special issues

B. Site visit to data center

1. Review of methods for inventorying data received from clinics
2. Review of methods for data management and verification
3. Assessment of the adequacy of methods for filing and storing paper records received from clinics, including the security of the storage area and methods for protecting records against loss or unauthorized use
4. Review of available computing resources
5. Review of method of randomization and of safeguards to protect against breakdowns in the randomization process
6. Review of data editing procedures
7. Review of computer data file structure and methods for maintaining the analysis database
8. Review of programming methods both for data management and analysis, including an assessment of program documentation
9. Comparison of information contained on original study forms with that in the computer data file
10. Review of methods for generating analysis data files and related data reports
11. Review of analysis philosophy
12. Review of methods for backing up the main data file
13. Review of master file of key study documents, such as handbooks, manuals, data forms, minutes of study committees, etc., for completeness

# 18 Community and International Studies

## Norman Hearst and Stephen B. Hulley

**M**ost clinical research takes place in university medical centers or other academic institutions. Such sites offer many advantages for conducting research, including the obvious one of having experienced researchers. An established culture, reputation, and infrastructure for research facilitate the work of everyone from novice investigator to tenured professor. Success breeds more success, thus concentrating clinical research in centers of excellence. This chapter, in contrast, deals with research that takes place outside of these centers.

The term **community research** (or **community-based research**) has been used in many ways. The term is imprecise; after all, almost any group of people might be considered a community. We define **community research** as research that takes place outside the usual university or medical center setting and that is designed to meet the needs of the communities where it is conducted.

**International research,** particularly in the developing world, can involve many of the same challenges of establishing a research program where none existed before. Like community research, international research often involves collaboration between local investigators and colleagues from an established research center. Such collaboration can be productive and highly advantageous for all involved, but it is challenging because of the distances and cultural differences involved.

## ■ WHY COMMUNITY AND INTERNATIONAL RESEARCH?

Community research has advantages that often make it the best or the only way to address certain research questions. These have to do with the questions that can be asked and the populations that can be studied. Furthermore, participation in the research process has benefits for a community that go beyond the value of the information collected in a particular study.

### Local Questions

Many research questions require answers available only through local research. Data from elsewhere may be an imperfect indicator of the incidence and prevalence of disease, and of the distribution of risk factors in the investigator's community. Interventions, especially those designed to change behavior, may not have the same effect in different settings. For example, an AIDS prevention program that

| ■ **TABLE 18.1** |
| :--- |
| Examples of Research Questions Requiring Local Research |

What are the rates of child car seat and seat belt use in a low-income neighborhood of Chicago?

What are the patterns of antimicrobial resistance of tuberculosis isolates in Uganda?

What is the impact of a worksite-based AIDS prevention campaign for migrant farmworkers in Texas?

What proportion of coronary heart disease among women in Brazil is associated with cigarette smoking?

is effective for sex workers in the United States may not work in India (1). Finding approaches that fit local needs requires local research (Table 18.1).

Biologic data on the pathophysiology of disease and the effectiveness of treatments are usually generalizable to a wide variety of populations and cultures. But even here there can be racial differences or differences based on disease etiology. The efficacy of antihypertensive drugs is different in Africans from that in Europeans (2). The causative agents and patterns of antimicrobial sensitivity for pneumonia are different in Bolivia from those in Boston.

## Greater Generalizability

Community research is sometimes useful for producing results that are more generalizable. For example, patients with back pain who are seen at referral hospitals are very different from patients who present with back pain to primary care providers. Studies of the natural history of back pain or response to treatment at a tertiary care center therefore may be of limited use for clinical practice in the community.

Partly in response to this problem, several practice-based research networks have been organized in the past two decades (3) in which physicians from community settings work together to study research questions of mutual interest. An example is the response to treatment of patients with carpal tunnel syndrome in primary care practices (4). Most patients improved with conservative therapy; few required referral to specialists or sophisticated diagnostic tests. This contrasted with the previous literature on the disease from academic medical centers, which had indicated that the majority of patients with carpal tunnel syndrome require surgery.

## Building Local Capacity

Clinical research should not be the exclusive property of academic medical centers in a few cities of the developed world. The priorities of researchers in these sites are bound to reflect the issues they encounter in their daily practice or that they believe are of general scientific or economic importance. Conducting research in the community setting ensures that questions of local importance will also be addressed.

The value of participation in research goes beyond the specific information collected in each study. Conducting research has a substantial positive ripple effect by raising local scholarly standards and encouraging creativity and independent thinking. Each project builds skills and confidence that allow local researchers to see themselves as full participants in the scientific process, not just consumers of knowledge produced elsewhere. This in turn encourages more research. Furthermore, participating in research can bring intellectual and financial resources to a community and help to encourage local empowerment and self-sufficiency.

# ■ COMMUNITY RESEARCH

In theory, community research is much like any other research. The general approach outlined in this book applies just as well in a small town in rural America or Kathmandu as it does in San Francisco or London. In practice, the greatest challenge is finding experienced colleagues or mentors with whom to interact and learn. Such help may not be available locally. This often leads to an important early decision for would-be local investigators: to work alone or in collaboration with more established investigators based elsewhere.

## Starting on Your Own

Getting started in research without the help of a more experienced colleague is like teaching oneself how to swim: it is not impossible, but it is difficult. Sometimes, however, it is the only option. Following a few rules may make the process easier.

1. **Start simple.** It is seldom a good idea to begin research in a community with a randomized controlled trial. Small descriptive studies producing useful local data may make more sense—better a small success than a large failure. More ambitious projects can be saved for later. For example, a descriptive study of condom use among young men in Uganda conducted by a novice local researcher served as a first step toward a larger intervention trial on AIDS prevention in that community (5).
2. **Think of local comparative advantage.** What questions can an investigator answer in his local setting better than anyone else? This usually means leaving the development of new laboratory techniques and treatments to the academic medical centers and drug companies of the world. It is often best for a young investigator to focus on health problems or populations that are unusual elsewhere, but common in his community.
3. **Network.** As discussed in Chapter 2, networking is important for any investigator. A new investigator should make whatever contact he can with scientists elsewhere who are addressing similar research questions. If formal collaborators are not available, it may at least be possible to find someone to give feedback on a draft of a research protocol, a questionnaire, or a manuscript. Attending a scientific conference in one's field of interest is a good way to make such contacts. Contacts can also be made at a distance through telephone, letters, and e-mail. Complimenting a person's work (if not overdone) can be a good way to initiate such a contact.

## Collaborative Research

Because it is difficult to get started on one's own, a good way to begin research in a community is often in collaboration with more experienced researchers based elsewhere. There are two main models for such collaboration: top-down and bottom-up (6).

The **top-down** model refers to studies that originate in an academic center and involve community investigators in the recruitment of patients and the conduct of the study. This occurs, for example, in large multicenter trials that invite hospitals and clinics to enroll patients into an established research protocol. This approach has the great advantage that it comes with built-in senior collaborators who are usually responsible for obtaining the necessary resources to conduct the study. It can be a good way to get started in research, and such collaboration often benefits everyone.

Although one can gain valuable experience through this sort of collaboration, opportunities to develop as a researcher may be limited. Just as important, the potential benefit to one's community may be no greater than if the study had been done elsewhere. Once the study is over, the academic center or drug company may cut off involvement quickly with little or nothing left behind in the community.

In the **bottom-up** model, established investigators provide guidance and technical assistance to local investigators and communities developing their own research agendas. This can be ideal for building local research capacity, especially when such a partnership is sustained on a long-term basis. But establishing an institutional relationship of this type is not easy. Supporting bottom-up community research can be time-consuming and therefore expensive. Most agencies are more interested in sponsoring specific research projects than in building local research capacity. Even when funding to cover expenses is available, experienced investigators may prefer to spend their time conducting their own research rather than helping others get started.

Community researchers need to take advantage of the potential incentives they can offer to more established investigators with whom they would like to work. In the top-down model, the most important thing they can offer is access to subjects. In the bottom-up model, the incentives can include the intrinsic scientific merit of a study in the community, co-authorship of resulting publications, and the satisfaction of helping a less experienced colleague in a worthwhile endeavor.

To start a new research program, the ideal option may be to form a long-term partnership with an established research institution. Collaboration under such a structure can include a combination of top-down and bottom-up projects. It must be remembered, however, that good research collaboration is fundamentally between individual investigators. The best an institution can do is to provide the climate, the structure, the resources, and the long-term commitment that encourage individual collaboration.

# ■ INTERNATIONAL RESEARCH

International research may involve collaboration between groups with different levels of experience and resources, and thus involve some of the same issues as community research. However, international research is subject to additional challenges. The issues described below are especially important.

## Barriers of Distance, Language, and Culture

Because of the **distances** involved, opportunities for face-to-face communication and site visits between international colleagues are likely to be limited. Fortunately, fax and e-mail have made international communication easier, faster, and less expensive than it used to be. Good communication is possible at any distance, but it requires special time and effort on both sides. The most modern methods of communication are of no help if they are not used regularly. Lack of frequent communication and prompt response to queries made on either side is a sign that a long-distance collaboration may be in trouble.

**Language** differences are often superimposed on the communication barriers caused by distance. If the first language spoken by investigators at all sites is not the same, it is important that there be a language that everyone can use. Expecting all interactions to be in English tends to place investigators in developing countries at a disadvantage. Foreign investigators who do not speak the local language are unlikely to have more than a superficial understanding of the country's culture and cannot participate fully in many key aspects of a study, including questionnaire development and conversations with study subjects and research assistants. This is especially important in studies with behavioral components.

Even when linguistic barriers are overcome, **cultural** differences can cause serious misunderstandings between investigators and their subjects or between investigators. Literal word-by-word translations of questionnaires may have different meanings, be culturally inappropriate, or omit key local factors. Institutional norms may be different. For example, in some settings, a foreign collaborator's department chief who had little direct involvement in a study might expect to be first author of the resulting publication. Such issues should be anticipated and clearly laid out in advance, preferably in writing, as part of the important process of gaining high-level local institutional support for the project. Patience, good will, and flexibility on all sides can usually surmount problems of this type. Frequent, clear, and open communication and prompt clarification of any questions or confusion are essential. When dealing with cultural and language differences, it is better to be repetitive and risk stating the obvious than to make incorrect assumptions about what the other person thinks.

## Issues of Funding

Because of economic inequities, collaboration between institutions in developed and developing countries is generally only possible with funding originating from donors in the developed country or, less often, with funding from other developed countries or international organizations. Usually, such funding tends to flow through the institution in the developed country, reinforcing the subordinate position of the developing country institution. As in any situation with an unequal balance of power, this creates a potential for exploitation. When investigators from developed countries control the purse strings, it is not uncommon for them to treat their counterparts in the developing country more like employees than like colleagues. International donors and funding agencies need to be especially careful to discourage this and instead to promote true joint governance of collaborative activities.

Different practices of financial management are another potential area for conflict between cultures. Developed country institutions may attempt to impose accounting standards that are difficult or impossible to meet locally. Developing country institutions may charge high overhead or load budgets with computers and other equipment that they expect to keep after the study is over. While this is understandable given their needs and lack of alternative funding sources, it is important that any subsidies beyond the actual cost of conducting the research be clearly negotiated and that the potential for diversion of funds by institutions or individuals be minimized.

## Ethical Issues

International research raises **ethical issues** that must be faced squarely. All the general ethical issues for research apply (Chapter 14). Because international research presents an enhanced potential for exploitation, it also requires additional considerations and safeguards.

What, for example, is the appropriate comparison group when testing new treatments in a developing country where conventional treatment is unavailable? Placebo controls are unethical when other effective treatments are the standard of care in a community. But what is the "standard of care" in a community where most people are too poor to afford proven treatments? On the one hand, it may not be possible for investigators to provide state-of-the-art treatment to every participant in a study. On the other hand, allowing placebo controls simply because people are poor may encourage drug companies and others to test their new treatments in the developing world without proper protections and benefits for volunteers. Studies in poor countries of expensive antiretroviral drugs have drawn new attention to these concerns (7,8).

A related issue has to do with testing treatments that, even if proven effective, are unlikely to be economically accessible to the population of the host country. Are such studies ethical, even if they follow all the usual rules? If not, what proportion of study subjects should be able to afford the new treatment to make the study ethical? These questions do not have simple answers. Established international conventions governing ethical research, such as the Declaration of Helsinki, have been challenged and are subject to multiple interpretations (9,10).

A key test may be to consider why the study is being conducted in a developing country in the first place. If the true goal is to gather information to help the people of that country, this should weigh in the study's favor. If, on the other hand, the goal is expediency or to avoid obstacles to doing the study in a developed country, the study should be subject to all ethical requirements that would apply in the sponsoring country.

For this and other reasons, studies in developing countries that are directed or funded from elsewhere should be approved by ethical review boards in both countries. But while such approval is necessary, it does not guarantee that a study is ethical. Systems for ethical review of research in many developing countries are weak or nonexistent and can sometimes be manipulated by local investigators or politicians who stand to benefit from a study. Conversely, review boards in rich countries are sometimes ignorant of or insensitive to the special issues involved in international research. Official approval does not remove the final responsibility for the ethical conduct of research from the investigators themselves.

Less talked about but also important are ethical issues in the treatment of collaborators from developing countries. Several issues must be agreed upon in advance. Who owns the data that will be generated? Who needs whose permission to conduct and publish analyses? Will developing country investigators get the support they need to prepare manuscripts for international publication without having to pay for this by giving up first authorship? How long a commitment is being made on both sides? A recent multinational trial of voluntary counseling and testing to prevent HIV infection in the developing world abruptly dropped its collaborating site in Indonesia (11). According to the investigators, this was because the outcome variable of interest (HIV seroconversion) turned out to be less common at that site than projected in the study's power calculations. Even though this decision made practical sense, it was perceived by the Indonesians as a breach of faith.

Finally, an explicit goal of all international collaboration should be to increase local research capacity. What skills and equipment will the project leave behind

■ **TABLE 18.2**
Strategies to Improve International Collaborative Research

Developing country scientists
  Choose collaborators carefully
  Learn English (or other language of collaborators)
  Become familiar with the international scientific literature in area of study
  Be sure that collaboration will build local research capacity
  Clarify administrative and scientific expectations in advance

Developed country scientists
  Choose collaborators carefully
  Learn the local language and culture
  Be sensitive to local ethical issues
  Encourage local collaboration in all aspects of the research process
  Clarify administrative and scientific expectations in advance

Funding agencies
  Set funding priorities based on public health need
  Recognize the importance of building local research capacity
  Encourage true collaboration rather than a ``top–down'' model

when completed? What training activities will take place for project staff? Will local researchers participate in international conferences? Will this be only for high-level local investigators who already have many such opportunities, or will junior colleagues have a chance as well? Will the local researchers be true collaborators, or are they simply being hired to collect data? Scientists in developing countries should ask and expect clear answers to all these questions. As summarized in Table 18.2, good **communication** is a recurring theme in successful international collaborative research.

## Risks and Frustrations

Researchers from developed countries who contemplate becoming involved in international research need to start with a realistic appreciation of the difficulties and risks involved. Launching such work is usually a long, slow process. Bureaucratic obstacles are common on both ends. In countries that lack infrastructure and political stability, years of work can be vulnerable to major disruption from natural or manmade catastrophe. In extreme cases, these can threaten the safety of project staff or investigators. For example, important collaborative AIDS research programs that had been built over many years were completely destroyed by recent civil wars in Rwanda and the Congo. Less catastrophic and more common are the daily hardships and health risks that expatriate researchers may face, ranging from unsafe water and malaria to smog, common crime, and traffic accidents.

Another frustration for researchers in developing countries is the difficulty in applying their findings. Even when new strategies for preventing or treating disease can be successfully developed and proven to be effective, lack of political will and resources often thwarts their widespread application. Researchers need to be realistic in their expectations, gear their work toward investigating strategies that would be feasible to implement if found effective, and be prepared to act as advocates for improving the health of the populations they study.

## The Rewards

Despite the difficulties, the need for more health research in many parts of the world is overwhelming. Many investigators in major academic centers wonder how much difference their work really makes. It often seems that there are plenty of other qualified people who could do the job just about as well as they do. By participating in international research, an investigator in a developed country can sometimes have a far greater and more immediate impact on people's lives than would be possible by staying within the walls of his own university.

Many of the potential problems with international research have their positive aspects. While funding is harder to obtain, the same amount of money can go much farther. Cross-cultural collaboration is as rewarding as it is difficult. The chance to have meaningful involvement and make a real contribution in a foreign land is a rare privilege. Furthermore, it can teach unexpected lessons that enrich careers and lives at home. All stand to gain through increased collaboration and expanding the traditional settings for research. Keeping a broad perspective is the best way to serve science and the public good.

## ■ SUMMARY

1. Community research is necessary to discover **regional differences** in such things as the epidemiology of a disease or the cultural and behavioral factors that determine which interventions will be effective.
2. Although the theoretical issues involved in research are broadly applicable, practical issues, such as **acquiring funding or a mentor,** are more difficult when trying to begin research in a community setting.
3. Collaboration between academic medical centers and community researchers can follow a **top-down model** (community investigators conduct studies that originate from the academic center) or **a bottom-up model** (investigators from the academic center help community investigators conduct their own research).
4. International research involves many of the same issues as community research with additional challenges related to **communication, cultural differences, funding, unequal balance of power,** and **ethics.**
5. Overcoming these challenges can bring the rewards of **helping people in need, a large public health impact,** and **rich cross-cultural experiences.**

## EXERCISES

1. You wish to study the characteristics and clinical course of patients with abdominal pain of unclear etiology. You plan to enroll patients with abdominal pain in whom no specific cause can be identified after a standard battery of tests. There are two options for recruiting study subjects: 1) the G.I. clinic at your university medical center or 2) a local network of community clinics. What are the advantages and disadvantages of each approach?
2. You have been assigned to work with the Chinese Ministry of Health in a new program to prevent smoking-related diseases in China. Of the following research questions, to what degree does each require local research as opposed to research done elsewhere?

**a.** What is the prevalence and distribution of cigarette smoking in China?
**b.** What diseases are caused by smoking?
**c.** What strategies are most effective for encouraging people to quit smoking?

## References

1. Hearst N, Mandel J, Coates TJ. Collaborative AIDS prevention research in the developing world: the CAPS experience. *AIDS* 1995;9(Suppl 1):S1–5.
2. Drugs for hypertension. *Med Lett Drugs Ther* 1999;41:23–28.
3. Nutting PA, Beasley JW, Werner JJ. Practice-based research networks answer primary care questions. *JAMA* 1999;281:686–8.
4. Miller RS, Ivenson DC, Fried RA, et al. Carpal tunnel syndrome in primary care: a report from ASPN. *J Fam Pract* 1994;38:337–44.
5. Kamya M, McFarland W, Hudes ES, et al. Condom use with casual partners by men in Kampala, Uganda. *AIDS* 1997;11(Suppl 1):S61–6.
6. Hearst N, Mandel J. A research agenda for AIDS prevention in the developing world. *AIDS* 1997;11(Suppl 1):S1–4.
7. Lurie P, Wolfe SM. Unethical trials of interventions to reduce perinatal transmission of the human immunodeficiency virus in developing countries. *N Engl J Med* 1997;337:853–6.
8. Perinatal HIV Intervention Research in Developing Countries Workshop Participants. Science, ethics, and the future of research into maternal-infant transmission of HIV-1. *Lancet* 1999;353:832–5.
9. Brennan TA. Proposed revisions to the Declaration of Helsinki: will they weaken the ethical principles underlying human research? *N Engl J Med* 1999;341:527–31.
10. Levine RJ. The need to revise the Declaration of Helsinki. *N Engl J Med* 1999;341:531–4.
11. Kamenga MC, Sweat MD, De Zoysa I, et al. The voluntary HIV-1 counseling and testing efficacy study: design and methods. *AIDS and Behavior* 2000;4:5–14.

# 19 Writing and Funding a Research Proposal

## Steven R. Cummings, Elizabeth A. Holly, and Stephen B. Hulley

**T**he **protocol** is the detailed written plan of the study. Writing the protocol forces the investigator to organize, clarify, and refine all the elements of the study, and this enhances the scientific rigor and the efficiency of the project. Thus even if the investigator does not require funding for a study, a protocol is necessary for guiding the work.

A **proposal** is a document written for the purpose of obtaining funds from granting agencies. It contains the study protocol, the budget, and other administrative and supporting information that is required by the specific agency or board. This chapter will focus on the structure of a proposal and on how to write one that will be successful.

## ■ WRITING PROPOSALS

The task of preparing a proposal generally requires several months of organizing, writing, and revising. The following steps can help the project to get off to a good start.

1. **Decide where the proposal will be submitted.** Every **funding agency** has its own unique process and requirements for proposals. Thus the investigator should start by deciding where the proposal will be submitted, determining the limit on amounts of funding, and obtaining detailed guides about how to craft the proposal for that particular agency.

2. **Organize a team and designate a leader.** Most proposals are written by a team of several people who will eventually carry out the study. This team may be small (just the investigator and his mentor) or large (including collaborators, a biostatistician, a fiscal administrator, and support staff). It is important that this team include or have access to the main expertise needed for designing and implementing the study.

One member of the team must assume the responsibility for leading the effort. Generally this is the **principal investigator** (PI), the individual who will have ultimate authority and accountability for the study. For National Institutes of Health (NIH) proposals (and most other types) the PI should generally be an experienced scientist whose knowledge and wisdom are useful for design decisions and whose track record with previous studies increases the likelihood of funding (reviewers give considerable weight to the value of experience). Some studies also have a project director, a junior scientist who will serve as the day-to-day manager of the study and who can coordinate the proposal-writing effort.

Sometimes the project director comes to assume the PI title and role. Either the PI or the project director must exert steady leadership, delegating responsibilities for writing and other tasks, setting deadlines, conducting periodic meetings of the team, and ensuring that all the necessary tasks are completed on time.

3. **Follow the guidelines of the funding agency.** All funding sources provide written **guidelines** that the investigator must carefully study before starting to write the proposal. This information includes an outline for organizing the proposal, page limits, information on the amount of money that can be requested, and elements that must be included in the proposal.

However, these guidelines do not contain all the important information that the investigator needs to know about the operations and the preferences of the funding agencies. The National Institutes of Health (NIH) and private foundations have **scientific administrators** whose job is to help investigators tailor their proposals to be more responsive to the agency's funding policies. Early in the development of the proposal it is a good idea to discuss the plan with the individual at the agency who will coordinate the review of the applications. This will clarify what the agency prefers (such as budgetary limits and the scope and detail required in the proposal) and confirm that the research plan is within the bounds of the agency's interests. The initial contact can be made by e-mail or letter, but a telephone call or visit is often a better way to establish a relationship and get information that will lead to a fundable proposal.

It is useful to make a **checklist** of details that are required for proposals and to carefully review the checklist before sending the proposal. NIH, for example, requires that applications use no more than a certain number of characters per inch, and cover sheets require several signatures. Rejection of an otherwise excellent proposal for lack of adherence to details is a frustrating and avoidable experience.

4. **Establish a timetable and meet periodically**. A schedule for completing the writing tasks keeps gentle pressure on team members to meet their obligations on time. In addition to addressing the scientific components specified by the funding agency, the timetable should take into account the administrative requirements of the institution that will sponsor the research. Universities often require a time-consuming review of the budget and submission to the local Institutional Review Board before a proposal can be submitted to the funding agency. Leaving these details to the end can precipitate a last-minute crisis that damages an otherwise well-done proposal.

A **timetable** generally works best if it specifies deadlines for written products and if each individual participates in setting his own assignments. The timetable should be reviewed at periodic meetings of the writing team to check that the tasks are on schedule and the deadlines still realistic.

5. **Find a model proposal.** It is helpful to borrow from a colleague a copy of a successful recent proposal to the agency from which funding is being sought. Successful applications illustrate in a concrete way the format and content of a good proposal. The investigator can adapt the best ideas from the model and then design and write a proposal that is even clearer, more logical, and more persuasive. It is also a good idea to borrow examples of written criticisms that have been provided by the agency for either successful or unsuccessful proposals. This will illustrate the key points that are important to the scientists who will be reviewing the proposal.

Although the process may be time-consuming, any funded prior federal application can also be obtained from the investigators or from NIH via the Freedom of Information Act. Proposals of interest can be identified by using the Internet to search the NIH "CRISP" database of funded grants. The NIH Web site and

**■ TABLE 19.1**
Elements of a Proposal, Based on the NIH Model

Title
Abstract
Table of contents
Budget
Biosketches of investigators (2-page curricula vitae)
Resources, equipment, and physical facilities
Specific aims
Significance
Preliminary studies and experience of the investigators
Methods
  Overview of design
    Time frame and nature of control
  Study subjects
    Selection criteria
    Design for sampling
    Plans for recruiting subjects
  Measurements
    Main predictor variables (intervention, if an experiment)
    Outcome variables
    Potential confounding variables
  Pretest plans
  Statistical issues
    Approach to statistical analyses
    Hypotheses and sample size estimates
  Quality control and data management
  Timetable and organizational chart
Ethical considerations
Consultants and arrangements between institutions
References
Appendices

individual institutes have information about how to obtain copies of funded proposals.

6. **Work from an outline.** Begin by setting out the proposal in outline form (Table 19.1). This provides a starting point for writing and is useful for organizing the tasks that need to be done. If several people will be working on the grant, the outline helps in assigning responsibilities for writing parts of the proposal. One of the most common road blocks to creating an outline is the feeling that an entire plan must be worked out before starting to write the first sentence. The investigator should put this notion aside and let his thoughts flow onto paper, creating the raw material for editing, refining, and getting specific advice from colleagues.

7. **Review, pretest, and revise repeatedly.** Writing a proposal is an iterative process; there are usually many versions, each reflecting new ideas, advice, and pretest experiences. Before the final draft is written, the proposal should be critically reviewed by colleagues who are familiar with the subject matter and funding agency. Particular attention should go to the quality of the research question, the validity of the design and methods, and the clarity of the writing. It is better to have sharp and detailed criticism before the proposal is submitted than to have the project rejected because of failure to anticipate and address potential problems. When the proposal is nearly ready for submission, the final step is to review it carefully for internal consistency, format, adherence to agency guidelines, and typographical errors.

# ■ ELEMENTS OF A PROPOSAL

The elements of a **proposal** are set out in Table 19.1 in the sequence required by the NIH (1). Some funding institutions may require less information or a different format, and the investigator should organize the proposal according to the guidelines of the agency that will receive the proposal (generally available on the Web). The scientific elements (the study protocol) are emphasized in boldface type in Table 19.1; these should be written out for all studies, including those that do not need funding.

## The Beginning

The **title** should be descriptive and concise. It provides the first impression and a lasting reminder of the content and design of the study. A good title manages to summarize these elements, achieving brevity by avoiding unnecessary phrases like "A study to determine the. . . ." In an NIH grant application, the choice of words in the title is particularly important because it can influence the decision on which study section (review group) and institute will receive the protocol (2).

The **abstract** is a concise summary of the protocol that should begin with the research question, then set out the design and methods, and conclude with a statement of the importance of potential findings of the study (3). Most agencies require that the abstract be kept within a limited number of words, so it is best to use efficient and descriptive terms. The abstract will generally be written after the other protocol elements are settled, and it should go through enough revisions to ensure that it is first rate. This will be the only page read by some reviewers, and a convenient reminder of the major features of the proposal for everyone else. It must therefore stand on its own, incorporating all the features of the proposed study and persuasively revealing the strengths.

The **table of contents** is an essential aid to the reader. It may be useful to include a more detailed table of contents than the summary version suggested in the NIH instructions. This is especially true for proposals that are large or have complex or unusual sections. The items in the table of contents should correspond to prominently labeled headings or subheadings in the text.

## The Administrative Parts

Almost all agencies require an administrative section that includes a budget and a description of the qualifications of personnel and the institution and access to equipment, space, and expertise.

The **budget** section is generally organized according to guidelines from the funding institution. The NIH, for example, has a prescribed format that requires a detailed budget for the first 12-month period and a summary budget for the entire proposed project period (usually 3 to 5 years). The detailed 12-month budget includes the following categories of expenses: personnel (including names and positions of all persons involved in the project, the percent of time each will devote to the project, and the dollar amounts of salary and fringe benefits listed separately for each individual); consultant costs; equipment (itemized); supplies (itemized); travel (itemized); patient care costs; alterations and renovations; consortium/contractual costs; and other expenses (e.g., the costs of telephones, mail, copying, illustration, publication, books, and fee-for-service contracts).

The budget should not be left until the last minute. Many elements require time (to get good estimates of the cost of space, equipment, and personnel). The best approach is to notify a knowledgeable administrator as soon as possible about the plan to submit a proposal and schedule regular meetings with him to review progress and a written timeline for finishing the administrative section. An administrator can begin working as soon as the outline of the proposal is formulated, recommending the amounts for budget items. Institutions have regulations that must be followed and deadlines to meet, and an experienced administrator can help the investigator anticipate institutional rules, pitfalls, and potential delays. The administrator can also be very helpful in drafting the text of the sections on budget and resources, and in collecting the biosketches, appendixes, and other supporting materials.

The need for the amounts requested for each item of the budget must be fully explained in a **budget justification.** Salaries will generally comprise most of the overall cost of a typical clinical research project, so it is important to show the need for each person, and his effort, in the payroll. Carefully conceived job descriptions for the investigators and other members of the research team should leave no doubt in the reviewers' minds that the estimated effort of each individual is essential to the success of the project.

Reviewers often look at the percentages of time committed by key members of the project. Occasionally, proposals may be criticized because key members of the research team have only a very small (5%) commitment of time listed in the budget and a large number of other studies listed in their other support (implying that they have too many other commitments to be able to devote the necessary energy to the proposed study). On the other hand, the reviewers may also balk at percentages that are inflated beyond the requirements of the job description.

Even the best-planned budgets change as the needs of the study change or there are unexpected expenses and savings. In general, once the grant is awarded the investigator is allowed to spend money in different ways from those specified in the budget, provided that the changes are modest and the expenditures are all appropriate to the study. When the investigator wants to move money across categories or to make a substantial change (up or down) in the effort of key investigators, he will need to get approval from the funding agency. Agencies generally approve reasonable requests for rebudgeting so long as the investigator is not asking for an increase in total funds.

The **biosketches** of investigators are two-page resumes that include academic degrees, current and previous employment, honors, and Federal Government committee service. The biographical sketch also should list in chronological order the titles, all authors, and complete references to all publications during the past 3 years and to representative earlier publications pertinent to the application. A senior investigator with a lengthy curriculum vitae should pick the most important positions and a recent set of publications that are relevant to the research project.

The **resources** available to the project, including computer and technical equipment and office and laboratory space, should be fully described. Components of these sections are usually available in prior grant proposals written by colleagues in the investigator's institution.

## The Aims and Significance Sections

The **specific aims** are statements of the research question using a format that specifies in concrete terms the desired outcome. Each aim should be described in one or two sentences. Most research proposals have several aims and these should be presented in a logical sequence. Sometimes this means putting them in order of importance, and sometimes in chronological order (objectives served by baseline data first, then those related to follow-up). Sometimes, as in the following example, the most logical approach is to present the descriptive aims first, then the analytic aims:

1. To recruit 400 healthy men, 40–59 years old and evenly divided between caucasian and African American.
2. To carry out a randomized blinded trial comparing the effects of testosterone and placebo on risk factors for heart disease, prostate cancer, and fractures.

The specific aims section can also serve as an outline for organizing later sections; the components of the significance and methods sections should follow a parallel sequence.

When a study has many facets, it is tempting to impress the reader with a long and detailed listing of specific aims. This strategy may backfire, creating a proposal that is overly ambitious or cluttered. When numerous specific aims are possible, it is best to propose only the most important and interesting ones. In general, this should not exceed one page.

The **significance** section sets the proposal in context, describing the background in the field under study. It should be written, as much as possible, in a way that is comprehensible to someone who is not an expert in that field. Enough information should be given to make clear what this particular study will accomplish and why it is important. How, specifically, will the study findings advance understanding, change clinical practice, or influence policy?

The purpose of this section is to demonstrate that the investigator understands what has been accomplished, what the problems are, and what needs to be done. The appropriate breadth or detail of the review depends on the scope of the specific aims, the complexity of the field, and the expectations of the review panel. Usually, a critical review of the best and most recent 20 or 30 references will suffice.

The **preliminary studies** and **previous work** of the investigators section should describe relevant previous work by the investigator, making reference to detailed reports and preprints in the appendices. Emphasis should be placed on the importance of the previous work and on the reasons it should be continued or extended. This is also a good place to put one or two paragraphs about each investigator, emphasizing background, previous research experience, and skills pertinent to the proposed research.

Pilot studies that support the research question and the feasibility of the study are important to many types of proposals, especially when the research team has little previous experience in the area to be studied, when the question is novel, and when there may be doubts about the feasibility of the proposed procedures or recruitment of subjects. Results of these studies should be highlighted here, with details provided in the appendices.

## The Scientific Methods

The **methods** section generally receives close scrutiny from reviewers, and it will later serve as the basis for the operations manual for carrying out the study. Weakness in the technical methods is a common reason that proposals fail to be approved or funded by the NIH (4). For these reasons, this section deserves careful attention to detail.

The first concern is how to organize the section. Sometimes agencies provide guidelines about how to organize the methods. If not, we recommend the components and sequence listed in Table 19.1. A detailed table of the contents of the

■ **TABLE 19.2**

Example of a Study Timeline for a Randomized Trial of the Effect of Testosterone Administration on Risk Factors for Heart Disease, Prostate Cancer, and Fractures

|  | Baseline | 3 Months | 6 Months | 12 Months | 24 Months |
|---|---|---|---|---|---|
| Medical history | X |  | X | X | X |
| Blood pressure | X | X | X | X | X |
| Prostate exam | X |  |  | X | X |
| Free-PSA | X |  |  | X | X |
| LDL, HDL cholesterol | X | X | X | X | X |
| Electrocardiogram | X |  |  |  | X |
| Bone density | X |  |  | X | X |

methods section can be very helpful at this point, and an overview of the design, sometimes accompanied by a schematic diagram or table, is essential for orienting the reader (Table 19.2).

The other specific components of the methods section have been discussed in other parts of this book. The subjects and measurements (Chapters 3 and 4) and the pretest plans, data management, and quality control (Chapters 16 and 17) are the centerpiece of the proposal, and require sufficient detail so that sophisticated reviewers will understand exactly how the study will be performed and the reasons for the design choices. Long descriptions of some techniques, such as the details of biochemical assays or of questionnaires, can be put into an appendix.

The **statistical section** should usually begin with the plans for analysis. This can be set out in the logical sequence, first the descriptive tabulations and then the approach to analyzing associations among variables. This will lead to the topic of sample size (Chapters 5 and 6), which should begin with a statement of the null hypotheses and the choice of statistical test before giving the sample size and power estimates at the specified alpha, beta, and effect size. Most NIH review panels attach considerable importance to the statistical section, so it is a good idea to involve a statistician in writing, or at least in reviewing, this component of the proposal.

The proposal must provide a realistic work plan and **timetable,** including dates when each major phase of the study will be started and completed (Fig. 19.1).

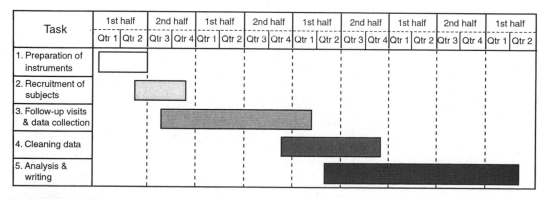

■ **FIGURE 19.1**

A hypothetical timetable.

Similar timetables can be prepared for staffing patterns and other components of the project. An organizational chart describing the research team should indicate levels of authority and accountability, and show how the team will function (Fig. 19.2).

## Final Pieces

The **human subjects** section is devoted to the ethical issues raised by the study, setting forth the issues of safety, privacy, and confidentiality. This section should indicate the specific plans to inform potential subjects of the risks and benefits, and to obtain their consent to participate (Chapter 14). NIH has six points that need to be carefully addressed in their human subjects section. This section is an appropriate place to describe the inclusion of women, children, and participants from minority groups, as required of NIH proposals, expanding on information provided in the methods section.

The proposed use and value of each **consultant** should be described, accompanied by a letter of agreement from that individual and a copy of his biosketch. (Investigators with effort listed in the budget do not need to provide letters.) An explanation of the programmatic and administrative arrangements between the applicant organization and **collaborating institutions** should be included, accompanied by letters of support from responsible officials addressed to the investigator.

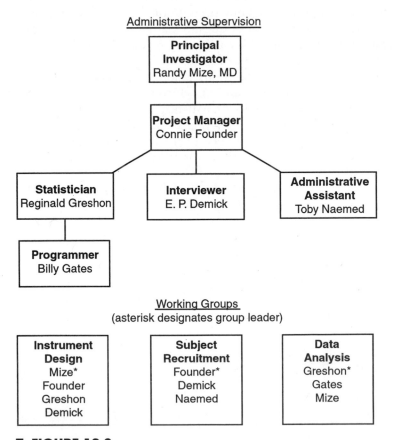

**■ FIGURE 19.2**

A hypothetical organizational chart.

The **references** send a message about the investigator's familiarity with a field. They should be comprehensive and balanced, but an exhaustive and unselected list is not necessary. Each reference should be cited accurately; errors in these citations or misinterpretation of the work can be irritating to reviewers who are familiar with the field of research.

Technical and supporting material can be placed in **appendixes.** Examples are reports of previous work in the area by the investigators, letters of support, and detailed questionnaires and instruments for making measurements that are particularly important to the plans.

# ■ CHARACTERISTICS OF GOOD PROPOSALS

A good proposal has several attributes. First is the **scientific quality of the research plan:** It must be based on a good research question, use a design and methods that are rigorous and feasible, and have a research team with sufficient experience, skill, and commitment to carry it out.

A second attribute is the **technical quality of the proposal** itself. Clarity of presentation is one of the most important determinants of the fate of NIH grant applications. Even if the research question is important and the study plan excellent, a poor presentation can leave the reviewer confused and uninterested. The proposal should be concise and engaging, and not lose the attention of the reviewer with writing that wanders vaguely through peripheral topics. A proposal that is well organized, thoughtfully written, attractively presented, and free of errors reassures the reader that the conduct of research is likely to be of similar quality.

When writing a proposal, it is essential to keep the circumstance of the reviewer in mind. Reviewers are often overwhelmed by a large stack of lengthy proposals, so the merits of the project must stand out in a way that will not be missed even with a quick and cursory reading. Clear outlines, short sections with meaningful subheadings, brief point-by-point summaries, concise tables, and simple diagrams can guide the reviewer's understanding of the most important features of the proposal. It is good to leave some white space on the pages.

Most reviewers are sophisticated and are easily put off by overstatement and other heavy-handed forms of grantsmanship. Proposals that exaggerate the importance of the project or overestimate what it can accomplish will generate skepticism. Writing with enthusiasm is a good idea, but the investigator should be realistic about the limitations of the project. Most reviewers are adept at identifying potential problems in the design or feasibility of a research project.

Rather than ignore potential flaws, an investigator can address them explicitly, discussing the advantages and disadvantages of the various trade-offs in reaching the chosen plan. It is a mistake to overemphasize these problems, however, for this may lead a reviewer to focus disproportionately on the weaker aspects of the proposal and to overlook its strengths. The goal is to reassure the reviewer that the investigator has anticipated the potential problems and has a realistic and thoughtful approach to dealing with them. If the investigator thinks of issues that are not fully resolved in the main body of the proposal, it may be useful to pose these as questions with thoughtful and balanced answers in a "**Questions and Issues**" section at the very end of the methods section.

Finally, the investigator should leave time in the last week or two before the deadline to have someone with excellent language skills read the proposal for clarity, grammatical errors, and spelling errors that are missed by word-processing spell- and grammar-check programs. The editor need not be an expert in the field to provide useful suggestions that increase the clarity and professional appearance of the document.

# ■ FINDING SUPPORT FOR RESEARCH

Investigators should be alert to opportunities to conduct good research without formal proposals for funding. For example, a beginning researcher may be able to analyze data sets that have been collected by others or make use of small amounts of unrestricted funds to conduct studies. Conducting research without funding of formal proposals is generally quicker and simpler but has disadvantages that the projects must be inexpensive and limited in scope. Furthermore, academic institutions often base decisions about advancement in part on a faculty member's track record of garnering external funding for research.

There are four main sources of funds for medical research: (a) the government (notably the NIH), (b) private nonprofit institutions (notably foundations), (c) private profit-making corporations (notably pharmaceutical companies), and (d) intramural resources (e.g., from the investigator's university). Getting support from one of these sources is a complex and competitive process that favors investigators with experience and tenacity.

## NIH Grants and Contracts

It takes 9 to 10 months from the time a successful application is submitted to NIH until it receives funding. During this time the application goes through a process of initial administrative review, **peer review,** final decision by a Council of an institute, and, if successful, administrative procedures to set the final budget and arrange for payments. In this process, NIH staff function as administrators and the funding decisions are largely made by scientists selected from universities not involved in the application. This peer review process, although laborious, is reasonably fair and tends to enhance the quality of medical research in the same way that journal reviewers enhance the quality of the medical literature.

The NIH funds many types of research proposals. The largest number of grants are "RO-1s," conceived by the investigator on a topic of his choosing or written in response to a publicized request by one of the institutes at NIH (Fig. 9.3). "K" awards (so named by the abbreviations, such as K-08 or K-23 awards) are sponsored by individual institutes and designed to help train and develop the careers of junior or midlevel investigators. **Institute-initiatives** proposals are designed to stimulate research in areas designated by NIH advisory committees, and take the form of either Requests for Proposals (RFPs) or Requests for Applications (RFAs). RFPs and RFAs differ from each other chiefly in the type of agreement: under an RFP, the investigator contracts to perform certain research activities determined by the NIH. Under an RFA, the investigator conducts research in a topic area defined by the NIH, but the specific research question and study plan are proposed by the investigator. RFPs use the **contract** mechanism to reimburse the contractor for the costs involved in achieving the planned objectives, and RFAs use the **grant** mechanism to support activities that are more open-ended.

RO-1 applications are usually reviewed by one of many NIH "**study sections.**" Each of these deals with projects on several topics and is composed of experts in those areas drawn from institutions around the country. A list of the study sections and their current membership is available on the NIH Web site, and many investigators use this information to make sure their applications will be responsive to the particular individuals who may provide their peer review. Proposals for K-

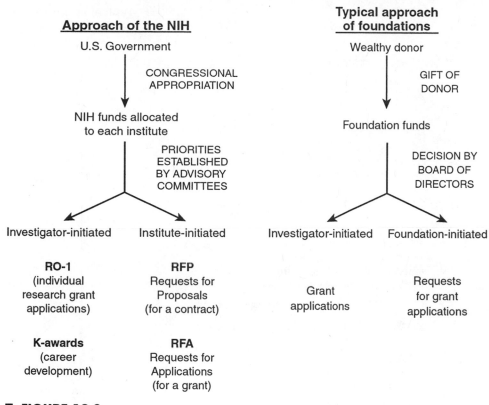

**Approach of the NIH**

U.S. Government

CONGRESSIONAL APPROPRIATION

NIH funds allocated to each institute

PRIORITIES ESTABLISHED BY ADVISORY COMMITTEES

Investigator-initiated          Institute-initiated

**RO-1**
(individual research grant applications)

**RFP**
Requests for Proposals
(for a contract)

**K-awards**
(career development)

**RFA**
Requests for Applications
(for a grant)

**Typical approach of foundations**

Wealthy donor

GIFT OF DONOR

Foundation funds

DECISION BY BOARD OF DIRECTORS

Investigator-initiated     Foundation-initiated

Grant applications

Requests for grant applications

■ **FIGURE 19.3**

Overview of NIH and foundation funding sources and mechanisms.

awards are usually reviewed by experts in a general area of research sponsored by the Institute. Proposals sent in response to an RFA or RFP are usually reviewed by ad hoc committees of peers that follow the same procedures as the study sections in passing on the merits of a proposal.

When an investigator submits an RO-1 or K-series grant application to the NIH, it is assigned by the Center for Scientific Review (CSR) to a particular study section (Fig. 19.4). After review and discussion, each member of the study section assigns a priority score of 1 to 3 for each of the applications judged to be in the upper half. (A few applications are deferred to the next cycle 4 months later, pending clarification by the investigator on points that were unclear.) This is done by secret ballot, and the average is computed and multiplied by 100 to yield a score from 100 (best) to 300 (worst). This score is compared with other scores from the study section to generate a percentile rank. The first percentile is the top and virtually certain to receive funding.

The CSR also assigns each grant application to a particular institute at NIH. Each institute then funds the grants assigned to it, in order of priority score (tempered by an advisory council review and by the institute director), until the budget it has received from Congress is exhausted. If an application is of interest to more than one institute, a "secondary" institute may provide funds if the primary institute cannot, or the institutes may share funding.

The investigator should decide in advance, with advice from senior colleagues, on the outcome he prefers for the two key assignments that are made by the

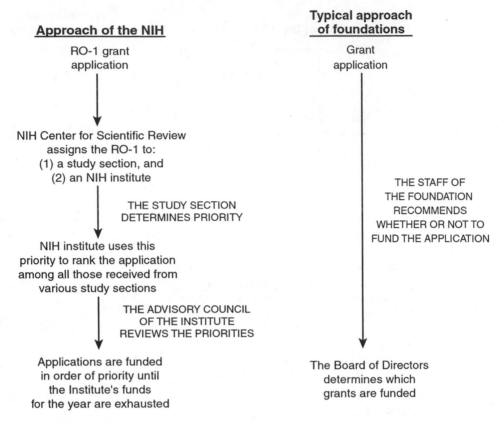

**■ FIGURE 19.4**
NIH and foundation procedures for reviewing grant applications.

CSR—to a study section and to an institute. Study sections vary a great deal not only in topic area but also in the stringency and nature of their review, and there is a considerable difference among institutes in the extent and quality of the competition. Although the assignments are not fully controllable (2), the investigator can influence them by (a) choosing words in the title and abstract that make it obvious what the best assignment would be; (b) stating his preference in the cover letter for the application; (c) asking the NIH scientist in charge of the study section of choice (the "scientific review administrator") or the NIH scientist who will handle the grant at the institute of choice (the "scientific program director") for advice on how to steer the application.

After an application has been reviewed by the appropriate committee, the investigator receives written notification of the committee's action. This **summary statement** includes detailed comments and criticisms from the committee members who reviewed the application.

Applications that are not funded, as is often the case for the first submission, can be revised and submitted again, as many as three times within 2 years. If the reviewers' criticisms suggest that the application can be made more acceptable to the committee, then a thoughtfully revised version may have an excellent chance of obtaining funding when it is resubmitted. An investigator need not automatically make all the changes suggested by reviewers, but he should adopt revisions that will satisfy the reviewer's criticisms wherever possible and justify any decision not to do so. A good format for the resubmission is to begin with an introduction that quotes each major criticism from the summary statement and briefly states the corresponding response and changes in the proposal.

## Grants from Foundations and Specialty Societies

**Private foundations** generally restrict their funding to specific areas of interest. Some disease-based foundations and **specialty societies,** such as the American Heart Association, also sponsor small research programs, many of which are designed to support junior investigators. The total amount of research support is far smaller than that provided by NIH, and most foundations have the goal of using this money to fill the gaps, funding projects of merit that for one or another reason would not be funded by NIH. Decisions about funding follow procedures that vary from one institution to another but that usually respond rapidly to relatively short proposals. The decisions are made by an executive process rather than by peer review. Typically, the staff of the foundation makes a recommendation that is ratified by a board of directors (Fig. 19.4).

To determine whether a foundation might be interested in a particular proposal, an investigator should consult with his senior advisors or check foundation Web sites and published directories of foundations. These sources will describe the goals and purposes of individual foundations and often list projects that have recently been funded. If it appears that the foundation might be an appropriate source of support, it is best to contact the appropriate staff member of the foundation to describe the project, determine their potential interest, and get guidance about how to submit a proposal. Many foundations ask that investigators send a short (three- to five-page) letter describing the background and principal goals of the project, the qualifications of the investigators, and the approximate duration and costs of the research. If the proposal is of sufficient interest, the foundation may request a more detailed proposal.

## Corporate Support

Support for studies of how well a drug or a piece of equipment works can be sought by contacting the research director of the manufacturer. Corporations that make drugs and devices (referred to as "industry") are a major source of funding, especially for randomized trials of new treatments. However, support from profit-making companies can be challenging. Companies often work under severe time pressure to submit results to the Food and Drug Administration (FDA) to get products to market as soon as possible, and may demand that investigators meet challenging timelines for recruiting participants and producing clean data. Another concern is the potential channeling of the research and analyses to meet the corporate and marketing goals. This can, at least in subtle ways, infringe on the objectivity of the work or reporting of results.

However, all medical research (regardless of the source of support) is susceptible to various extra-scientific influences. Because society places a premium on a favorable result, negative results are dull and hard to publish, even though we all recognize that a conclusive negative finding is often as important as a conclusive positive one. Investigators can create some safeguards against undue influence of financial and social pressures. It is important that contracts with companies include clear terms protecting the right to publish. Studies that involve several investigators can have manuscripts reviewed by publication committees, most of whose members are scientists not affiliated with the company.

One advantage of corporate support is that it is the only practical way to address some research questions. There would be no other source of funds, for example, for testing a new antibiotic that is not yet on the market. Another advantage is the relative speed with which this source of funding can be acquired; drug companies are often eager to sign up additional physicians and clinics to participate in their multicenter clinical trials. Additionally, most pharmaceutical companies place a high premium on maintaining a reputation for integrity (which enhances their dealings with the vigilant FDA), and the research expertise, measurement instruments, and statistical support they provide can improve the quality of the research.

## Intramural Support

Universities often have local research funds for their own investigators that can be discovered through the dean's office. Grants from these intramural funds are generally limited to small amounts, but they are usually available much more quickly (weeks to months) and to a higher proportion of applicants than grants from the NIH or private foundations. Intramural funds may be restricted to special purposes, such as pilot studies that may lead to external funding, or the purchase of equipment that will permit a study to be done by scientists whose salary is supported by training funds. Such funds are often earmarked for junior faculty members or fellows and provide a unique opportunity for a beginning investigator to acquire the experience of leading a funded project.

## ■ SUMMARY

1. The **protocol** is the detailed written plan of the study. It is the scientific component of a **proposal** for funding, which also contains administrative and supporting information required by the funding agency.
2. An investigator who has developed a research question and a one- to two-page outline of the study plan should begin by getting advice from senior colleagues about the choice of **funding agency.** The next steps are to study that agency's written **guidelines** and to contact the **scientific administrator** in the agency for advice.
3. The process of writing a proposal, which often takes much longer than expected, includes organizing a **team** with the necessary expertise, designating a **project leader,** establishing a **timetable** for written products, finding a **model proposal, outlining the proposal** along agency guidelines, and reviewing progress at regular **meetings.** The proposal should be **reviewed** by knowledgeable colleagues, revised often, and polished at the end with attention to details.
4. A **good proposal** requires not only a good research question, study plan, and research team, but also a good presentation: The proposal must communicate clearly and concisely, following a logical outline and indicating the advantages and disadvantages of the trade-offs in the study plan. The merits of the proposal should stand out so that they will not be missed by a busy reviewer.
5. There are four main sources of support for clinical research:
   a. The **NIH and other governmental sources** are the largest providers of support, using a complex system of peer and administrative review that moves slowly but encourages good science.
   b. **Foundations and societies** are often interested in research questions that would not be funded at NIH and have review procedures that are quicker and more partial than those of NIH.

   c. **Manufacturers of drugs and devices** are a very large source of support that is usually channeled to tests of specific new drugs and medical devices.

   d. **Intramural funds** can provide small amounts of money quickly and are suitable for pilot studies and beginning investigators.

## References

1. Instruction Sheet for Grant Application Form PHS 398. U.S. Department of Health and Human Services, OMB No. 0925–0001.
2. Stallones RA. Research grants: advice to applicants. *Yale J Biol Med* 1975;48:451–8.
3. Cremmins ET. *The art of abstracting.* Philadelphia: ISI Press, 1982.
4. Cuca JM. NIH grant applications for clinical research: reasons for poor ratings or disapproval of clinical research. *Clin Res* 1983;31:453–63.

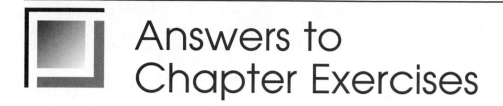

# Answers to Chapter Exercises

## ■ CHAPTER 1

1. a. **Research question:** Does treatment with vitamin D increase leg muscle strength in healthy people 70 years of age or greater? **Study design:** Randomized blinded trial

   b. **Research question:** Does estrogen replacement therapy in postmenopausal women increase risk for breast cancer? **Study design:** Cohort study

   c. **Research question:** Do psychotropic medications increase risk for hip fracture among elderly men and women? **Study design:** Case-control study

   d. **Research question:** What is the state of knowledge about AIDS among schoolchildren in Zimbabwe? **Study design:** Cross-sectional descriptive study.

## ■ CHAPTER 2

1. The possibility that "depression" and "health status" are related is interesting, but the question is vague and may not be possible to answer. To answer this question, these two concepts would need to be operationally defined. How will depression and health status be measured? Even with good operational definitions, it will be difficult to establish causality; that is, does depression lead to worse health or vice versa? There is also the likelihood that the answer to the question depends on the population being studied. A more defined and feasible question might be, "Among college freshmen, does depression assessed by the CES-D questionnaire predict health status measured by the Rand General Health Questionnaire four years later?"

2. This is an interesting research question that also needs to be made more specific. What is meant by red meat? Does veal qualify? What is meant by cancer? Any cancer, including skin cancer? The research question could be rewritten as follows: "Is the amount of beef consumed per week among middle-aged women associated with occurrence of breast cancer over the next several decades?" This question is less vague, but it may not be feasible to produce a scientifically rigorous answer. If the research design is a case-control study (generally the most feasible for cancer etiology), subjects may have difficulty remembering how many servings of red meat they ate during different periods in their lifetime. Such approaches are not novel—there have already been several studies of the association of eating meat and breast cancer, generally suggesting a small increase in risk among women who eat meat. Better data on meat consumption could be obtained by performing a prospective cohort study, but this would require a very large number of subjects followed for many years.

3. This question is vague and could be rewritten as follows: "Does dietary restriction of cholesterol and saturated fat reduce the incidence of myocardial

infarction in middle-aged men with total serum cholesterol over 260 mg/dL?" This question is more specific, but the trial that is implied is neither novel nor feasible. There have been several trials of dietary intervention among middle-aged men with high serum cholesterol. None has had the power to show a significant difference between treated and (nonblinded) control groups in the incidence of coronary heart disease events, and the weak effect of diet on blood cholesterol makes it unlikely that an adequately powered trial is feasible. A feasible version of this research question could be framed for lipid-lowering drugs, which are more effective than diet and permit drug treatment to be compared with blinded placebo, yielding stronger causal inference. But it would not be novel; numerous randomized blinded trials have demonstrated effectiveness in lowering coronary heart disease (CHD). There are still some populations in which such a drug trial with disease end points would be novel (e.g., young adults [but too few events to be feasible] and the very old [bingo!]).

4. This question is probably not relevant or important enough to answer. Many women are anxious about having a mammogram and therefore delay or avoid the procedure. It is not the discomfort of the procedure itself, but the fear that a breast cancer will be diagnosed that creates anxiety. The relaxation exercise is unlikely to reduce this fear of finding cancer. In addition, such relaxation training will not be useful in getting more women to have a mammogram, because the intervention occurs only after the woman has already made the decision to have the test.

5. This question could be rewritten: "Among female sexual partners of HIV-infected men, do those randomized to receive contraceptive vaginal sponges have a lower sero-conversion rate than those who receive placebo sponges." The question is important and relevant, since there is some evidence that nonoxynol-9 might reduce sexual transmission of the HIV virus. However, there are ethical concerns about the implementation of this study. Randomization of women to use of two different types of vaginal sponge might encourage these women to believe that they are protected from HIV infection and thus not use condoms, which are currently the only proven protection against HIV infection. An alternative might be to distribute condoms to all participants and encourage their use. However, if all couples in the study comply with this advice, feasibility is compromised because the transmission rate will be too low to detect any difference between the nonoxynol-9 users and nonusers.

# ■ CHAPTER 3

1. The target population (all eleventh graders, or more broadly, all high school students) may not be appropriate to the research question. If the antecedents of smoking take place at an earlier age, it might be better to study junior high students.

   The study sample (the students at this one high school) may not represent the target population; the causes of smoking differ in various cultural settings, and a better sample might be drawn from several high schools randomly selected from the whole region. Moreover, the sampling design (calling for volunteers) is likely to attract students who are not representative of the accessible population in their smoking behavior.

2. The unrepresentative sample could have resulted from random error, but this would have been unlikely unless it was a very small sample. If the sample

numbered 10, a 7:3 disproportion would occur fairly often as a result of chance; in fact, the probability of finding at least seven heads in 10 tosses of a coin is 17% (plus another 17% chance of finding seven tails). But if the sample size were 100, the probability of finding at least 70 heads is less than 0.01%. This illustrates the fact that the investigator can estimate the magnitude of the random component of sampling error once the sample has been acquired and that she can reduce it to any desired level by enlarging the sample size.

The unrepresentative sample could also have resulted from systematic error. The large proportion of females could have been due to different rates of participation among boys and girls. The strategies for preventing nonresponse bias include the spectrum of techniques for enhancing recruitment discussed in Chapter 3. The large proportion of females could also represent a technical mistake in enumerating or selecting the names to be sampled. The strategies for preventing mistakes include the appropriate use of pretesting and quality control procedures that will be discussed in Chapter 17.

3. a. Random sample (probability)
   b. Stratified random sample (probability), with a threefold oversampling of women, perhaps because the investigator anticipated that few women would attend the concert
   c. Systematic sample (nonprobability)
   d. Cluster sample (probability)
   e. Consecutive sample (nonprobability)
   f. Convenience sample (nonprobability)
   g. Judgmental sample (nonprobability)

# ■ CHAPTER 4

1. a. Dichotomous
   b. Continuous
   c. Dichotomous
   d. Ordered discrete (continuous)
   e. Dichotomous
   f. Ordered discrete
   g. Ordinal
   h. Continuous
   i. Dichotomous

   Power is increased by using an outcome variable that contains ordered information; that is, (d) has more power than (e). As to (i), use of blood cholesterol level as a continuous outcome would offer far more power (carry far more information) than presence or absence of hypercholesterolemia.

2. a. This situation will lead to loss of both accuracy and precision. Accuracy will suffer because the observer's hold on the baby will likely alter the observed weight; depending on technique, this might tend to consistently increase the observed weight or to consistently decrease it. This is primarily a problem with the subjects and could probably be solved by weighing the parent with and without the baby, and taking the difference.
   b. This is primarily a problem with precision, because the pointer on the scale will vary around the true weight (if the scale is accurate). The problem is with the subjects, who need to be quiet and calm for the measurement. Same solution as in (a).

c. This is a problem of precision. It is most likely due to a defect in the scale, which may need refurbishing or replacing. The problem could also be due to observer error if the person reading the scale does not let the pointer on the scale come to rest before reading the weight. This problem could be corrected by proper training and testing of the observer.

d. This is a problem with accuracy. It is most likely due to measurement device error and can usually be corrected by properly calibrating the scale.

e. This is mainly a problem with precision, since the babies' weights will vary, depending on whether or not they ate and wet their diapers before the examination. The problem is subject variability and could be controlled by giving the mothers instructions not to feed the babies for 3 hours before the examination, and weighing all babies naked.

# ■ CHAPTER 5

1. Sample size = the expected number of subjects in a study

Null hypothesis = a statement of the research hypothesis that indicates that there is no difference between the groups being compared

Alternative hypothesis = a statement of the research hypothesis that indicates that there is a difference between the groups being compared

Power = the likelihood of detecting a statistically significant difference between the groups being compared (with a given sample size, at a given level of statistical significance) if the real difference in the population equals the effect size

Level of statistical significance = the preset chance of falsely rejecting the null hypothesis

Effect size = the minimum size of the difference in the two groups being compared that the investigator wishes to detect

# ■ CHAPTER 6

1. $H_0$: There is no difference in the height of stomach cancer cases and controls.

$H_A$ (two-sided): There is a difference in the height of stomach cancer cases and controls

Height is a continuous variable and case-control is dichotomous, so a $t$-test should be used.

> Effect size = 5 cm
> Standard deviation (SD) = 10 cm
> $E/S = 0.5$

From Appendix 6.A,

> If alpha = 0.05, beta = 0.20, then 63 subjects are needed per group.
> If alpha = 0.05, beta = 0.10, then 84 subjects are needed per group.
> If alpha = 0.01, beta = 0.20, then 93 subjects are needed per group

Extra credit: Suppose the investigator only had access to 40 cases. What could she do?

Most strategies for increasing power will not help:

a. Use a continuous variable—height is already being measured as a continuous variable.

b. Use a more precise variable—height is a very precise variable, the standard deviation being composed almost entirely of between-individual variation, which cannot be reduced.

c. Use paired measurements—not applicable; "change" in height is not relevant

d. Use a more common outcome—not applicable.

e. Use unequal group sizes—the $N$ of controls can be increased, as it is easy to find subjects without stomach cancer. If the number of controls is increased fourfold to 160, one can use the approximation formula on page 79:

$$n' = ([c + 1] \div 2c) \times n$$

where $n'$ represents the "new" number of cases, $c$ represents the control-to-case ratio (in this example, 4), and $n$ represents the "old" number of cases (assuming a control per case). In this example,

$$n' = ([4 + 1] \div 8) \times 63 = (5/8) \times 63 = 40,$$

which is just the number of cases that are available. Thus a study with 40 cases and 160 controls will have similar power as one with 63 cases and 63 controls.

2. $H_0$: There is no difference in mean strength between the DHEA-treated and placebo-treated groups.

$H_A$: There is a difference in mean strength between the DHEA-treated and placebo-treated groups.

> alpha = 0.05 (two-sided); beta = 0.10
> test = $t$ test
> effect size = 10% × 20 kg = 2 kg
> standard deviation = 5 kg

The standardized effect size $(E/S)$ is 0.4 (2 kg/5 kg). Looking at Appendix 6.A, go down the left column to 0.40, then across to the fifth column from the left, where alpha (two-sided) = 0.05 and beta = 0.10. Approximately 131 subjects per group would be needed. If a one-sided test is justified, then the sample size would be 107 per group. If beta = 0.20 (in addition to using a one-sided test), then the sample size is only 77 per group.

3. $H_0$: There is no difference in the mean change in strength between the DHEA-treated and placebo-treated groups.

$H_A$: There is a difference mean change in strength between the DHEA-treated and placebo-treated groups.

> alpha = 0.05 (two-sided); beta = 0.10
> test = $t$ test
> effect size = 10% × 20 kg = 2 kg
> standard deviation = 2 kg

The standardized effect size $(E/S)$ is 1.0 (2 kg/2 kg). Looking at Appendix 6.A, go down the left column to 1.0 then across to the fifth column from the left where alpha (two-sided) = 0.05 and beta = 0.10. Approximately 21 subjects per group would be needed.

4. $H_0$: There is no difference in frequency of left-handedness in dyslexic and nondyslexic students.

$H_A$: There is a difference in frequency of left-handedness in dyslexic and nondyslexic students.

alpha = 0.05 (two-sided); beta = 0.20
test = chi-squared test (both variables are dichotomous)
effect size = odds ratio of 2.0

Given that the proportion of nondyslexic students who are left-handed ($P_2$) is about 0.1, the investigator wants to be able to detect a proportion of dyslexic students who are left-handed ($P_1$) that will yield an odds ratio of 2.0. The sample size estimate will use a chi-squared test, and one needs to use Appendix 6.B. However, that appendix is set up for entering the two proportions, not the odds ratio, and all that is known is one of the proportions ($P_2 = 0.1$).

To calculate the value for $P_1$ that gives an odds ratio of 2, one can use the formula on p. 69:

$$P_1 = OR \times P2 \div ([1 - P_2] + [OR \times P_2]).$$

In this example:

$$P_1 = (2 \times 0.1) \div ([1 - 0.1] + [2 \times 0.1]) = 0.18$$

So $P_1$ is 0.18 and $P_2$ is 0.1. $P_1 - P_2$ is 0.08. The table in Appendix 6.B.2 reveals a sample size of 294 per group.

Extra credit: Try this using the formula on page 87; just slog on through, carrying 6 places after the decimal.

5. Standard deviation of RO-1 scores = 100
   Total width of the confidence interval = 40 (20 above and 20 below)
   Confidence level = 99%
   Standardized width of the confidence interval = total width/standard deviation $W/S = 0.40$
   Using Table 6.D, go down the $W/S$ column to 0.40, then across to the 99% confidence level. About 166 RO-1 NIH grant application scores would need to be averaged to obtain a mean score with the specified confidence interval.

# ■ CHAPTER 7

1. a. Measure serum vitamin D levels in a cohort of white women more than 70 years of age and without a history of hip fractures and analyze the association with incident hip fractures observed over the next 5 years. (Choice of study subjects is based on the fact that hip fracture is most common in white women; the age cutoff is somewhat arbitrary, but based on the age at which hip fracture incidence rises rapidly and to substantial levels.) The use of reported dietary intake of vitamin D instead of the serum level might be more expensive because dietary histories take a lot of time to collect and score and would certainly be a less precise and less accurate measurement.

   b. Advantages of the prospective cohort design for studying vitamin D and hip fractures:

   ■ Temporal sequence (i.e., the hip fracture follows the vitamin D deficiency) helps establish a cause-effect relationship. Women who fracture their hips might become vitamin D deficient after the fracture because they must stay in bed to recuperate and vitamin D is produced from cholesterol in the skin in the presence of sunlight.

- The prospective design allows you to design good methods for measuring the predictor variable (i.e., serum vitamin D).

- The cohort design avoids the sampling bias that is always a possibility in case-control studies if the women with fractures come from a different accessible population than those without fractures.

Disadvantage of the prospective cohort design:

- A prospective cohort study will require many subjects followed for multiple years. The study will therefore be very expensive.

c. A retrospective cohort study could be done if you could find a cohort with stored serum or records on dietary vitamin D intake and with reasonably complete follow-up to determine who developed hip fracture. The main advantage of this design is that it would be less time-consuming and expensive. The major drawback is that measurements of vitamin D in the serum might be altered by the storage and that measurements of potential confounders (such as age, race, physical activity, cigarette smoking, etc.) may not be available.

# ■ CHAPTER 8

1. a. The cases might consist of all women between 30 and 75 years of age with ovarian cancer reported to the Northern California Cancer Center Tumor Registry. This tumor registry has been shown to include nearly 100% of incident ovarian cancer cases in five San Francisco Bay Area counties.
   b. The controls might be a random sample of all women between 30 and 75 years of age from the same five counties in the San Francisco Bay Area. The random sample might be obtained by using random-digit dialing.
   c. The methods outlined for choosing cases and controls are aimed at obtaining all cancer cases and a random sample of those at risk in the target population (women 30 to 75 years old in five Bay Area counties). However, it is possible, since ovarian cancer requires intensive therapy and is deadly, that some cases may be unwilling to enroll in your study or may already be dead. If family history of ovarian cancer is related only to aggressive forms of ovarian cancer, then you might underestimate the association of family history and ovarian cancer. It is also possible that healthy women who have a family member with ovarian cancer will be more interested in the study and more likely to enroll as a control when you contact them than women who do not have a family member with ovarian cancer. In this case, the prevalence of family history of ovarian cancer in the control group will be artificially high, and your estimate of the risk for ovarian cancer due to family history will be falsely low. You might minimize this problem by not telling the potential control subjects exactly what your research question is or exactly which cancer you are studying.

d. Family history of ovarian cancer is generally measured by asking subjects if any members of their family have had ovarian cancer. Recall bias is the most likely problem with this approach. Women with ovarian cancer, who are searching for a reason for their having developed cancer, may be more likely to remember a relative with ovarian cancer than a healthy woman. In this case, your estimate of the association between family history and ovarian cancer may be falsely high.

In addition, many women confuse the gynecologic cancers (cervical, uterine, and ovarian) and confuse benign gynecologic tumors that require surgery with malignant tumors. This may cause misclassification (some women without a family history of ovarian cancer will report having the risk factor and be misclassified). If misclassification occurs equally in the cases and controls, your estimate of the association between family history and ovarian cancer will be falsely low. If this type of misclassification is more common in cases (who may be more likely to misinterpret the type of cancer or the reason for surgery in relatives), then your estimate of the association between family history and ovarian cancer will be falsely high. Misclassification could be decreased by checking pathologic records of family members who are reported to have ovarian cancer to verify the diagnosis.

e. Since the predictor (family history of ovarian cancer) is dichotomous (present or absent) and the outcome is dichotomous (ovarian cancer present or absent), the best measure of association is the odds ratio, which approximates the relative risk when the outcome (such as ovarian cancer) is rare. Chi square is the appropriate test of statistical significance.

f. The case-control design is a reasonable way to answer this research question despite the problems of sampling bias, recall bias, and misclassification. The chief alternative would be a large cohort study, but because ovarian cancer is so rare, a cohort design is probably not feasible.

2. a. The study is cross-sectional because the potential predictors (maternal height and weight) are measured at the same time as the outcome (infant birthweight).

b. Causal inference in cross-sectional studies depends on the time sequence of the predictor and outcome variables. In this study, the mother's weight was measured just after delivery and reflects a combination of the mother's weight before she became pregnant and the amount of weight that she gained during pregnancy. Since the amount of weight gained during pregnancy may depend on the weight of the fetus, it is not clear which variable is the predictor. However, the mother's height measured just after delivery probably does not differ from her height if it had been measured before conception. It is reasonable therefore to conclude that maternal height is likely to be a predictor of birthweight.

# ■ CHAPTER 9

1. There are five possible explanations for the association between diet and CHD:

a. Chance—the finding that people with CHD eat fewer fruits and vegetables was due to random error. Recall from Chapter 5 that the probability of falsely rejecting the null hypothesis when it is true was called alpha, the "type I" error rate. Alpha is set during the design phase when the sample size is estimated. Alpha can be reduced by increasing the sample size or decreasing the power of the study. Strategies to increase power include increasing the precision of the measurements (e.g., choosing the more time-consuming instrument for assessing usual intake for the past month, rather than the faster 24-hour recall). In the analysis phase, the $P$-value is used to compare the magnitude of the association observed with what might have been expected by chance alone.

b. Bias—there was a systematic error (a difference between the research question and the way the study plan was carried out) with regard to the sample, predictor variable, or outcome variable. For example, the sample may be biased if the controls were HMO patients attending an annual health maintenance examination, as such patients may be more health conscious (and hence eat more fruits and vegetables) than the entire population at risk for CHD. The measurements of diet could be biased if people who have had a heart attack are more likely to recall poor dietary practices than controls (recall bias) or if unblinded interviewers asked the questions or recorded the answers differently in cases and controls. The likelihood of bias can be reduced by consulting with colleagues and carefully considering major design decisions such as selection of study subjects, and by blinding measurements wherever possible.

c. Effect-cause—it is possible that having a heart attack reduced people's appetites, so that they ate less food in general (including less fruits and vegetables). The possibility of effect-cause can often be addressed by designing variables to examine the historical sequence—for example, by asking the cases if they changed their diet after their heart attack. In this instance, a strategy would be to express fruit and vegetable intake as percentage of total intake rather than as the absolute intake.

d. Confounding—there may be other differences between those who eat more fruits and vegetables and those who eat fewer, and these other differences may be the actual cause of the lower rate of CHD. For example, people who eat more fruits and vegetables may exercise more. The strategies for addressing the latter possibility are as follows:

| Design Phase | Plan | Advantages | Disadvantages |
|---|---|---|---|
| Specification | Enroll only people who report no regular exercise | Simple | Will limit the pool of eligible subjects, making recruitment more difficult. The study may not generalize to people that exercise. |
| Matching | Match each case to a control with similar exercise level | Eliminates the effect of exercise as a predictor of CHD, often with a slight increase in the precision (power) to observe diet as a predictor. | Requires extra effort to identify controls to match each case. Will waste cases if there is no control with a similar exercise level. Eliminates the opportunity to study the effect of exercise on CHD. Requires a matched statistical analysis model. |

| | Plan | Advantages | Disadvantages |
|---|---|---|---|
| **Analysis Phase** | | | |
| Stratification | For the analysis, group the subjects into three or four exercise strata | Easy, comprehensible, and reversible | Can only reasonably evaluate a few strata and a few confounding variables before you find no cases (or controls) in a cell. Will lose some of the information contained in fitness measured as a continuous variable by switching to a categorical variable, and this may result in incomplete control of confounding. |
| Statistical adjustment (modeling) | Use logistic regression model to control for fitness as well as other potential confounders | Can reversibly control for all the information in fitness as a continuous predictor variable, while simultaneously controlling for other potential confounders such as age, race, and smoking | The statistical model might not fit the data, resulting in incomplete control of confounding and potentially misleading results. For example, the effect of diet or physical fitness may not be the same in smokers and non-smokers. The important potential confounders must have been measured in advance. Sometimes it is difficult to understand and describe the results of the model, especially when variables are not dichotomous. |

In addition to these four strategies for controlling confounding in observational studies, there is the ultimate solution: designing a randomized blinded trial.

e. Cause-effect—the fifth possible explanation is the jackpot—that eating fruits and vegetables really does reduce the rate of CHD events. This explanation is made likely partly by a process of exclusion, reaching the judgment that each of the other four explanations is unlikely and partly by seeking other evidence to support the causal hypothesis. An example of the latter is to consider the biologic evidence that a component of many fruits and vegetables (e.g., antioxidants) is antiatherogenic.

# ■ CHAPTER 11

1. a. Design 5-year randomized blinded trial of vitamin D versus placebo in white women more than 70 years of age, with hip fracture incidence as the outcome.

Advantages of the randomized blinded trial for studying vitamin D and hip fractures:

■ Show cause-effect more conclusively.

- Randomization and blinding eliminate confounding and co-interventions.
- A trial makes it possible to determine the effectiveness of a treatment program (i.e., reversibility/preventability of the vitamin D deficiency disorder with treatment begun late in life).

  Disadvantages of the randomized blinded trial:
- Large, expensive, and time-consuming study.
- Ethical issues must be considered. This study should come last, after observational studies indicate treatment is promising, but do not establish whether benefits are real and outweigh harms.
- Problem of choosing the dosage of vitamin D for the randomized blinded trial, a problem you do not have with observational designs.

   b. Run-in design to improve compliance and thereby increase power/reduce sample size.

     Factorial design—consider running another randomized blinded trial in the same cohort (e.g., effect of aspirin on cardiovascular disease).

     Develop a surrogate for the outcome that will improve efficiency (question 1c).

     Group randomization, perhaps with vitamin D in the food or beverage at some institutions and not at others.

   c. Measure coordination and strength as outcome variables. When there is a rapidly responsive and continuous outcome variable, a much smaller and shorter study can be designed.

# ■ CHAPTER 12

   1. a. The best way to sample subjects for a diagnostic test is generally to sample patients at risk of a disease, before it is known who has the disease and who does not. In this case, sampling women who present acutely to a clinic or emergency room with signs and symptoms consistent with pelvic inflammatory disease (PID) would probably be best. Comparing the erythrocyte sedimentation rates (ESRs) of women hospitalized with PID to those of a healthy control population (nurses, medical students) would be the worst approach, because both the spectrum of disease and especially the spectrum of nondisease are not representative of the groups in whom the test would be used clinically. (Those hospitalized for PID probably have more severe disease than average, and healthy volunteers are much less likely to have high ESRs than women with abdominal pain due to causes other than PID.)

     b. If those assigning the final diagnosis used the ESR to help decide who had PID and who did not, both the sensitivity and specificity might be falsely high. The more those assigning the diagnosis relied on the ESR, the greater the bias in the study.

     c. This is a bit of a trick question. Which cutoff to use depends on the prior probability and the consequences of false-negative and false-positive results. The best answer is that you should not use any particular cutoff for defining an abnormal result. Rather, you should graphically display the trade-off between sensitivity and specificity using an ROC curve and present likelihood ratios for various ESR intervals rather than sensitivity and specificity at different cutoffs.

2. a. This problem illustrates the common error of excluding people from the numerator, without excluding them from the denominator. Although it is true that there were only two children with "unexpected" intracranial injuries, the denominator for the yield must be the number of children with normal neurologic examinations and mental status—probably a much smaller number than 200.

   b. Unless the finding of an intracranial injury leads to changes in management and there is some way to estimate the effects of these management changes on outcome, it will be very hard to know what yield is sufficient to make the test worth doing. It would be better to use "intracranial injury requiring intervention" as the outcome in this study, although this will require some consensus on what injuries require intervention and some estimate of the effectiveness of these interventions for improving outcome.

   c. The first advantage is the ability to examine possible benefits of normal results. For example, a normal CT scan might change the management plan from "admit for observation" to "send home." In diagnostic yield studies, normal results are generally assumed to be of little value. Second, as mentioned earlier, abnormal CT scan results might not lead to any changes in management (e.g., if no neurosurgery was required and the patient was going to be admitted anyway). Studying effects of tests on medical decision-making helps to determine how much new information they provide, beyond what is already known at the time the test is ordered.

# ■ CHAPTER 13

1. Three possibilities:
   a. Analyze data from the National Health and Nutrition Examination Survey (NHANES). These national studies are conducted periodically and their results are available to any investigator at a nominal cost. They contain data from population-based samples that include variables on self-reported clinical history of gallbladder disease and the results of abdominal sonography.

   b. Analyze Medicare data on frequency of gallbladder surgery in patients more than 65 years of age in the United States or National Hospital Discharge Survey data on the frequency of such surgery for all ages. Both data sets contain a variable for race. Denominators could come from census data. Like the NHANES, these are very good population-based samples but have the problem of answering a somewhat different research question (i.e., what are the rates of surgical treatment for gallbladder disease). This may be different from the actual incidence of gallbladder disease due to factors such as access to care.

   c. Check local coroner records on the relation between gallbladder disease (as an incidental finding on autopsy) and race. Such a sample, however, may have biases due to who gets autopsied.

2. a. Using the Multiple Risk Factor Intervention Trial (MRFIT) data set made it feasible, inexpensive, and relatively quick to answer the fellow's research question. Also, the outcome variable for the fellow's research question (coronary heart disease events) was measured very carefully in the MRFIT study because it was also the main outcome of that trial.

   b. In this real example, several specific limitations developed. Unfortunately, the predictor variable (serum triglycerides) was only measured once at baseline in the MRFIT and the precision offered by multiple measurements has proved to be important. Because the MRFIT trial had been completed several years before the fellow began his project, there was no longer a statistician or data analyst working on the study and it was hard to get exactly the analyses that the fellow wanted from the new set of researchers who had access to the database. Finally, the intervention (low-fat diet) complicated the analysis and interpretation of the association of serum triglycerides (measured at the beginning of the trial) and coronary heart disease events.

# ■ CHAPTER 14

1. a. Performing your study in a nursing home has the advantage that the population of participants is stable and easily accessible, particularly for follow-up. If your study shows that the new device is more comfortable and less likely to cause urinary tract infection, this might eventually benefit the subjects. Because your intended study population is dependent and may not be mentally capable of giving informed consent, several ethical issues must be addressed. Some of the nursing home population will have Alzheimer's or other forms of dementia so that they will not be able to understand the purpose of the study or its potential risks and benefits. The protocol should specify how it will be determined that potential subjects have the capacity to make informed decisions. As a dependent and vulnerable population, nursing home residents may feel coerced into participating in the study and be unable to express reservations for fear of jeopardizing their care. Measurement of outcome may be biased if patients are unable to provide an assessment of comfort. In this case, generalizability of the study results to other populations requiring indwelling catheters may be limited. Can the study be carried out in a less vulnerable population (e.g., patients with stroke or spinal cord injury living at home)?

   b. Institutional review board approval is always required for an experimental study involving human subjects. Informed consent must also be obtained, since a new and invasive procedure will be used that may have unexpected adverse effects, including more discomfort or more urinary tract infections.

   c. If there is any possibility that a potential participant is unable to give informed consent, a brief test of mental competence, such as the Mini-Mental State Questionnaire, could be administered. Potential subjects who cannot provide informed consent should be excluded.

2. a. Each Institutional Review Board makes its own specific decisions on a case-by-case basis, but some general guidelines have come into widespread use. New therapies for serious diseases must be compared with other therapies that are already accepted and in use ("standard of care"). Thus you must demonstrate that the standard of care for patients with inoperable lung cancer is no active therapy, rather than any chemotherapy or radiation therapy. There should also be some evidence (from animal studies, Phase I studies, clinical practice, or observational studies) that the new therapy will improve survival. However, there should not be convincing evidence that the new therapy is superior. This uncertainty as to whether the new therapy will result in a better outcome is called *equipoise*. Recruitment must not overrepresent the possible benefits or minimize the dangers of the new

therapy. Study data should be examined periodically during the trial using prespecified stopping rules to determine if the trial should be stopped early because either the benefits or the adverse effects of the drugs are unexpectedly large and clearcut.

b. Informed consent should include: (1) the nature of its study, indicating that it is not known whether the new therapy is better than no active therapy; (2) a description of the study that includes number and length of visits, procedures during each visit (such as filling out questionnaires and drawing blood), the new chemotherapeutic treatment regimen (medications, dosage, route, and timing); (3) a description of what randomization means; (4) a description of the potential adverse effects of the new regimen and the likelihood that they will occur, how these will be monitored, and what symptomatic relief will be provided; (5) a description of the potential benefits of the trial; (6) a description of therapies such as chemotherapy and radiation therapy that are available outside the trial; (7) notification that the participant is not obligated to take part in the study and can withdraw at any time; (8) notification that confidentiality will be protected to the extent possible; and (9) notification that any questions will be answered before enrollment and throughout the study.

c. The people obtaining informed consent should have a thorough understanding of the research question, the study design and protocol (including both the new chemotherapy and palliative care), and the potential side effects of the new regimen. The person obtaining consent should be able to explain these components to the patients in clear lay language and answer any questions. The person should be impartial in the presentation of the advantages and disadvantages of enrolling in the study and be able to explain the process of randomization. A detailed operations manual for the study should be available to study personnel obtaining informed consent. Training should be specific and detailed, including practice discussions. Administration of informed consent should be periodically monitored by investigators and peers, and feedback should be provided. There should be no conflict of interest on the part of those administering informed consent.

3. a. A particular physician may recruit more participants because he is more interested in the study and describes it to more of his patients than other physicians. He may also be able to recruit more participants because he has more patients, better rapport with patients, or patients who are more compliant, educated, or interested than those in other practices. Alternatively, this physician may be misrepresenting the potential benefits of the new medication or pressuring patients to participate by making them feel that refusing will jeopardize their continued medical care. He may even be enrolling ineligible subjects or fabricating the data.

b. In general, it is a better study design to have independent project staff recruit subjects (rather than the personal physician) to reduce the potential conflict of interest and enhance uniformity of recruitment procedures. Periodic site-visits are essential for monitoring recruitment and enrollment procedures. In this case a sample of enrolled subjects could also be interviewed by the investigators to be sure they really exist, and to determine if they understand the study, the risks and benefits, and whether they feel that they have been pressured to enroll. If conflict of interest is detected, corrective actions should be reviewed by the Institutional Review Board.

# ■ CHAPTER 15

1. a. "Or" is confusing—there are three different drinks but only one response option.

   b. There is no way to respond if the subject is drinking more than 8 drinks per day.

   c. There is no definition of how big a "drink" is.

   d. The question does not specify time—weekdays versus weekend, every day versus less than daily.

   e. It may be better to specify a particular time frame (e.g., in the past 7 days).

2. 1. Which of the following statements best describes how <u>often</u> you drank alcoholic beverage during the past year? An alcoholic beverage includes wine, liquor or mixed drinks.  Select one of the 8 categories.

   |  |  |  |  |
   |---|---|---|---|
   | ☐ | Every day | ☐ | 2−3 times per month |
   | ☐ | 5−6 days per week | ☐ | About once a month |
   | ☐ | 3−4 days per week | ☐ | Less than 12 times a year |
   | ☐ | 1−2 days per week | ☐ | Rarely or not at all |

   2. During the past year, <u>how many</u> drinks did you <u>usually</u> have on a <u>typical day when you drank alcohol</u>? A drink is about 12 oz. of beer, 5 oz. of wine, or 1 1/2 oz. of hard liquor.          _____drinks

   3. During the past year, what is the <u>largest number</u> of alcoholic drinks you can recall drinking <u>during one day</u>?          _____drinks

   4. About how old were you when you first started drinking alcoholic beverages?
      _____years old.  (If you have never consumed alcoholic beverages, write in "never" and go to question #7)

   5. Was there ever a period when you drank quite a bit more than you do now?

   ☐ No
   ☐ Yes ➤

   > If Yes, which of the following statements best describes how often you drank during that period? Select one of the 8 categories
   >
   > 5a. | | | |
   > |---|---|---|---|
   > | ☐ | Every day | ☐ | 2−3 times per month |
   > | ☐ | 5−6 days per week | ☐ | About once a month |
   > | ☐ | 3−4 days per week | ☐ | Less than 12 times a year |
   > | ☐ | 1−2 days per week | ☐ | Rarely or not at all |
   >
   > 5b. During that period, how many drinks did you usually have on a typical day when you drank alcohol? _____ drinks
   >
   > 5c. For about how many years did you drink more than you do now? _____ years

   6. Have you ever  had what might be considered a drinking problem?    ☐ No
   ☐ Yes

3. a. Obtaining data through interviews requires much more staff training and staff time than a self-administered questionnaire and is therefore much more expensive.

   b. Some subjects do not like to tell another person the answer to sensitive questions in the area of sexual behavior.

   c. Unless the interviewers are well trained and the interviews are standardized, the information obtained may vary.

   d. However, interviewers can repeat and probe in a way that improves comprehension and produces more accurate and complete responses in some situations than a self-administered questionnaire.

# ■ CHAPTER 17

1. a. (■ Not enough)
   - Identify all missing and outlying values and recheck the paper forms to make sure that the data were entered correctly.

   - Retrieve missing data from charts.

   - Collect missing interview data from surviving patients (but this will not help for those who died and for those whose responses might have changed during the follow-up period).

   - Make a special effort to find subjects who had been lost to follow-up, and at least get a telephone interview with them.

   - Obtain vital status, using the National Death Index or a firm that finds people.

   b. ■ Collect less data.
   - Check forms on site immediately after collecting the data to be certain that all items are complete and accurate.

   - Use interactive data entry with built-in checks for missing and out-of-range values. This is best done shortly after data collection so that missing data can be collected before the patient leaves the hospital (or dies).

   - Use duplicate data entry.

   - Periodically tabulate the distributions of values for all items during the course of the study to identify missing values and potential errors.

   - Hold periodic team meetings to review progress.

   - Tape record interviews as a safety net.

# ■ CHAPTER 18

1. The G.I. Clinic
   a. **Advantages:** This is likely to be a convenient and accessible source of patients. The clinic staff probably has experience participating in research. Implementing a standard battery of diagnostic tests for patients with abdominal pain should not be difficult.

   b. **Disadvantages:** Patients in this clinic might be a highly selected subset of all patients presenting with abdominal pain. Your results may therefore have limited generalizability.

Community Clinics

   a. **Advantages:** Here you can identify patients at first presentation without the selection and delay caused by the referral process. Community physicians may benefit from the opportunity to participate in research.

   b. **Disadvantages:** These are mainly logistic. Identifying participating physicians and patients and implementing a standard research protocol will be a major organizational task.

2. a. This can only be answered with local data. Research elsewhere will not help you.

   b. This is well known from the international literature. Repeating such research in China is unlikely to be an efficient use of resources.

   c. For this question, the generalizability of research from elsewhere is likely to be intermediate. Strategies for smoking cessation proven successful in other countries may serve as a basis for strategies to be tried in China, but you cannot be sure they will have the same success in China without local research. Previous studies in populations elsewhere with cultural ties to China, such as recent Chinese immigrants to the United States, may be especially helpful.

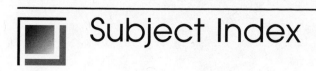

# Subject Index

Note: Page numbers in italics indicate figures; those followed by t indicate tables.